Sports Biomechanics and Medicine

Sports Biomechanics and Medicine

Edited by **Pablo De Souza**

Callisto Reference
New York

Published by Callisto Reference,
106 Park Avenue, Suite 200,
New York, NY 10016, USA
www.callistoreference.com

Sports Biomechanics and Medicine
Edited by Pablo De Souza

International Standard Book Number: 978-1-63239-690-7 (Hardback)

Printed in China.

Contents

Preface

This book aims to highlight the current researches and provides a platform to further the scope of innovations in this area. This book is a product of the combined efforts of many researchers and scientists from different parts of the world. The objective of this book is to provide the readers with the latest information in the field.

This book is a compilation of chapters that discuss the most vital concepts and emerging trends in the fields of sports biomechanics and medicine. Sports biomechanics is a branch of biomechanics that applies the law of mechanics, physics and principles of biology on human movement and actions especially related to sports. It understands the cause and effect relationship of the human body movement. Sports medicine on the other hand deals with curing and preventing sports injuries as quickly as possible. Both of them try to optimize the performance of an athlete by providing the required guidance, equipment and drugs. While understanding the long-term perspectives of the topics, this book makes an effort in highlighting their impact as a modern tool for the growth of the discipline. The topics covered herein offer the readers new insights in the field of sports biomechanics. It covers theoretical and experimental studies in this field which elucidate some of the crucial and unexplored concepts. Researchers and students involved in the area of sports biomechanics will be assisted by this book.

I would like to express my sincere thanks to the authors for their dedicated efforts in the completion of this book. I acknowledge the efforts of the publisher for providing constant support. Lastly, I would like to thank my family for their support in all academic endeavors.

Editor

1

The Association between Anthropometric Variables, Functional Movement Screen Scores and 100 m Freestyle Swimming Performance in Youth Swimmers

Daisy Bond [1], Laura Goodson [1], Samuel W. Oxford [1], Alan M. Nevill [2] and Michael J. Duncan [1,*]

[1] Centre for Applied Biological and Exercise Sciences, Coventry University, Coventry CV1 5HB, UK; E-Mails: bondd3@coventry.ac.uk (D.B.); goodsonl@coventry.ac.uk (L.G.); s.oxford@coventry.ac.uk (S.W.O.)

[2] Faculty of Education, Health and Well-Being, University of Wolverhampton, Walsall WS1 3BD, UK; E-Mail: a.m.nevill@wlv.ac.uk

* Author to whom correspondence should be addressed; E-Mail: michael.duncan@coventry.ac.uk

Academic Editor: Eling Douwe de Bruin

Abstract: This study examined the association between anthropometric variables, Functional Movement Screen (FMS) scores and 100 m freestyle swimming performance in early adolescent swimmers. Fifty competitive, national level, youth swimmers (21 males, 29 females, mean age ± SD = 13.5 ± 1.5 years, age range 11–16 years) performed an "all-out" 100 m freestyle (front crawl) swim as fast as they could in a 50 m pool. A median divide for 100 m timed swim was also used to divide the sample into faster or slower groups. Height, body mass, skinfolds and limb lengths were also assessed. Maturation was calculated by proxy using anthropometric measures and participants also undertook the FMS as a measure of functional performance. Backwards linear regression indicated a significant model ($p = 0.0001$, Adjusted $R^2 = 0.638$) explaining 63.8% of the variance in swim performance with total sum of skinfolds, upper leg length, lower leg length, hand length and total height significantly contributing to the model. Swimmers who were classed as fast had lower total sum of skinfolds ($p = 0.005$) and higher total FMS score ($p = 0.005$) compared to their slower peers. In summary, this study indicates that anthropometric variables significantly explained the variance in 100 m freestyle swimming performance in youth swimmers.

Keywords: pediatric; skinfolds; limb length; functional performance

1. Introduction

Understanding the physical and anthropometric factors that underpin performance in the sport of swimming is important in relation to talent development and targeting training programs effectively [1]. The use of anthropometry and physical testing is prevalent in many talent identification and talent development programmes including those of the Federation Internationale De Natation (FINA) [2]. As such examining the impact of anthropometric variables on swimming performance in pediatric swimmers is of interest to scientists and coaches alike. A body of literature has documented how anthropometric and other variables might predict pediatric swimming performance [3–7]. Anthropometry alone, however, may not be best suited for monitoring pediatric swimmers. For example, Geladas *et al.* [7] reported that 100 m freestyle swimming performance was best predicted by a combination of anthropometric and physical tests ($r = -0.22$ to -0.31) in a sample of 263, 12–14 year old swimmers. Thus, there is a need to better understand how these factors might influence swimming performance in adolescent swimmers.

In recent years there has been an increase in the use of pre-participation movement screens as a means to quantify functional movement as well as predicting injury risk and sports performance [8]. The Functional Movement Screen (FMS) [8]), is one such measure which is predictive of injury risk [9] and has been shown to improve following online video-based compared to fully supervised resistance exercise in adolescent basketball athletes [10]. Recent work by Paszkewicz *et al.* [11] has also reported that the FMS can discriminate between levels of pubescence and detect alterations during the pubertal growth cycle in children and adolescents aged 8–14 years old. The FMS comprises seven movement tests that employ a variety of positions and movements closely related to normal growth and development [12]. It is conceptualised that fundamental movements, such as those tested by the FMS, operate as the basis of more complex movement patterns used in common daily activities [8,9]. As such the use of the FMS offers a practical way by which to evaluate the functional movement patterns that underpin all aspects of human movement. Recent longitudinal research with 121 track and field athletes has also supported the efficacy of this method. Chapman *et al.* [13] reported that athletes who scores a FMS composite score of 14 or higher had a significantly greater performance improvement in their disciplines over the following year compared to athletes who scored less than 14 on the FMS. Conversely, data presented by Parchman and McBride [14] reported no significant association between FMS scores, golf club head speed, and various fitness tests in 25 adult golfers. Other research with a non-athletic child population has also reported that FMS scores were significantly related to body mass index [15], with higher BMI being associated with poorer FMS performance. Despite this data, few studies have examined how these functional movement patterns develop in adolescents generally and no studies to date have examined if and how FMS performance might be associated with anthropometric factors and performance in adolescent athletes.

The aim of this study was to examine the association between anthropometric variables, functional movement screen scores and 100 m freestyle swimming performance in trained adolescent swimmers.

We hypothesized that both anthropometric variables and functional movement screen scores would be significant predictors of 100 m freestyle swimming performance.

2. Method, Results, Discussion

2.1. Method

2.1.1. Participants

Following institutional ethics approval, informed consent and parental informed consent, 50 competitive youth swimmers aged 11–16 years (21 males, mean age ± SD = 13.6 ± 1.7 years and 29 females, ages 11–16 years, mean age ± SD = 13.4 ± 1.3 years) participated in this study. The swimmers were currently competing at national level and were part of an Amateur Swimming Association beacon squad. Individual participants were currently engaged in 4 to 9 formal training sessions per week (mean ± SD of training sessions per week = 6.9 ± 1.2 sessions/week). Participants were recruited via formal approach to coaches at Amateur Swimming Association swimming clubs in the West Midlands, UK with inclusion criteria being currently competitively included in a national level beacon squad.

2.1.2. Anthropometry

Height (cm) and body mass (kg) were assessed using a SECA stadiometre and weighing scales (±0.1 cm and 0.1 kg, respectively; SECA Instruments Ltd., Hamburg, Germany). Skinfolds were taken on the right hand side of the body using Harpenden skinfold callipers (±0.2 mm Harpenden Instruments, Cambridge, UK) from the triceps, biceps, subscapular, iliac crest, supraspinale, mid abdominal, front thigh and medial calf sites. Individual skinfolds were summed to create a total sum of skinfolds measure to reflect overall adiposity [16]. Limb lengths were assessed using a non-stretchable tape measure and consisted of measures of upper arm, lower arm and hand lengths and upper leg, lower leg and foot lengths. Anthropometric measurements were collected by an experienced anthropometrist, following guidelines from the International Society for the Advancement of Kinanthropometry (ISAK) [16]. In addition, physical maturation was assessed using the predictive equation of Mirwald *et al.* [17] based on age, height, leg length and sitting height by predicting the age at peak height velocity (APHV). Mean ± SD of APHV was 14.56 ± 0.83 years).

2.1.3. Functional Movement Assessment

Each participant also underwent functional movement assessment using the FMS™ screening system (see functionalmovement.com). The FMS consists of seven tests; Deep squat, in-line lunge, hurdle step, shoulder mobility, stability push-up, rotational stability and active straight leg raise, which challenge an individual's ability to perform basic movement patterns that reflect combinations of muscle strength, flexibility, range of motion, coordination, balance and proprioception [8,18]. The FMS was administered by a trained rater using standardised procedures, instructions and scoring [8,18]. Each participant was given 3 trials on each of the seven tests (deep squat, hurdle step, in-line lunge, shoulder mobility, active straight leg raise, trunk-stability push-up and rotary stability) in accordance with recommended guidelines [8,18]. Each trial was scored from 0 to 3 with higher scores reflecting better functional movement. For each test, the highest score from the three trials was recorded and used to generate an overall composite FMS score with a maximum value of 21 and in accordance with recommended protocols [8,13]. Comprehensive instructions for each movement are also provided elsewhere [18] and readers are referred to these for in-depth detail on the development and functional basis for the FMS. A pilot study was also conducted with 10 participants to determine test re-test (two-week) agreement between the investigators conducting the FMS rating in the present study. Kappa values revealed excellent test re-test agreement for total composite score and individual FMS tests (Kappa = 0.97 to 1). Intraclass correlation coefficient (ICC) for the three attempts at each of the seven tests taken were also high with all ICCs >0.9.

2.1.4. Measures of Swimming Performance

The participant's coaching staff provided information regarding each participant's 100 m freestyle personal best swim time. Participants also undertook a timed 100 m freestyle swim. In the timed 100 m swim, participants were requested to perform an "all-out" 100 m freestyle (front crawl) swim at maximal speed in a 50 m pool. Participants started the timed swim, diving in from the side of the pool and performing normal turning action at the end of each length. Prior to the trial, swimmers performed a 400-m warm-up swim, followed by a 10 min passive resting period before the 100-m all-out trial, consistent with procedures used previously by Latt *et al.* [19]. Moreover, timed freestyle swim performance was significantly related to individual personal best times ($r = -0.967$, $p = 0.0001$) for the swimmers.

2.1.5. Statistical Analysis

Pearson's product moment correlations were employed to examine the association between timed freestyle swim performance, FMS score, APHV and anthropometric variables. Backwards linear regression was then employed to examine the amount of variance in timed swim performance that could be explained from FMS score, APHV and anthropometric variables. A fully saturated model was employed where all variables were included in the analysis in the first instance and variables removed until a parsimonious model was determined. A median split for timed freestyle swim performance was also used to divide the sample into faster or slower groups. A series of 2 Gender (*i.e.*, male *vs.* female) by 2 swim speed (*i.e.*, faster *vs.* slower) ways analysis of covariance (ANCOVA) controlling for APHV were used, employing backwards elimination to achieve a parsimonious solution, to examine any differences in FMS score and anthropometric variables as a result of gender or timed freestyle swim performance. The use of ANCOVA in this way allows for any independent differences (main effects) in swim speed between boys and girls and faster and slower swimmers to be determined whilst also allowing any interactive effects between gender and faster and slower swimmers to be determined. In addition, the inclusion of APHV as a covariate provides a mean to determine the independent association between APHV and FMS or anthropometric variables and also any interaction effects between APHV and gender and APHV and fast *vs.* slow swimmers to be determined (See Field [20] for an overview). The statistical package for social sciences (Version 20, SPSS Inc., Amonk, NY, USA, 2011) was used for all analysis.

2.2. Results

Pearson's product moment correlations indicated significant relationships between timed freestyle swim performance and all the dependent variables except for lower leg length (all $p < 0.05$, $r = -0.264$ to 0.654, see Table 1). Backwards linear regression indicated a significant model (F 5.49 = 18.3, $p = 0.0001$, Adjusted $R^2 = 0.638$) explaining 63.8% of the variance in swim performance with total sum of skinfolds ($\beta = 0.041$, $p = 0.05$), upper leg length ($\beta = 0.428$, $p = 0.005$), lower leg length ($\beta = 0.858$, $p = 0.001$), hand length ($\beta = -1.709$, $p = 0.0001$), and total height ($\beta = -0.67$, $p = 0.0001$), significantly contributing to the model.

Results from ANCOVA analysis, controlling for maturation indicated significant gender main effects for foot length ($F = 20.6$, $p = 0.0001$), lower leg length ($F = 5.6$, $p = 0.018$) and hand length ($F = 6.5$, $p = 0.019$) with boys having higher mean values than girls (See Table 2). Boys however, had significantly ($F = 8.2$, $p = 0.005$, see Table 2) poorer total FMS score compared to girls. Significant main effects for swim speed (fast *vs.* slow) were also evident for total sum of skinfold ($F = 11.1$, $p = 0.005$, See Table 2) and Total FMS score ($F = 9.4$, $p = 0.005$, See Table 2). Swimmers who were classed as fast swim speed had lower total sum of skinfolds and higher total FMS score compared to their slower swim speed peers. There were also significant gender X fast *vs.* slow interactions for height ($p = 0.013$, See Table 3) and body mass ($p = 0.0001$, See Table 3). Boys who were classed as fast swim speed were significantly taller and had significantly greater body mass than girls who were classed as fast swim speed. There were no significant differences in height or body mass between boys and girls who were classed as slow swim speed swimmers. There were no significant main effects or interactions for upper leg length ($p > 0.05$). Maturation (APHV) was not significant in any of the analysis, ($p > 0.05$). There were also no significant differences in APHV between boys and girls or those classed as fast or slow for swim speed (all $p > 0.05$).

2.3. Discussion

The main findings of this study are: (1) that anthropometric variables (total sum of skinfolds, upper leg length, lower leg length, hand length and total height) were able to explain 63.8% of the variance in 100 m maximal freestyle swimming performance; (2) that swimmers classed as faster, based on a median split, had lower total sum of skinfolds and exhibited better functional movement patterns than their slower peers, after controlling for APHV; (3) Boys had larger foot, lower leg and hand length and poorer functional movement performance than girls.

Table 1. Pearson's product moment correlations (r) between 100 m timed swim performance, anthropometric variables and Functional Movement Screen (FMS) score in competitive youth swimmers.

Performance variable	Height (m)	Mass (kg)	Upper arm length (cm)	Lower arm length (cm)	Hand length (cm)	Upper leg length (cm)	Lower leg length (cm)	Foot length (cm)	Sum of skinfolds (mm)	Total FMS (0–21)
100 m freestyle timed swim	−0.654 **	−0.543 **	−0.561 **	−0.483 **	−0.626 **	−0.350 *	−0.264	−0.494 **	0.410 **	−0.333 *

* and ** $p < 0.05$ and 0.01 respectively.

Table 2. Mean (±SE) of anthropometric variables and total FMS score between boys and girls and swimmers classified as faster or slower ([a] $p = 0.019$ compared to girls, [b] $p = 0.018$ compared to girls, [c] $p = 0.0001$ compared to girls, [d] $p = 0.005$ compared to girls, [e] $p = 0.005$ compared to slow).

Sample	Timed freestyle swim performance (s)	Height (cm)	Body mass (kg)	Upper arm length (cm)	Lower arm length (cm)	Hand length (cm)	Upper leg length (cm)	Lower leg length (cm)	Foot length (cm)	Sum of skinfolds (mm)	Total FMS (0–21)
Pooled data ($n = 50$)	68.8 (1.0)	164 (1.5)	54.4 (1.4)	32.2 (0.43)	25.5 (0.59)	18.4 (0.19)	52.2 (0.62)	49.2 (0.62)	24.9 (0.32)	94.2 (4.8)	15.9 (1.4)
Boys ($n = 21$)	68.7 (1.1)	169 (2.9)	58.9 (2.7)	32.9 (0.47)	25.3 (0.68)	18.8 (0.24) [a]	52.9 (0.81)	50.6 (0.86) [b]	26.1 (0.31) [c]	84.6 (6.3)	15.2 (0.26) [d]
Girls ($n = 29$)	69.9 (0.93)	161 (0.9)	51.2 (1.2)	31.6 (0.39)	25.6 (0.61)	18.1 (0.20)	51.7 (0.70)	47.8 (0.71)	23.8 (0.38)	98.3 (5.1)	16.3 (0.22)
Fast ($n = 24$)	63.9 (0.9)	169 (2.1)	58.5 (2.2)	32.8 (0.41)	26.3 (0.53)	18.9 (0.27)	52.3 (0.77)	49.2 (0.78)	25.3 (0.33)	77.7 (6.4) [e]	16.4 (0.24) [e]
Slow ($n = 26$)	74.7 (1.1)	161 (1.2)	54.4 (1.0)	31.4 (0.48)	24.1 (0.61)	18.0 (0.25)	52.3 (0.82)	49.7 (0.84)	24.7 (0.36)	106.4 (6.9)	15.2 (0.27)

Table 3. Mean (±SE) of anthropometric variables and total FMS score between fast and slow boys and fast and slow girls (^{a} $p = 0.0001$ compared to slow boys, ^{b} $p = 0.021$ compared to fast girls, ^{c} $p = 0.0001$ compared to slow girls, ^{d} $p = 0.001$ compared to slow boys, ^{e} $p = 0.003$ compared to fast girls, ^{f} $p = 0.001$ compared to slow girls).

Sample	Timed freestyle swim performance (s)	Height (cm)	Body mass (kg)	Upper arm length (cm)	Lower arm length (cm)	Hand length (cm)	Upper leg length (cm)	Lower leg length (cm)	Foot length (cm)	Sum of skinfolds (mm)	Total FMS (0–21)
Fast boys ($n = 14$)	61.4 (1.3)	176 (2.7) ^{a,b,c}	64.2 (2.7) ^{d,e,f}	35.3 (0.78)	27 (0.49)	19.8 (0.34)	55.2 (0.99)	52.7 (1.01)	27.1 (0.51)	73.0 (4.7)	16.1 (0.51)
Slow boys ($n = 7$)	75.9 (1.9)	157.5 (3.9)	49.9 (3.8)	30.4 (1.4)	22.8 (1.0)	18.1 (0.55)	50.7 (1.8)	48.9 (2.0)	25.5 (0.89)	114.9 (20.1)	14.5 (0.429)
Fast girls ($n = 12$)	66.4 (1.4)	162 (0.88)	52.0 (1.6)	31.6 (0.35)	25.7 (0.81)	18.4 (0.31)	51.2 (1.2)	47.1 (1.1)	24.2 (0.5)	87.6 (7.4)	16.5 (0.26)
Slow girls ($n = 17$)	73.5 (1.2)	158.3 (1.2)	50.6 (1.8)	30.7 (0.43)	25.2 (0.67)	17.6 (0.17)	51.1 (0.74)	48.0 (0.84)	23.2 (0.29)	107.9 (7.4)	16.1 (0.23)

Although anthropometric predictors of swim performance have been examined in prior literature [4–8] no studies to date have examined how functional movement relates to swim performance in either adults or youth swimmers. As swimmers start heavy training at a relatively young age it is important to assess which parameters may be the best predictors of sprint swimming performance to enhance youth development programmes [19,21]. For coaches such data is useful in highlighting the key anthropometric variables that might best relate to 100 m freestyle performance in early adolescent swimmers after controlling for any impact of physical maturation. It is however important to note that the results presented here are only indicative of anthropometric profiles at one given point in time. If such anthropometric profiling were to be used for talent identification a longitudinal design alongside monitoring of training loads within a periodised programme would need to be undertaken to better understand predictors of swimming performance. Furthermore, as faster swimmers had better FMS scores, this study highlights potential utility of the FMS in swimming. However, there was a greater spread of FMS scores seen in boys (fast boys = 16.1; slow boys = 14.5) compared to girls (fast girls = 16.5; slow girls = 16.1). This variance might explain why anthropometric variables significantly contributed to the regression model whereas FMS score did not. This point is however speculative and the reason for the variance of FMS scores in boys in not known. Subsequent a posteriori analysis of data that APHV values were higher for fast boys (14.5 ± 0.2 years) compared to slow boys (14.1 ± 0.3 years). Although there was no significant difference in APHV, this may have contributed to the higher FMS scores in fast boys compared to their slower counterparts. However, the cross sectional nature of the data presented here do not allow any insight as to whether those athletes with better functional movement pattern swim faster or whether those athletes with greater swim performance develop better functional capability. Further research, including longitudinal investigation of functional movement development, in youth swimmers is therefore needed.

Our results are supportive of prior research that has also identified anthropometric variables as important predictors in swimming [6,7,19,22]. In particular, prior studies have suggested that taller swimmers glide better through the water [5,23] and also have a larger arm span, benefitting swimming efficiency (via a larger stroke length) [24].

We acknowledge however that only anthropometric variables relating to leg and arm length and total body fatness were examined in the present study. Future research with youth swimmers would therefore be useful which also assesses other anthropometric variables such as arm span and arm and leg volume to provide a more comprehensive anthropometric profile of competitive youth swimmers.

By categorizing swimmers regarding their swim speed, this study also evidenced that "faster" young swimmers displayed better functional movement patterns compared to their "slower" counterparts. This is an important and novel finding with practical applications. Prior research with adults has suggested lower FMS scores are related to increased injury risk in adults [25]. While investigating the association between FMS score and injury risk/history was beyond the scope of the present study, this appears an interesting avenue for future research. The research findings presented in the present study are supportive of research that has identified that higher FMS scores are related to enhanced performance in adult track and field athletes [13]. However, it is difficult to compare the present study with the prior work as few studies have presented FMS data in young people and none to date appear to have presented FMS scores in youth athletes. It is also important to note that only the total FMS score was utilised in the present study. The total FMS score provides an indication of overall functional movement performance [8,13].

Examining how scores on the individual tests within the FMS relates to athletic performance would be useful in developing the understanding of the FMS-performance relationship in youth athletes. However, in order to accomplish this, a far larger sample size than that in the present study would be required. Access to such a sample size of national level youth swimming performers is logistically difficult to obtain. Consequently, this is a direction for future research. It is also not possible within the present study to assert whether improving FMS leads to enhanced swimming performance or whether those who are better swimmers exhibit better functional movement patterns.

3. Conclusions

The present study indicates that anthropometric variables (63.8%) significantly explained the variance in 100 m freestyle swimming performance in early adolescent swimmers. Moreover, after adjusting for physical maturation, swimmers classed as faster had lower sum of skinfolds and better functional movement patterns than swimmers classed as slower. While gender differences were logically observed for anthropometrical variables, boys displayed lower functional movement ability than girls.

Author Contributions

Daisy Bond, Laura Goodson, Michael J. Duncan and Samuel W. Oxford designed the study, Daisy Bond and Laura Goodson collected the data. Michael J. Duncan, Alan M. Nevill and Samuel W. Oxford analysed and interpreted the data. Michael J. Duncan, Samuel W. Oxford and Alan M. Nevill wrote the manuscript. All authors critically reviewed, contributed to and approved the manuscript.

Conflicts of Interest

The authors declare no conflict of interest.

References

1. Mevaloo, S.F.; Shahpar, F.M. Talent identification programmes. In Proceedings of the 17th FINA World Sport "Medicine Congress. Enhancing Performance: The Healthy Aquatic Athlete", Manchester, UK, 7–8 April 2008.
2. FINA: Federation Internationale De Natation. Talent Identification programmes, 2014. Available online: http://www.fina.org/ (accessed on 7 January 2015).
3. Morais, J.E.; Jesus, S.; Lopes, V.; Garrido, N.; Silva, A.; Marinho, D.; Barbosa, T.M. Linking selected kinematic, anthropometric and hydrodynamic variables to young swimmer performance. *Pediatr. Exerc. Sci.* **2012**, *24*, 649–664.
4. Jürimäe, J.; Haljaste, K.; Cicchella, A.; Lätt, E.; Purge, P.; Leppik, A.; Jürimäe, T. Analysis of swimming performance from physical, physiological and biomechanical parameters in young swimmers. *Pediatr. Exerc. Sci.* **2007**, *19*, 70–81.
5. Lätt, E.; Jürimäe, J.; Haljaste, K.; Cicchella, A.; Purge, P.; Jürimäe, T. Longitudinal development of physical and performance parameters during biological maturation of young male swimmers. *Percep. Mot. Skills* **2009**, *108*, 297–307.

6. Zuniga, J.; Housh, T.J.; Mielke, M.; Hendrix, C.R.; Camic, C.L.; Johnson, G.O.; Housh, D.J.; Schmidt, R.J. Gender comparisons of anthropometric characteristics of young sprint swimmers. *J. Strength Cond. Res.* **2011**, *25*, 103–108.
7. Geladas, N.D.; Nassis, G.P.; Pavlicevic, S. Somatic and physical traits affecting sprint swimming performance in young swimmers. *Int. J. Sports Med.* **2005**, *26*, 139–144.
8. Kiesel, K.; Plisky, P.J.; Voight, M.L. Can serious injury in professional football be predicted by a preseason functional movement screen? *N. Am. J. Sports Phys. Ther.* **2007**, *2*, 147–158.
9. Lisman, P.; O'Connor, F.G.; Deuster, P.A.; Knapik, J.J. Functional movement screen and aerobic fitness predict injuries in military training. *Med. Sci. Sports Exerc.* **2013**, *45*, 636–643.
10. Klusemann, M.J.; Pyne, D.B.; Fay, T.S.; Drinkwater, E.J. Online video-based resistance training improves the physical capacity of junior basketball athletes. *J. Strength Cond. Res.* **2012**, *26*, 2677–2684.
11. Paszkewicz, J.R.; McCarty, C.W.; VanLunen, B.L. Comparison of functional and static evaluation tools among adolescent athletes. *J. Strength Cond. Res.* **2013**, *27*, 2842–2850.
12. Cook, G.; Burton, L.; Kiesel, K. *Movement: Functional Movement Systems: Screening, Assessment, Corrective Strategies*; On Target Publications: London, UK, 2011.
13. Chapman, R.F.; Laymon, A.S.; Arnold, T. Functional movement scores and longitudinal performance outcomes in elite track and field athletes. *Int. J. Sports Physiol. Perf.* **2014**, *9*, 203–211.
14. Parchmann, C.J.; McBride, J.M. Relationship between functional movement screen and athletic performance. *J. Strength Cond. Res.* **2011**, *25*, 3378–3384.
15. Duncan, M.J.; Stanley, M. Functional movement is negatively associated with weight status and positively associated with physical activity in British primary school children. *J. Obes.* **2012**, *697563*, 2012.
16. Stewart, A.; Marfell-Jones, M.; Olds, T.; de Ridder, H. *International Standards for Anthropometric Assessment*; ISAK: Lower Hutt, New Zealand, 2011.
17. Mirwald, R.L.; Baxter-Jones, A.; Bailey, D.A.; Beunen, G.P. An assessment of maturity from anthropometric measurements. *Med. Sci. Sports Exerc.* **2002**, *34*, 689–694.
18. Cook, G.; Burton, L.; Hoogenboom, B. Pre-participation screening: The use of fundamental movements as an assessment of function—Part 2. *N. Am. J. Sports Phys. Ther.* **2006**, *1*, 132–139.
19. Lätt, E.; Jürimäe, J.; Mäestu, J.; Purge, P.; Rämson, R.; Haljaste, K.; Keskinen, K.L.; Rodriguez, F.A.; Jürimäe, T. Physiological, biomechanical and anthropometrical predictors of sprint swimming performance in adolescent swimmers. *J. Sports Sci. Med.* **2010**, *9*, 398–404.
20. Field, A. *Discovering Statistics Using SPSS*; SAGE: London, UK, 2008.
21. Kjendlie, P.L.; Ingjer, F.; Madsan, O.; Stallman, R.K.; Stray-Gundersen, J. Differences in the energy cost between children and adults during front crawl swimming. *Eur. J. Appl. Physiol.* **2004**, *91*, 473–480.
22. Silva, A.J.; Costa, A.M.; Oliveira, P.M.; Reis, V.M.; Saavedra, J.; Perl, J.; Rouboa, A.; Marinho, D.A. The use of neural network technology to model swimming performance. *J. Sports Sci. Med.* **2007**, *6*, 117–125.
23. Toussaint, H.; Hollander, P. Energetics of competitive swimming: Implications for training programmes. *Sports Med.* **1994**, *18*, 384–405.

24. Saavedra, J.M.; Escalante, Y.; Rodriguez, F.A. A multivariate analysis of performance in young swimmers. *Pediatr. Exerc. Sci.* **2010**, *22*, 135–151.

25. Kiesel, K.; Plisky, P.J.; Butler, R. Functional movement test scores improve following a standardized off-season intervention program in professional football players. *Scand. J. Med. Sci. Sports* **2011**, *21*, 287–292.

2

Physiological Responses Underlying the Perception of Effort during Moderate and Heavy Intensity Cycle Ergometry

Kristen C. Cochrane *, Terry J. Housh, Ethan C. Hill, Cory M. Smith, Nathaniel D.M. Jenkins, Joel T. Cramer, Glen O. Johnson and Richard J. Schmidt

Department of Nutrition and Health Sciences, 211 Ruth Leverton Hall, University of Nebraska-Lincoln, Lincoln, NE 68583, USA; E-Mails: thoush1@unl.edu (T.J.H.); ethan.hill@unl.edu (E.C.H.); csmith@unl.edu (C.M.S.); nathaniel.jenkins@unl.edu (N.D.M.J.); jcramer@unl.edu (J.T.C.); gojohnson22@gmail.com (G.O.J.); rscmidt1@unl.edu (R.J.S.)

* Author to whom correspondence should be addressed; E-Mail: kcochrane@unl.edu

Academic Editor: Eling Douwe de Bruin

Abstract: This study examined patterns of responses for physiological and perceptual variables during cycle ergometry at a constant rate of perceived exertion (RPE) within the moderate and heavy exercise intensity domains. Nineteen (mean age 21.3 ± 0.5 years; 43.4 ± 2.0 mL·kg^{-1}·min^{-1} $\dot{V}O_{2Peak}$) moderately trained cyclists performed an incremental test to exhaustion and two 60 min constant RPE rides at the RPE corresponding to the gas exchange threshold (RPE_{GET}) and 15% above the GET ($RPE_{GET+15\%}$). Oxygen consumption ($\dot{V}O_2$), respiratory exchange ratio (RER), heart rate (HR), minute ventilation ($\dot{V}_E$), breathing frequency ($\mathcal{F}_b$), and power output (PO) were monitored throughout the rides. Polynomial regression analyses showed $\dot{V}O_2$, RER, HR, and $\dot{V}_E$ (correlation = −0.85 to −0.98) tracked the decreases in PO required to maintain a constant RPE. Only $\mathcal{F}_b$ tracked RPE during the moderate and heavy intensity rides. Repeated measures ANOVAs indicated that $\dot{V}O_2$ during the 60 min rides at RPE_{GET} was not different ($p > 0.05$) from $\dot{V}O_2$ at GET from the incremental test to exhaustion. Thus, monitoring intensity using an RPE associated with the GET is sustainable for up to 60 min of cycling exercise and a common mechanism may mediate $\mathcal{F}_b$ and the perception of effort during moderate and heavy intensity cycle ergometry.

Keywords: gas exchange threshold; perception; respiration; exercise intensity

---

1. Introduction

The gas exchange threshold (GET) and respiratory compensation point (RCP) have been used to demarcate the exercise intensity domains (moderate, heavy, or severe) [1–3]. It has been suggested that the GET demarcates the moderate from heavy domains [1,3], while the RCP demarcates the heavy from severe domains [2]. During constant power output (PO), cycle ergometry within the moderate domain, oxygen consumption ($\dot{V}O_2$), heart rate (HR), and blood lactate concentration ($([La^-]_b)$) reach steady state within 3 min [1,3]. In the heavy domain, however, $(La^-)_b$ appearance exceeds its rate of removal for the first 10–20 min then reaches a steady state [1]. Thus, each domain is characterized by unique patterns of physiological responses.

A number of studies have examined the physiological and perceptual responses during continuous, constant PO cycle ergometry [1,2,4,5] within both moderate and heavy exercise intensity domains. During fatiguing constant PO exercise there are predictable time-dependent patterns of responses for $\dot{V}O_2$, HR, rating of perceived exertion (RPE), breathing frequency ($\mathcal{F}_b$), and minute ventilation ($\dot{V}_E$) that are, in part, dependent upon the exercise intensity associated with the task. There are, however, different patterns of responses for various physiological variables when continuous exercise is maintained at a constant physiological or perceptual parameter instead of PO [6–10]. For example, Stoudemire *et al.* [8] reported increases in $(La^-)_b$ and HR, but decreases in $\dot{V}O_2$ and velocity during treadmill running at RPE levels within the moderate and heavy domains. In addition, Lajoie *et al.* [7] reported increases in $\dot{V}O_2$, HR, and RPE during 60 min of cycling exercise while maintaining maximal lactate steady-state, which is related to the anaerobic threshold. More recently, Cochrane *et al.* [6] reported dissociations among RPE, $\dot{V}O_2$, HR, $\dot{V}_E$, and respiratory exchange ratio (RER) during cycle ergometry at a constant RPE, 20% below the GET (within the moderate domain). To explain these patterns of fatigue-related responses, Cochrane *et al.* [6] made some hypotheses regarding the applicability of fatigue models [11–15]. It was hypothesized [6] that small nerve afferents associated with respiratory muscles responsible for mediating $\mathcal{F}_b$ were the likely mediators of the perception of effort during constant RPE cycle ergometry within the moderate domain. No previous study, however, has investigated whether the dissociations among physiological and perceptual variables are dependent upon the exercise intensity of the task, as seen during constant PO exercise. Intensity dependent dissociations may further explain mediators of perception during both moderate and heavy intensity exercise.

Although specific metabolic, cardiovascular, and respiratory responses have been documented during constant PO exercise, less is known regarding pacing strategies associated with these responses and how responses may differ during exercise at a constant perception of effort. It has been theorized [16,17] that there is some level of brain involvement in the perception and manifestation of fatigue, with some theories suggesting the brain is responsible for conscious and unconscious integration of feedback from the working muscles and external stimuli (environment and time) [15], those that suggest the brain performs regulation without peripheral feedback [13], and others advocating a greater influence of unconscious "reflexes" on responses during exercise [11,12,14]. However, there is still debate regarding which, if any, of these theories best explains pacing and the onset of fatigue during dynamic exercise. There may be a dual contribution from automatic "reflex" actions as well as large metabolic disturbances to the conscious integration of the perception of effort that helps form an individual's pacing strategy. The mechanisms underlying this conscious awareness of physiological responses are not fully understood. Thus, by controlling the sense of effort (RPE), dissociations among physiological and perceptual responses may point to potential mediators of both conscious and unconscious interpretations of effort and the awareness that determines pace.

It is hypothesized that the variable(s) that track RPE are associated with similar underlying mediators and/or mechanisms, and those that are experimentally uncoupled from perception (*i.e.*, they do not follow the same pattern of responses as RPE), may not contribute to the perception of effort during moderate and/or heavy intensity cycle ergometry exercise. Based on the findings of previous studies [6,11], it is also hypothesized that variables related to respiration may be the most potent mediators of perception during prolonged cycling exercise. If specific variables can be identified which may mediate perception, a framework can be provided to athletes and coaches to improve pacing strategies, training programs, and athlete performance during prolonged, aerobic exercise. No previous study, has investigated the patterns of responses for these metabolic, cardiovascular, and respiratory variables during prolonged (>30 min) cycle ergometry maintained at a constant perceptual intensity within both the moderate and heavy domains. Like constant PO cycle ergometry, there may be an effect of intensity on the patterns of responses for identified variables, and therefore, there may be mediators of perception that are dependent upon the intensity at which exercise is performed. In addition, it is unclear how controlling perception affects pacing and the metabolic cost of exercise ($\dot{V}O_2$) across an extended period of time (>30 min). Therefore, the purposes of this study were to (1) examine the metabolic ($\dot{V}O_2$ and RER), cardiovascular (HR), respiratory ($\dot{V}_E$ and $\mathcal{F}_b$), and work intensity (PO) responses during continuous, constant RPE cycle ergometry within the moderate and heavy domains; and (2) to determine the level of agreement and sustainability of two perceptually grounded exercise intensities (RPE_{GET} and $RPE_{GET+15\%}$) to corresponding $\dot{V}O_2$ values (GET and 15% above GET) from an incremental and continuous cycling test.

2. Methods

2.1. Participants

Ten women and nine men (mean ± SD age 21.3 ± 0.5 years; body mass 71.9 ± 2.6 kg; $\dot{V}O_{2Peak}$) 43.4 ± 2.0 mL·kg^{-1}·min^{-1}) (Table 1) volunteered for this study and visited the laboratory on four occasions, with 24–48 h between visits. The participants were moderately trained cyclists who participated in cycling related exercise between 3 and 6 h per week for the past six months leading up to the study [18]. During the first visit, the participants signed a written informed consent and were familiarized with the Borg 6–20 perceptual scale according to standard instruction [19–21]. All subjects were read a standard script and given standard instructions for creating anchors. In addition, during familiarization, all subjects completed 3–4 short cycling bouts (<5 min) using the scale on the calibrated cycle ergometer to ensure their ratings matched the load at which they worked.

Borg 6–20 Instructions: "While performing physical activity, we want you to rate your perception of exertion. This feeling should reflect how heavy and strenuous the exercise feels to you, combining all sensations and feelings of physical stress, effort, and fatigue. Do not concern yourself with any one factor such as leg pain or shortness of breath, but try to focus on your total feeling of exertion. The rating scale below ranges from 6 to 20, where "6" means "no exertion at all" and 20 means "maximal exertion". Choose the number below that best describes your level of exertion. This will give you a good idea of the intensity level of your activity, and you can use this information to provide feedback to the experimenter to either increase or decrease the workload at which you cycle to reach your goal intensity rating" [21].

Table 1. Descriptive characteristics of the subjects (n = 19).

Variable	Mean ± SD	Range
Age (y)	21.3 ± 0.5	19.0–25.0
Body Mass (kg)	71.9 ± 2.6	56.8–92.7
$\dot{V}O_{2peak}$ (mL·kg^{-1}·min^{-1})	43.4 ± 2.0	29.1–61.8
GET (mL·kg^{-1}·min^{-1})	30.3 ± 1.5	21.3–47.1
GET +15% (mL·kg^{-1}·min^{-1})	34.9 ± 1.7	24.4–54.2
RCP (mL·kg^{-1}·min^{-1})	39.7 ± 1.7	28.6–52.6
RPE_{GET} (W)	167 ± 10	102–300
$RPE_{GET + 15\%}$ (W)	196 ± 12	125–349
RPE_{GET}	14 ± 0.5	12–17
$RPE_{GET + 15\%}$	16 ± 0.5	14–19
RPE_{GET} (%$\dot{V}O_{2peak}$)	70.1 ± 1.6	57.4–83.8
$RPE_{GET + 15\%}$ (%$\dot{V}O_{2peak}$)	80.8 ± 1.9	66.1–98.1

Note: PE was based on the Borg 6–20 scale (Borg 1982).

This study was approved by the University's Institutional Review Board for Human Participants and complied with the requirements stipulated in the Declaration of Helsinki.

2.2. Determination of GET, RCP, and Peak Values

At visit 2, each participant performed an incremental test to exhaustion on a calibrated Lode (Corval V3; Groningen, The Netherlands) electronically braked cycle ergometer at a pedal cadence of 75 rev·min^{-1}. The ergometer seat height was adjusted so that the participant's legs were near full extension at the bottom of the pedal revolution. Toe clips were used to maintain pedal contact throughout the test. Each participant wore a nose clip and breathed through a 2-way valve (Hans Rudolph 2700 breathing valve, Kansas City, MO, USA). Expired gas samples were collected and analyzed using a calibrated TrueMax 2400 metabolic cart (Parvo Medics, Sandy, UT, USA). The gas analyzers were calibrated with room air and gases of known concentration prior to all testing sessions. The O_2, CO_2, and ventilatory parameters were expressed as 20 s averages [22] and the participants were fitted with a Polar Heart Watch system (Polar Electro Inc., Lake Success, NY, USA). After 1 min of unloaded cycling, the test began at 50 W and the power was increased by 30 W every 2 min until voluntary exhaustion or when the participant's pedal cadence decreased below 70 rev·min^{-1} for more than 10 s, despite strong, verbal encouragement. The $\dot{V}O_{2Peak}$ was defined as the highest 20 s $\dot{V}O_2$ value recorded during the test. The GET and RCP were determined using the V-slope method described by Beaver, Wasserman, & Whipp [23] from the $\dot{V}CO_2$ *vs.* $\dot{V}O_2$ and $\dot{V}_E$ *vs.* $\dot{V}CO_2$ relationships, respectively. In addition, peak values for heart rate (HR_{Peak}), breathing frequency ($\mathcal{F}_{b\,Peak}$), minute ventilation ($\dot{V}_{EPeak}$), and respiratory exchange ratio (RER_{Peak}) were defined as the highest 20 s averages during the incremental test, while PO_{peak} and RPE_{peak} were defined as the highest PO and RPE from the last complete stage of the incremental test to exhaustion.

2.3. Determination of RPE_{GET} and $RPE_{GET+15\%}$

The $\dot{V}O_2$ values for each participant were plotted *vs.* PO from their incremental test and the $\dot{V}O_2$ values corresponding with the GET and 15% above GET were used to determine the PO at both thresholds (Figure 1a). Ratings of perceived exertion values were then plotted *vs.* PO from the incremental test to estimate the RPE_{GET} and $RPE_{GET+15\%}$ (Figure 1b,c). The GET and GET + 15% thresholds were chosen because they represented exercise intensities associated with the moderate and heavy exercise intensity domains. Pilot work indicated that intensities greater than 15% above the GET resulted in work at or above RCP, and therefore, did not represent an intensity that could be maintained. Furthermore, intensities less than 15% above the GET (GET + 5% and GET + 10%) did not result in RPE ratings different from those ratings at GET, and therefore, represented a similar perceptual intensity.

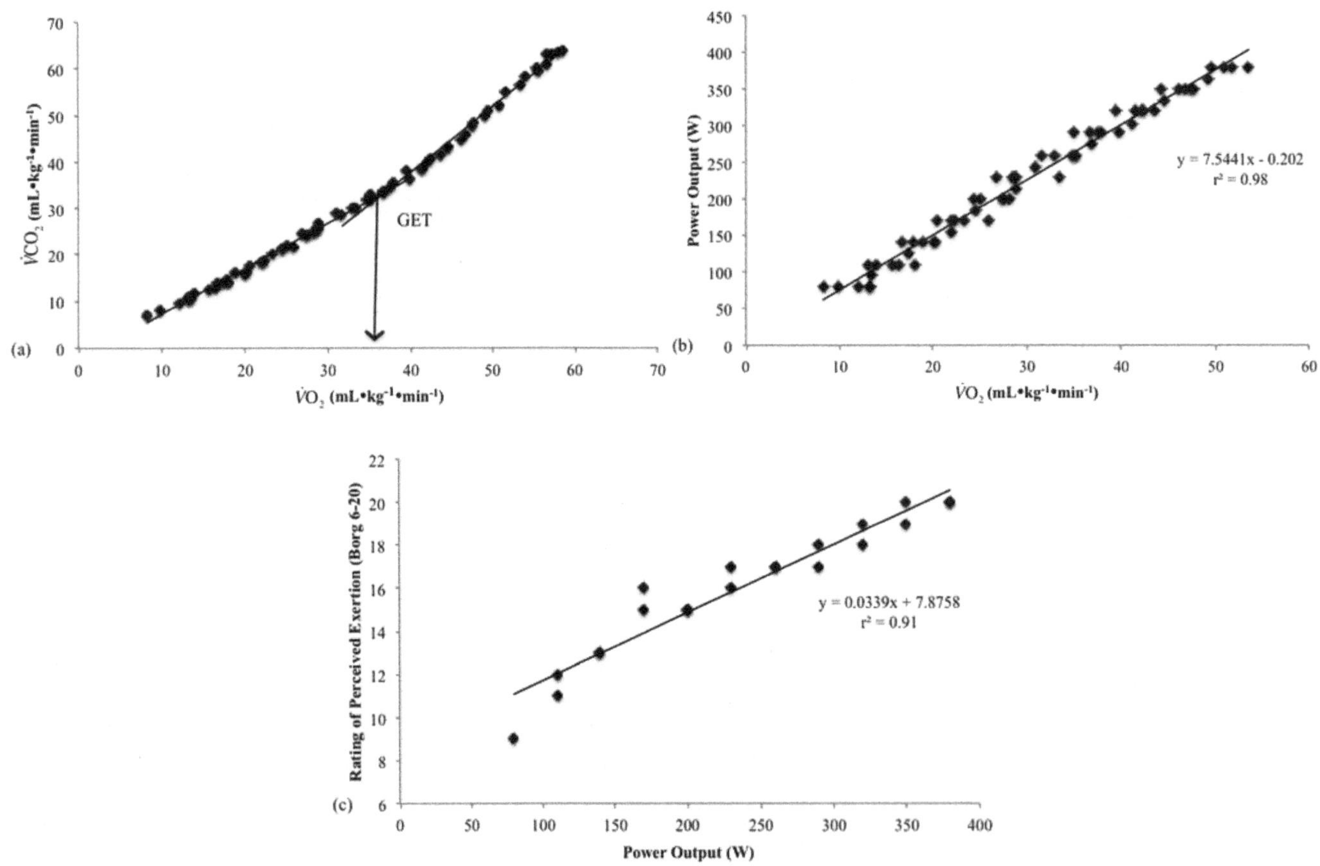

Figure 1. An example of the linear regression method used to determine the rating of perceived exertion (RPE) at the gas exchange threshold (GET): (**a**) $\dot{V}CO_2$ *vs.* $\dot{V}O_2$ relationship from the incremental test of participant 15; (**b**) Plot of the power output (PO) *vs.* $\dot{V}O_2$ relationship from the incremental test of participant 15; and (**c**) Estimation of the RPE that corresponded to the PO associated with GET determined from the RPE *vs.* PO relationship from the incremental test of participant 15.

2.4. Continuous 60 Min Rides

During the third and fourth visit, the participants rode for 60 min at either the RPE_{GET} or $RPE_{GET+15\%}$ (randomized, one during each visit). During the rides, $\dot{V}O_2$, HR, $\mathcal{F}_b$ $\dot{V}_E$, and RER values were recorded as 20 s averages every two min. The RPE was assessed every 30 s and PO was adjusted, as needed, to ensure that the RPE that corresponded to either the RPE_{GET} or $RPE_{GET+15\%}$ was maintained for the duration of the 60 min ride. Participants were unaware of the "goal" RPE until they produced their specific number during the 60 min ride(s). Once the "goal" RPE was achieved, participants were told to "maintain that feeling of exertion throughout the duration of the ride". The investigator controlled the change in PO necessary to maintain RPE. Pilot testing indicated that a change in 5 W was sufficient to elicit a change in RPE, however, during the rides at $RPE_{GET+15\%}$ greater increments (10 W) were required at the beginning of the ride to maintain the higher intensity. In addition, participants were unable to see the PO at which they worked and were only given feedback regarding time to completion at the 30 min mark. All participants were unaware of the absolute time and distance of the test until its completion. Although RPE was formally collected every 30 s, participants were instructed to voluntarily produce an RPE rating if their perception changed before the set 30 s production time point.

2.5. Statistical Analysis

The first 6 min of data collected during the 60 min rides were omitted to account for the initial cardiac and metabolic adjustments to exercise as well as adjustments in PO required to attain the RPE that corresponded to RPE_{GET} and $RPE_{GET+15\%}$. Each variable recorded during the constant RPE rides was normalized as a percentage of the value at $\dot{V}O_{2Peak}$ (*i.e.*, each value was divided by its value at $\dot{V}O_{2Peak}$ and multiplied by 100 to be expressed as a percentage). The mean, normalized $\dot{V}O_2$, HR, $\mathcal{F}_b$, $\dot{V}_E$, RER, and PO values were plotted at two min intervals from 7 to 60 min during the 60 min rides (Figures 2 and 3). Polynomial regression analyses were used to determine whether the individual and mean, normalized $\dot{V}O_2$, HR, $\mathcal{F}_b$, $\dot{V}_E$, RER, and PO *vs.* time relationships were best fit by a linear, quadratic, or cubic model. Oxygen consumption values from each ride were averaged according to four time points (7–19 min, 21–33 min, 35–47 min, and 49–60 min) across the 60 min ride, and two separate 1 × 5 Repeated Measures (RM) ANOVAs ($\dot{V}O_2$ incremental *vs.* $\dot{V}O_2$ 7–19 min *vs.* $\dot{V}O_2$ 21–33 min *vs.* $\dot{V}O_2$ 35–47 min *vs.* $\dot{V}O_2$ 49–60 min) were used to evaluate relative $\dot{V}O_2$ during the 60 min rides at RPE_{GET} and at $RPE_{GET+15\%}$, and how these values compared to the threshold value determined from the incremental test to exhaustion. Paired samples *t*-tests with Sidak-Bonferroni error correction were used to compare $\dot{V}O_2$ at GET *vs.* $\dot{V}O_2$ at GET + 15% at from the incremental test to that at 7–19 min, 21–33 min, 35–47 min, and 49–60 min of the 60 min rides. Partial eta squared (η_p^2) effect sizes were calculated for each RM ANOVA and Cohen d (*d*) effect sizes were calculated for each post hoc paired samples *t*-test. A type I error rate, set *a priori* at 5%, was considered statistically significant for all polynomial regression and RM ANOVAs analyses and an error rate of 1% was considered for all post hoc comparisons. The analyses were conducted using IBM SPSS Statistics v. 22 (Chicago, IL, USA).

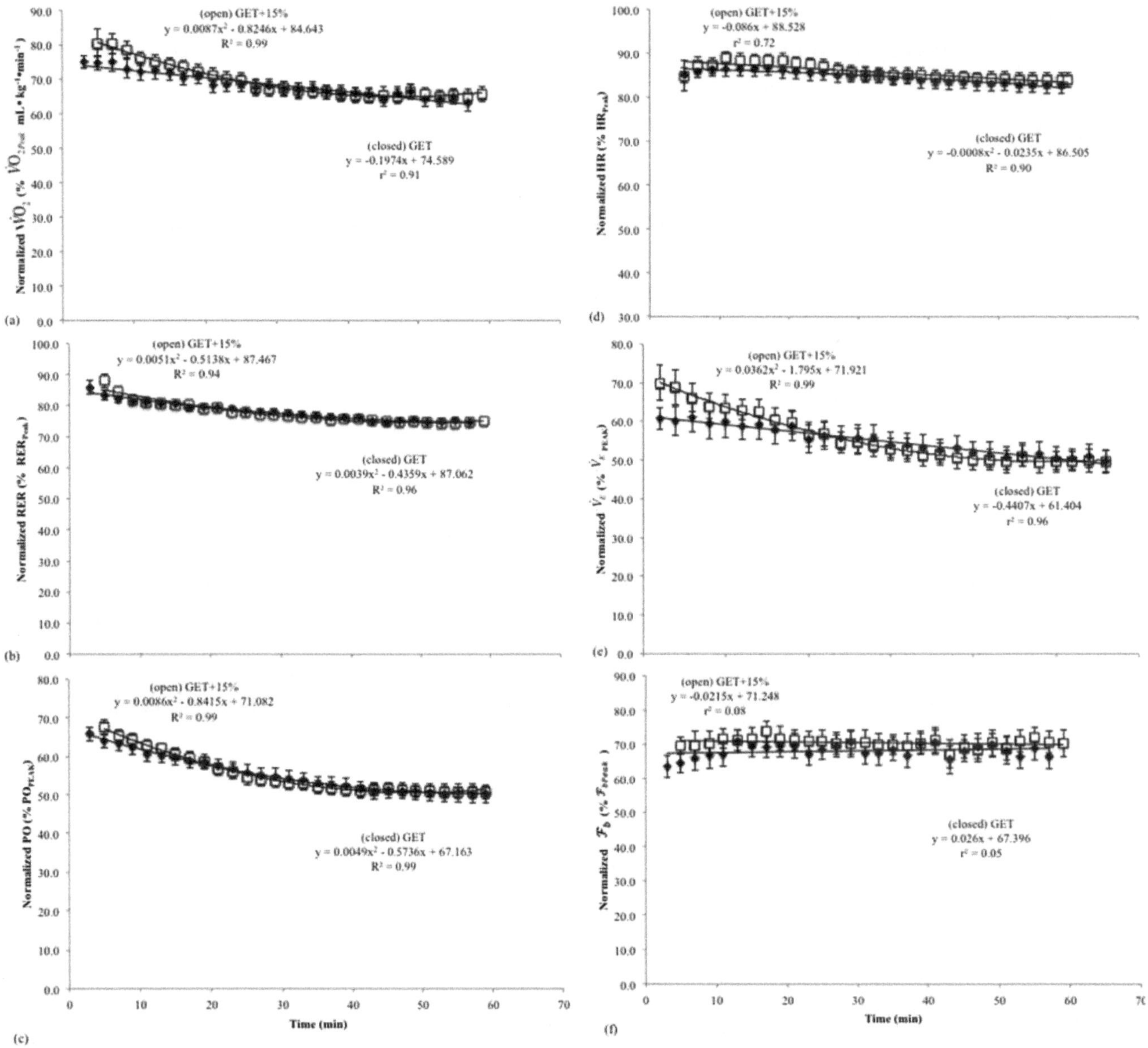

Figure 2. Normalized mean (±SD) values for the (**a**) oxygen consumption ($\dot{V}O_2$); (**b**) respiratory exchange ratio (RER); (**c**) power output (PO); (**d**) heart rate (HR); (**e**) minute ventilation ($\dot{V}_E$); and (**f**) breathing frequency ($\mathcal{F}_b$) *vs.* time relationships during the 60 min continuous rides at the rating of perceived exertion (RPE) at the gas exchange threshold (RPE_{GET}) and 15% above the GET ($RPE_{GET+15\%}$).

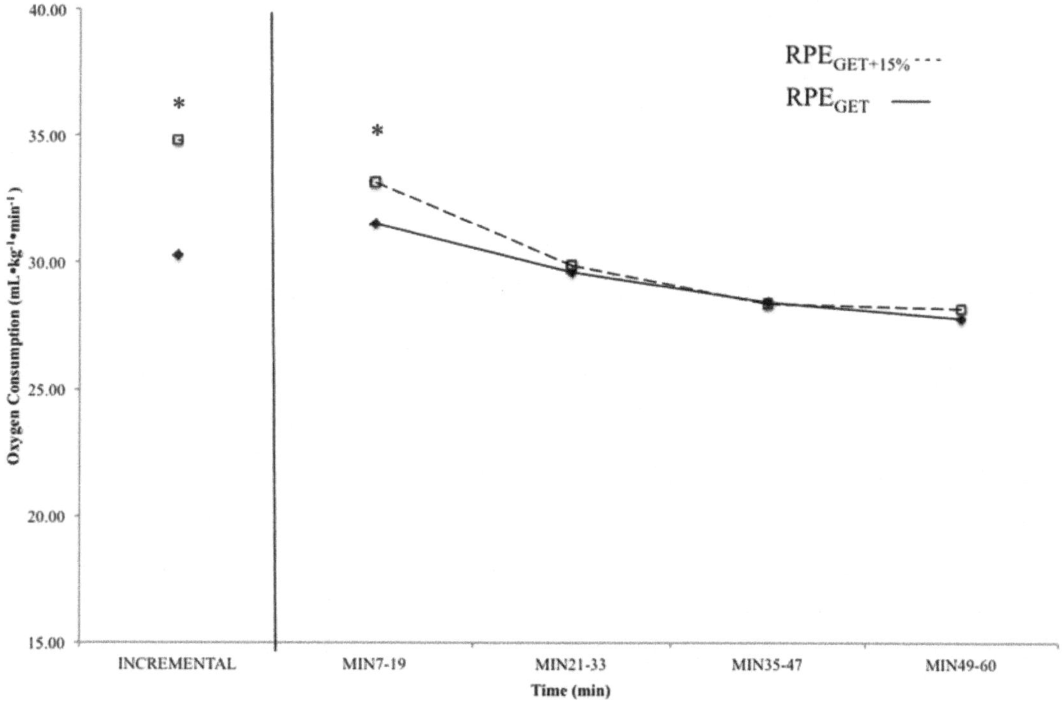

Figure 3. Mean, relative oxygen consumption values from the incremental test and 7–19 min, 21–33 min, 35–47 min, and 49–60 min from the 60 min continuous rides at the rating of perceived exertion (RPE) at the gas exchange threshold (RPE_{GET}---) and 15% above the GET ($RPE_{GET+15\%}$---). Data from the rides at the RPE corresponding with GET are displayed with solid boxes, while those from the rides at GET + 15% are open boxes. * indicates that oxygen consumption ($\dot{V}O_2$) was higher at the incremental test and 7–19 min in the $RPE_{GET+15\%}$ than RPE_{GET} condition ($p < 0.05$).

3. Results

The mean $\dot{V}O_2$ and PO values that corresponded to RPE_{GET} (RPE = 14 ± 0.5) and $RPE_{GET+15\%}$ (RPE = 16 ± 0.5) intensities were 30.3 ± 1.5 (167 ± 10 W) and 34.9 ± 1.7 mL·kg^{-1}·min^{-1} (196 ± 12 W), respectively. The results of the polynomial regression analyses (Figure 2a–f) indicated that during the 60 min rides at RPE_{GET}, there were significant, negative, linear relationships for mean, normalized $\dot{V}O_2$ (r^2 = 0.90) and $\dot{V}_E$ (r^2 = 0.96) *vs.* time; negative, quadratic relationships for mean, normalized HR (R^2 = 0.90), RER (R^2 = 0.96), and PO (R^2 = 0.98) *vs.* time; and no significant change for mean, normalized $\mathcal{F}_b$ (r^2 = 0.04) *vs.* time relationship. In addition, the results of the polynomial regression analyses during the 60 min rides at $RPE_{GET+15\%}$, indicated that there was a significant, negative, linear relationship for mean, normalized HR (r^2 = 0.72) *vs.* time; negative, quadratic relationships for mean, normalized $\dot{V}O_2$ (R^2 = 0.82), RER (R^2 = 0.92), $\dot{V}_E$(R^2 = 0.98), and PO (R^2 = 0.98) *vs.* time, and no significant change for the mean, normalized $\mathcal{F}_b$ (r^2 = 0.001) *vs.* time relationship.

The results of the RM ANOVA indicated that there was a significant main effect for $\dot{V}O_2$ during rides at RPE_{GET} (p<0.05; η_p^2 = 0.40). Follow-up pairwise comparisons revealed $\dot{V}O_2$ at 7–19 min was significantly (p<0.01) greater than $\dot{V}O_2$ at min 35–47 and at min 49–50. In addition, $\dot{V}O_2$ at 21–33 min was significantly (p<0.01) greater than that at min 35–47 and min 49–60. However, $\dot{V}O_2$ corresponding to GET from the incremental test to exhaustion was not significantly different from measured $\dot{V}O_2$ across the 60 min ride at RPE_{GET}. There was also a significant main effect for $\dot{V}O_2$ during rides at $RPE_{GET+15\%}$ ($p < 0.05$; $\eta_p^2 = 0.67$). Follow-up pairwise comparisons revealed that $\dot{V}O_2$ at min 7–19 was significantly greater than $\dot{V}O_2$ at all other time points (21–33 min, 35–47 min, and 49–60 min) during the 60 min ride at $RPE_{GET+15\%}$. Furthermore, there was no difference between $\dot{V}O_2$ at 35–47 min and 49–60 min, but $\dot{V}O_2$ during the last 25 min of the 60 min ride was significantly different ($p < 0.01$) from that collected during 7–19 min and 21–33 min. However, $\dot{V}O_2$ corresponding to 15% above GET from the incremental test to exhaustion was not significantly different from $\dot{V}O_2$ at 7–19 min, but differed from all other time points (21–33 min, 35–47 min, and 49–60 min).

The results of the paired samples *t*-tests indicated that the $\dot{V}O_2$ associated with the perceptual intensities, as calculated from the incremental test to exhaustion (GET and GET + 15%), were significantly different ($p < 0.01$; $d = 0.55$). In addition, comparison of the $\dot{V}O_2$ associated with the initial stage of each constant RPE ride indicated that subjects maintained a higher $\dot{V}O_2$ cost ($p < 0.01$; $d = 0.67$) during the first 20 min of rides at $RPE_{GET+15\%}$ than those at RPE_{GET}. There was no significant difference between RPE_{GET} and $RPE_{GET+15\%}$ for $\dot{V}O_2$ at min 21–33 ($p < 0.01$; $d = 0.10$), 35–47 min ($p < 0.01$; $d = 0.03$), or min 49–60 ($p < 0.01$; $d = 0.14$) (Figure 3).

4. Discussion

In the present study, RPE_{GET} and $RPE_{GET+15\%}$ were 70.1% ± 1.6% and 80.8% ± 1.9% of $\dot{V}O_{2Peak}$, respectively (Table 1). The GET typically occurs at between 70% and 80% of $\dot{V}O_{2Peak}$ in endurance-trained individuals [24], but at between 50% and 60% of $\dot{V}O_{2Peak}$ for those who are untrained [25]. The RCP, however, typically occurs at about 50% of the difference between $\dot{V}O_{2Peak}$ and GET (*i.e.*, 85%–90% of $\dot{V}O_{2Peak}$) in endurance-trained individuals [1]. Thus, in the present study, the RPE_{GET} and $RPE_{GET+15\%}$ corresponded to relative intensities similar to those of previous studies [1,6,24,25] and represented the demarcation of the moderate and heavy exercise intensity domain (RPE_{GET}), and an intensity within the heavy domain ($RPE_{GET+15\%}$).

During exercise at a constant perception of effort, there are dissociations among the patterns of responses for physiological and perceptual variables typical of constant PO exercise [6,8,9]. For example, Stoudemire *et al.* [8] reported that during treadmill running at a constant RPE corresponding with 2.5 mmol $(La^-)_b$ and 4.0 mmol $(La^-)_b$, there were dissociations among RPE, $(La^-)_b$, $\dot{V}O_2$, and velocity. To maintain RPE, velocity was reduced which resulted in a decreased metabolic cost and $\dot{V}O_2$ across time [8]. More recently, Cochrane *et al.* [6] reported dissociations among RPE, $\dot{V}O_2$, HR, $\dot{V}_E$, RER, and PO during continuous cycle ergometry at a constant RPE in the moderate domain. During the constant RPE rides, $\dot{V}O_2$, HR, $\dot{V}_E$, and RER tracked the time-dependent decreases in PO [6]. In the present study, there were similar dissociations among RPE *vs.* $\dot{V}O_2$, HR, $\dot{V}_E$, RER, and PO during continuous cycle ergometry at RPE_{GET} and $RPE_{GET+15\%}$. For example, $\dot{V}O_2$, HR, RER, $\dot{V}_E$, and PO decreased across time during both 60 min rides. Thus, the dissociations among RPE *vs.* $\dot{V}O_2$, HR, $\dot{V}_E$, RER, and PO in the present study were similar to those of previous studies [6,8] and further supported the hypothesis that metabolic, cardiovascular, and intensity related variables do not solely mediate the perception of effort during cycle ergometry at a constant RPE within the moderate or heavy exercise intensity domains.

The pattern of responses for both the mean, normalized HR and $\dot{V}_E$ differed between the rides at RPE_{GET} and $RPE_{GET+15\%}$. At RPE_{GET}, the mean, normalized HR and $\dot{V}_E$ responses exhibited quadratic and linear decreases, respectively, while at $RPE_{GET+15\%}$ the mean, normalized HR and $\dot{V}_E$ exhibited linear and quadratic decreases across the 60 min rides. Although the patterns for HR decline over time were different between the two rides, the mean, normalized HRs across the 60 min rides were similar (85.7% *vs.* 84.7% HR_{peak}). In addition, HR did not change proportionately with reductions in PO during the constant RPE rides. For example, at $RPE_{GET+15\%}$, greater reductions in PO were required at the initiation and throughout the 60 min rides, which likely explained the lack of a plateau and linear decline for HR during the more intense rides (Figure 2d). The participants, therefore, spent more time at their initial $\%HR_{peak}$ during the moderate intensity rides than during rides in the heavy domain. It has been reported [26] that during sustained, moderate intensity exercise (50%–75% $\dot{V}O_{2Peak}$), HR "drifts" upward as the intensity of exercise is maintained. This drift in HR has been attributed to increases in cutaneous blood flow due to increases in core temperature [26]. When riding at a constant RPE within the moderate exercise intensity domain, HR initially drifted up across time, but to a lesser degree than would be expected during constant PO cycle ergometry, due to reductions in PO, which resulted in an overall quadratic decrease across time. In the heavy domain ($RPE_{GET+15\%}$), however, HR exhibited a linear decrease across time, which was attributed to a more rapid initial reduction in PO. The patterns of response for HR in the present study differed from those of Stoudemire *et al.* [8] who reported a continuous rise in HR throughout two, 30 min runs at a constant RPE. Although the mechanisms responsible for the rise in HR over time during the constant RPE runs were not discussed [8], the dissociations for RPE and HR were consistent with the findings of the present study. That is, the uncoupling of HR and RPE indicates that HR did not mediate the perception of effort during constant RPE exercise within the moderate and heavy exercise intensity domains [8,27].

In the present study, the mean, normalized $\dot{V}_E$ exhibited a linear decrease across time during the constant RPE rides within the moderate intensity domain. During the rides within the heavy domain ($RPE_{GET+15\%}$), however, the mean, normalized $\dot{V}_E$ exhibited a quadratic decrease across time. Previous studies [4,28] have reported different time-dependent patterns of responses for $\dot{V}_E$ that are, in part, dependent upon the intensity of exercise as well as the parameter being held constant. For example, Dempsey [4] reported that during moderate intensity exercise at a constant PO, $\dot{V}_E$ typically increases as a function of tidal volume, whereas increases at higher intensities are mediated by increases in $\mathcal{F}_b$[4]. When cycling at a constant $\dot{V}_E$ within the moderate domain (50%–60% $\dot{V}O_{2Peak}$), however, tidal volume has been shown to decrease, while $\mathcal{F}_b$, core temperature, and RPE responses increased across time [28]. In the current study, both 60 min rides at RPE_{GET} and $RPE_{GET+15\%}$ resulted in decreases for metabolic ($\dot{V}O_2$ and RER) and work intensity (PO) related variables, which indicated a decrease in the metabolic cost of the exercise. Furthermore, RPE and $\mathcal{F}_b$ remained constant across time during the rides in the moderate and heavy exercise intensity domains. Thus, changes for the patterns of responses for $\dot{V}_E$ were not consistent with those of $\mathcal{F}_b$ or the perception of effort, but they tracked decreases in metabolic cost during the 60 min rides at a constant RPE.

During both moderate and heavy intensity rides, only $\mathcal{F}_b$ tracked RPE across time. The mean, normalized $\mathcal{F}_b$ response did not change across time during the rides at RPE_{GET} and $RPE_{GET+15\%}$. These findings were consistent with those of Cochrane *et al.* [6] who reported a close agreement between RPE and $\mathcal{F}_b$, but dissociations for both RPE and $\mathcal{F}_b$ *vs.* metabolic ($\dot{V}O_2$ and RER), cardiovascular (HR), and ventilatory ($\dot{V}_E$) responses during constant RPE cycle ergometry within the moderate intensity domain. It was hypothesized [6] that reflex actions associated with the exercise pressor reflex model of fatigue [12,29–31] best explained the similarity for RPE and $\mathcal{F}_b$ during the constant RPE rides. According to the exercise pressor reflex model [12,29–31], afferent signals from small group III (mechanical changes) and IV afferents (metabolic changes) from working thigh and respiratory muscles mediate the ventilatory, cardiovascular, and RPE responses during moderate and heavy intensity exercise [2,12,32,33]. It has also been suggested [11] that in addition to mediating cardioventilatory responses, group III and IV afferents may have a "critical role" in the regulation of the perception of effort during dynamic exercise. For example, a lower perception of effort was reported during exercise with an intact somatosensory feedback system, which incorporated both group III and IV afferents, than during exercise with blocked spinal receptors [11]. In the present study, it is unlikely that there was a continuous build-up of metabolic byproducts during either of the constant RPE rides, because of the decreases in metabolic cost ($\dot{V}O_2$ and RER) and work intensity (PO). For the rides beginning in the heavy exercise intensity domain, there may have been an increase in $(La^-)_b$ typical of heavy intensity exercise during the first 20 min of the rides, however, all participants ended the 60-min $RPE_{GET+15\%}$ rides below the GET (65.7% ± 2.2% $\dot{V}O_{2Peak}$) in the moderate domain. These findings did not support an increase in metabolic byproducts ($(La^-)_b$, H^+, K^+) or inadequate supplies of ATP [1,34,35]. In addition, there was likely a reduction in required central command due to the decreases in PO, which was tracked by reductions in HR and $\dot{V}_E$ across the 60 min rides. Previous studies [11,32,36] have suggested that group IV afferents may be linked to changes in central command and the cardiovascular system. It has been reported [11] that an increased rate of discharge from group IV afferents tracked increases in $\dot{V}_E$, HR, and central command during continuous, constant PO cycle ergometry. In the current study, there were reductions in HR, $\dot{V}_E$, and, potentially, a reduction in central command during the 60 min constant RPE rides, and therefore, group IV afferents may not have the same patterns of discharge during exercise at a constant RPE as those reported during constant PO exercise [11,28].

The results of the present study also have implications for the regulation of exercise intensity during prolonged cycling exercise. For example, there was no significant difference between the $\dot{V}O_2$ throughout the 60 min constant RPE rides at RPE_{GET} (Figure 3). There were differences, however, between the $\dot{V}O_2$ at 15% above the GET, as determined from the incremental test, and the $\dot{V}O_2$ during the last 40 min of the 60 min constant RPE ride at $RPE_{GET+15\%}$ (Figure 3). These findings indicated that the use of a perceptual intensity (RPE_{GET}) may be used for training at the gas exchange threshold, in place of more expensive monitoring methods such as $(La^-)_b$, heart rate, and oxygen consumption, during cycle ergometry exercise. However, cycling at a higher perceptual intensity (GET + 15%), such as that associated with the heavy exercise intensity domain, did not result in the same starting intensity ($\dot{V}O_2$) after 20 min, and therefore, prescribing exercise associated with a higher RPE may only be useful for the first 20 min of cycling exercise. Future studies should compare the effects of multiple training visits at a percentage of $\dot{V}O_2$ (GET and GET + 15%) and a perceptual intensity (RPE) on markers of aerobic performance.

The patterns of responses for physiological variables during exercise at a constant perceptual rating (RPE) within the moderate and heavy exercise intensity domains differ from those typically observed during constant power output exercise [1]. Given that it is not uncommon for cyclists to perform rides at varying workloads across time, these findings may provide applications for the prescription and tracking of performance. The finding that the $\dot{V}O_2$ corresponding with the GET, a commonly used threshold for tempo training exercises, was maintained by controlling perception during a 60 min cycling test also speaks to the ability of cyclists to maintain work at the demarcation point of the moderate and heavy exercise intensity domains. There is, however, a need to extend the findings of the present study on the effect of training at a constant RPE (RPE_{GET}) *vs.* a more traditional prescription ($\%HR_{peak}$ or $\%\dot{V}O_{2peak}$) on outcome variables associated with aerobic performance (onset of blood lactate, occurrence of GET, substrate utilization (RER), and $\dot{V}O_{2peak}$). Our study demonstrates that there may be a relationship between how one perceives exercise and the underlying mechanisms associated with breathing patterns and that the ability to regulate, or pace, cycling exercise at a constant RPE may be tied to the exercise intensity corresponding to the work bout.

In summary, the patterns of response for $\mathcal{F}_b$, which did not change across time but tracked RPE, were similar during both moderate and heavy intensity cycle ergometry exercise. In addition, the $\dot{V}O_2$ associated with an RPE grounded threshold corresponding to the GET appeared to be sustainable for up to 60 min of cycling exercise, while that above the GET could only be maintained for the first 20 min of exercise. The findings of the current study, as well as those of previous studies [6,10,15,18] supported the hypothesis that small group III afferents associated with mechanical distortions within the working thigh and respiratory muscles may influence both perceptual and respiratory responses associated with the frequency of breathing that were independent of changes in metabolic cost, cardiovascular, and ventilation responses. In addition, exercising at the RPE corresponding to the GET may be useful as a pacing or training tool.

Author Contributions

Kristen C. Cochrane was the primary manuscript writer, and carried out data acquisition, data analysis, and data interpretation. Ethan C. Hill, Cory M. Smith, and Nathaniel D.M. Jenkins were significant contributors to data acquisition, read and approved the final manuscript, and were manuscript reviewers/revisers. Joel T. Cramer, Glen O. Johnson, and Richard J. Schmidt were significant manuscript reviewers/revisers. Terry J. Housh was the primary manuscript reviewer/reviser, a substantial contributor to concept and design, and contributed to data interpretation.

Conflicts of Interest

The authors declare no conflict of interest.

References

1. Gaesser, G.A.; Poole, D.C. The slow component of oxygen uptake kinetics in humans. *Exerc. Sport Sci. Rev.* **1996**, *24*, 35–71.
2. Poole, D.C.; Ward, S.A.; Gardner, G.W.; Whipp, B.J. Metabolic and respiratory profile of the upper limit for prolonged exercise in man. *Ergonomics* **1988**, *31*, 1265–1279.
3. Whipp, B.J. Dynamics of pulmonary gas exchange. *Circulation* **1987**, *76*, 19–29.
4. Dempsey, J.A. Is the lung built for exercise. *Med. Sci. Sport Exerc.* **1986**, *18*, 143–155.
5. Housh, T.J.; Perry, S.R.; Bull, A.J.; Johnson, G.O.; Ebersole, K.T.; Housh, D.J.; de Vries, H.A. Mechanomyographic and electromyographic responses during submaximal cycle ergometry. *Eur. J. Appl. Physiol.* **2000**, *83*, 381–387.

6. Cochrane, K.C.; Housh, T.J.; Bergstrom, H.C.; Jenkins, N.D.M.; Johnson, G.O.; Schmidt, R.J.; Cramer, J.T. Physiological responses during cycle ergometry at a constant perception of effort. *Int. J. Sports Med.* **2015**, *36*, 466–473.
7. Lajoie, C.; Laurencelle, L.; Trudeau, F. Physiological responses to cycling for 60 min at maximal lactate steady state. *Can. J. Appl. Physiol.* **2000**, *25*, 250–261.
8. Stoudemire, N.M.; Wideman, L.; Pass, K.A.; McGinnes, C.L.; Gaesser, G.A.; Weltman, A. The validity of regulating blood lactate concentration during running by ratings of perceived exertion. *Med. Sci. Sport. Exerc.* **1996**, *28*, 490–495.
9. Lander, P.J.; Butterly, R.J.; Edwards, A.M. Self-paced exercise is less physically challenging than enforced constant pace exercise of the same intensity: Influence of complex central metabolic control. *Br. J. Sports Med.* **2009**, *43*, 789–795.
10. Ribeiro, J.P.; Hughes, V.; Fielding, R.A.; Holden, W.; Evans, W.; Knuttgen, H.G. Metabolic and ventilatory responses to steady state exercise relative to lactate threshold. *Eur. J. Appl. Physiol.* **1986**, *55*, 215–221.
11. Amann, M.; Blain, G.M.; Proctor, L.T.; Sebranek, J.J.; Pegelow, D.F.; Demsey, J.A. Group III and IV afferents contribute to ventilatory and cardiovascular responses to rhythmic exercise in humans. *J. Appl. Physiol.* **2010**, *109*, 966–976.
12. Kaufman, M.P.; Hayes, S.G. The exercise pressor reflex. *Clin. Auton. Res.* **2002**, *12*, 429–439.
13. Marcora, S.M. Do we really need a central governor to explain brain regulation of exercise performance. *Eur. J. Appl. Physiol.* **2008**, *104*, 929–931.
14. Mitchell, J.H.; Kaufman, M.F.; Iwamoto, G.A. The exercise pressor reflex: Its cardiovascular effects, afferent mechanisms, and central pathways. *Ann. Rev. Physiol.* **1983**, *45*, 229–242.
15. St. Clair Gibson, A.; Schabort, E.J.; Noakes, T.D. Reduced neuromuscular activity and force generation during prolonged cycling. *Am. J. Regul. Integr. Comp. Physiol.* **2001**, *281*, R187–R196.
16. Edwards, A.M.; Polman, R.C.J. Pacing and awareness: Brain regulation of physical activity. *Sport Med.* **2013**, *43*, 1057–1064.
17. Abbiss, C.R.; Laursen, P. Models to explain fatigue during prolonged endurance cycling. *Sport Med.* **2005**, *35*, 866–898
18. Pescatello, L.S.; Arena, R.; Riebe, D.; Thompson, P.D. *ACSM's Guidelines for Exercise Testing and Prescription*; Lippincott Williams & Wilkins: Philadelphia, PA, USA, 2014.
19. Borg, G.A. Perceived exertion as an indicator of somatic stress. *Scan. J. Rehab. Med.* **1970**, *2*, 92–98.
20. Borg, G.A. Psychophysical bases of perceived exertion. *Med. Sci. Sport. Exerc.* **1982**, *14*, 377–381.
21. Borg G. *Borg's Perceived Exertion and Pain Scales*; APA PsycNET: Champaign, IL, USA, 1998.
22. Robergs, R.A.; Dwyer, D.; Astorino, T. Recommendations for improved data processing from expired gas analysis indirect calorimetry. *Sport Med.* **2010**, *49*, 95–111.
23. Beaver, W.L.; Wasserman, K.; Whipp, B.J. A new method for detecting anaerobic threshold by gas exchange. *J. Appl. Physiol.* **1986**, *60*, 2020–2027.
24. Davis, J.A. Anaerobic threshold: Review of the concept and directions for future research. *Med. Sci. Sport Exerc.* **1985**, *17*, 6–18.
25. Davis, J.A.; Frank, M.H.; Whipp, B.J.; Wasserman, K. Anaerobic threshold alterations caused by endurance training in middle-aged men. *J. Appl. Physiol.* **1979**, *46*, 1039–1046.

26. Coyle, E.F.; Gonzalez-Alonso, J. Cardiovascular drift during prolonged exercise: New perspectives. *Exerc. Sport. Sci. Rev.* **2001**, *29*, 88–92.
27. Mihevic, P.M. Sensory cues for perceived exertion: A review. *Med. Sci. Sports Exerc.* **1981**, *13*, 150–163.
28. Martin, B.J.; Morgan, E.J.; Zwillich, C.W.; Weil, J.V. Influence of exercise hyperthermia on exercise breathing pattern. *J. Appl. Physiol.* **1979**, *47*, 1039–1042.
29. Amann M.; Proctor, L.T.; Sebranek, J.J.; Eldridge, M.W.; Pegelow, D.F.; Dempsey, J.A. Somatosensory feedback from the limbs exerts inhibitory influences on central neural drive during whole body endurance exercise. *J. Appl. Physiol.* **2008**, *105*, 1714–1724.
30. Amann, M.; Blain, G.M.; Proctor, L.T.; Sebranek, J.J.; Pegelow, D.F.; Dempsey, J.A. Implications of group III and IV muscle afferents for high-intensity endurance exercise performance in humans. *J. Appl. Physiol.* **2011**, *589*, 5299–5309.
31. Hayes, S.G.; Kaufman, M.P. Gadolinium attenuates exercise pressor reflex in cats. *Am. J. Physiol. Heart Circ. Physiol.* **2001**, *280*, H2153–H2161.
32. McCord, J.L.; Kaufman, M.P. Reflex Autonomic Responses Evoked by Group III and IV Muscle Afferents. In *Translational Pain Research: From Mouse to Man*; Kruger, L., Light, A.R., Eds.; CRC Press: Boca Raton, FL, USA, 2009.
33. Garland, S.J.; Kaufman, M.P. Role of muscle afferents in the inhibition of motoneurons during fatigue. *Adv. Exp. Med. Biol.* **1995**, *384*, 271–278.
34. Hug, F.; Faucher, M.; Kipson, N.; Jammes, Y. EMG signs of neuromuscular fatigue related to the ventilatory threshold during cycling exercise. *Clin. Physiol. Funct. Imag.* **2003**, *23*, 208–214.
35. Enoka, R.M.; Stuart, D.G. Neurobiology of muscle fatigue. *J. Appl. Physiol.* **1992**, *72*, 1631–1648.
36. Goodwin, G.M.; McCloskey, D.I.; Mitchel, J.H. Cardiovascular and respiratory responses to changes in central command during isometric exercise at constant muscle tension. *J. Physiol.* **1972**, *226*, 173–190.

3

A Comparison of Upper Body Strength between Rock Climbing and Resistance Trained Men

Kristina M. Macias [†], Lee E. Brown [†,*], Jared W. Coburn [†] and David D. Chen [†]

Human Performance Laboratory, Department of Kinesiology, California State University, Fullerton, 800 N State College Blvd, Fullerton, CA 92831, USA; E-Mails: Kristina.macias@gmail.com (K.M.M.); jcoburn@fullerton.edu (J.W.C.); dapchen@fullerton.edu (D.D.C.)

† These authors contributed equally to this work.

* Author to whom correspondence should be addressed; E-Mail: leebrown@fullerton.edu

Academic Editor: Eling de Bruin

Abstract: Studies have shown that advanced rock climbers have greater upper body strength than that of novice climbers or non-climbers. The purpose of this study was to compare upper body strength between rock climbing and resistance trained men. Fifteen resistance trained men (age 25.28 ± 2.26 yrs; height 177.45 ± 4.08 cm; mass 85.17 ± 10.23 kg; body fat 10.13 ± 5.40%) and 15 rock climbing men (age 23.25 ± 2.23 yrs; height 175.57 ± 8.03 cm; mass 66.66 ± 9.40 kg; body fat 6.86 ± 3.82%) volunteered to participate. Rock climbing (RC) men had been climbing for at least two years, 2–3 times a week, able to climb at least a boulder rating of V4–5 and had no current injuries. Resistance trained (RT) men had been total body strength training for at least two years, 2–3 times a week with no current injuries. Each participant performed pull-ups to failure, grip strength, and pinch strength. RT were significantly older and heavier than RC. RC performed significantly more pull-ups (19.31 ± 4.31) than RT (15.64 ± 4.82). RC had greater relative pinch strength (R 0.27 ± 0.10 kg/kg; L 0.24 ± 0.07 kg/kg) than RT (R 0.19 ± 0.04 kg/kg; L 0.16 ± 0.05 kg/kg) and greater relative grip strength (R 0.70 ± 0.10 kg/kg; L 0.65 ± 0.12 kg/kg) than RT (R 0.57 ± 0.14 kg/kg; L 0.56 ± 0.15 kg/kg). Overall, RC men demonstrated greater performance in tests involving relative strength when compared to RT men. Rock climbing can promote increased upper body strength even in thc absence of traditional resistance training.

Keywords: grip; finger; pinch; pull-ups; push-ups; relative

1. Introduction

Rock climbing involves lifting their body mass by pulling with their upper body musculature and using many different handholds and grips, including a wide 4-finger pinch and a small two finger pinch. This requires significant finger, grip and upper body strength. Balas [1] demonstrated that a higher climbing volume and an eight week training program resulted in increased grip and relative upper body strength of youth climbers. They also observed that hand-arm strength and endurance, body composition and climbing volume combined were predictors of climbing performance. Studies have also shown a significant difference in grip and pinch maximal voluntary contraction (MVC) in elite climbers when compared to recreational and non-climbers [2–6].

Predictors of climbing ability include upper body strength, grip and finger strength, along with high relative strength and lower body fat [7,8]. Elite climbers exhibit significantly greater strength than recreational climbers and non-climbers and this is seen even more prominent when the grip is more climbing specific [5,6,9]. Limonta *et al.* [2] observed a higher maximal voluntary contraction and a significant difference in endurance time between elite climbers and sedentary individuals during controlled fatiguing contractions in finger flexor muscles. Grant [4] determined that elite climbers had significantly greater flexibility (leg span), upper body strength (pull-ups and bent arm hang), and left and right pincer strength than recreational climbers and physically active non-climbers.

Based on the previous studies, rock climbing appears to have an important upper body strength component, which is derived from that training. Studies have observed significant differences in handgrip and pincer strength between climbers and sedentary individuals [3,4]. However, there is a paucity of research comparing strength of those involved in high-level rock climbing and traditional resistance training. Therefore, the purpose of this study was to compare upper body strength between rock climbers and resistance-trained men. We hypothesized that resistance trained men would exhibit significantly greater absolute grip due to their traditional training. Another hypothesis was that climbers would exhibit superior relative strength due to their experience with bodyweight support activity.

2. Materials and Methods

2.1. Participants

All participants were males between the ages of 20–29 with no injuries in the past six months that would prevent them from completing each task. Climbers had at least two years' experience, climbed indoors 2–3 times per week, outdoors at least once a month and did not participate in a structured resistance training program. Each participant was considered a self-reported "advanced" climber with at least a Hueco Scale rating of V4–5 (on a V0–16 scale) [10]. Resistance-trained men had at least two years' experience in full body lifting consisting of squats, deadlift, bench press and pull-ups. At the beginning of each visit, subjects signed a university IRB approved informed consent document. Then height and weight were recorded on a stadiometer (216, Seca Corporation, Ontario, CA, USA) and weight scale (ES200L, Ohaus Corporation, Pinebrook, NJ, USA).

2.2. Body Fat Percentage

Skinfold thickness was measured to the nearest .5mm using skinfold calipers (Lange, Santa Cruz, CA, USA). Two measurements were taken on the right side of the body (chest, abdomen and thigh) and the average of the values was recorded for analysis. Body fat percentage was estimated using the Jackson and Pollock equation [11].

2.3. Pull-Ups

For all performance tests, subjects performed at least three repetitions for warm-up and familiarization until they could execute the test per the specific guidelines, then rested for 2 min. Pull-ups and push-ups were counterbalanced. They completed the maximum number of pronated pull-ups possible in one minute [12]. They were positioned hanging from the bar with arms at full extension then pulled up so their chin reached the top of the bar then lowered themselves back down to full arm extension with their legs also fully extended [4]. If they used any momentum from their lower body as assistance the repetition was not counted. They were able to rest with arms at full extension, but if they let go of the bar the test was terminated.

2.4. Push-Ups

They laid prone on the floor and placed their thumbs at shoulder width, kept their body in a straight line and touched their chin to a tennis ball at the bottom of each repetition [13]. A cadence was set to 80 beats per minute (40 push-ups per minute) with a metronome and the test lasted a maximum of two min. When they were unable to keep the cadence or stopped due to fatigue, the test was terminated. [14].

2.5. Finger Strength

Participants rested for 5 min before finger strength tests were administered. A Flexiforce sensor (Model A201, South Boston, MA, USA) was used to measure finger strength between the thumb and all four fingers (1 = index, 2 = middle, 3 = ring, and 4 = little finger) [15]. They squeezed putty grip (Power putty) five times with each hand for warm-up, then rested 2 min. They were seated in an upright position with their arm placed on a table that was adjusted so that the elbow and shoulder joints were flexed to 90 degrees. Starting with the thumb and index finger, they placed the finger lightly over the sensor with the thumb opposed. The other fingers were curled under to prevent them from assisting when the sensor was squeezed. When signaled, they gradually squeezed the sensor for 5 s leading to maximal force. Next the thumb and middle finger were tested, with only the ring and little finger curled under. Then the ring finger was tested with only the little finger curled under. Finally, the little finger was tested last. Each finger on each hand was measured alternately three times with 15 s rest and the best of the three repetitions was recorded for analysis. Relative values were determined by dividing strength by body mass (kg/kg).

2.6. Pinch Strength

A handgrip dynamometer (T.K.K5401 Takei Koyo, Tokyo, Japan) was used to measure pinch strength. Participants squeezed putty grip (Power putty) five times with each hand for warm-up, then rested 2 min. The dynamometer was set to 4.5 cm wide [4]. They were seated in an upright position exactly the same as for finger strength with the dynamometer digital display facing away. They grasped the moveable arm of the dynamometer with four fingertips and the thumb opposed and braced around the immovable part of the device, while the administrator held the device stable [16]. Measurements were taken alternately between left and right hands with 15 s rest. Each hand was measured three times and the best of the three repetitions was recorded for analysis. Relative values were determined by dividing strength by body mass (kg/kg).

2.7. Grip Strength

The same handgrip dynamometer was used for measurement. The size of the grip was adjusted so that the second joint of the middle finger was positioned at 90 degrees. Participants were seated in an upright position on a box that was 47 cm tall, while holding the dynamometer in one hand, arm at their side with the digital display facing away. They squeezed the dynamometer for 5 s leading to maximal force then released [17]. Measurements were taken alternately between the left and right hands with 15 s rest. Each hand was measured three times and the best of the three repetitions was recorded for analysis. Relative values were determined by dividing strength by body mass (kg/kg).

2.8. Statistical Analyses

Two independent t-tests analyzed pull-ups and push-ups between groups. Multiple 2 × 2 (group × hand) mixed factor ANOVAs analyzed absolute and relative grip and absolute and relative pinch strength. Multiple 2 × 2 × 4 (group × hand × finger) mixed factor ANOVAs analyzed absolute and relative finger strength. Main effects were followed up with *t*-tests or LSD post hoc tests. Alpha level was set a-priori at 0.05.

3. Results

RT were significantly older and heavier than RC, but height and body fat percentage were not significantly different (Table 1).

Table 1. Mean ± SD of age, height, mass and body composition between resistance trained (RT) and rock climbing (RC) men.

Variable	RT	RC
Age (yrs)	25.28 ± 2.26*	23.25 ± 2.23
Height (cm)	177.45 ± 4.08	175.57 ± 8.03
Mass (kg)	85.17 ± 10.23*	66.66 ± 9.40
Body Fat (%)	10.13 ± 5.40	6.86 ± 3.82

Note: * Significantly (age $P = 0.02$; mass $P = 0.02$) greater than RC.

For pull-ups and push-ups, RC performed a significantly greater number of pull-ups than RT, but push-ups were not significantly different (Table 2).

Table 2. Mean ± SD of pull-ups and push-ups between resistance trained (RT) and rock climbing (RC) men.

Performance	RT	RC
Pull-ups (#)	15.64 ± 4.82	19.31 ± 4.31*
Push-ups (#)	38.28 ± 4.89	34.56 ± 8.13

Note: * Significantly ($P = 0.03$) greater than RT.

For absolute grip, there was no interaction or main effect for group but there was a main effect for hand with the right being stronger than the left. For relative grip, there was no interaction but there was a main effect for hand with the right being stronger than the left and a main effect for group with RC having significantly greater relative grip strength than RT (Table 3).

Table 3. Mean ± SD of left and right absolute and relative grip between resistance trained (RT) and rock climbing (RC) men and combined total for both groups.

Performance	RT	RC	Group Total
R grip (kg)	49.26 ± 14.16	46.15 ± 6.24	47.60 ± 10.61#
L grip (kg)	48.45 ± 15.42	43.16 ± 6.33	45.63 ± 11.60
R gripREL (kg/kg)	0.57 ± 0.14	0.70 ± 0.10	0.64 ± 0.14#
L gripREL (kg/kg)	0.56 ± 0.15	0.65 ± 0.12	0.61 ± 0.14
R&Lavg gripREL (kg/kg)	0.56 ± 0.14	0.67 ± 0.11*	-

Note: # Significantly (absolute $P = 0.03$; relative $P = 0.01$) greater than left; * Significantly ($P = 0.02$) greater than RT.

For absolute pinch, there was no interaction or main effect for group but there was a main effect for hand with the right being stronger than the left. For relative pinch, there was no interaction but there were main effects for group and hand. RC had significantly greater relative pinch strength than RT (Table 4).

Table 4. Mean ± SD of left and right absolute and relative pinch strength between resistance trained (RT) and rock climbing (RC) men and combined total for both groups.

Performance	RT	RC	Group Total
R pinch (kg)	16.07 ± 3.00	18.03 ± 7.01	17.11 ± 5.52#
L pinch (kg)	14.15 ± 4.65	16.11 ± 5.35	15.19 ± 5.05
R pinchREL (kg/kg)	0.19 ± 0.04	0.27 ± 0.10	0.23 ± 0.08#
L pinchREL (kg/kg)	0.16 ± 0.05	0.24 ± 0.07	0.20 ± 0.07
R&Lavg pinchREL (kg/kg)	0.18 ± 0.04	0.25 ± 0.08*	-

Note: # Significantly (absolute $P = 0.00$; relative $P = 0.00$) greater than left; * Significantly ($P = 0.00$) greater than RT.

For absolute and relative finger strength there were no significant three way or two-way interactions or main effects for group or hand. However, there was a main effect for fingers for both. Both absolute (Figure 1) and relative (Figure 2) finger strength were followed up with LSD post hoc tests for pairwise comparisons that showed the first finger was significantly stronger than fingers three and four. The second finger was significantly stronger than fingers one, three and four. The third finger was significantly stronger than finger four.

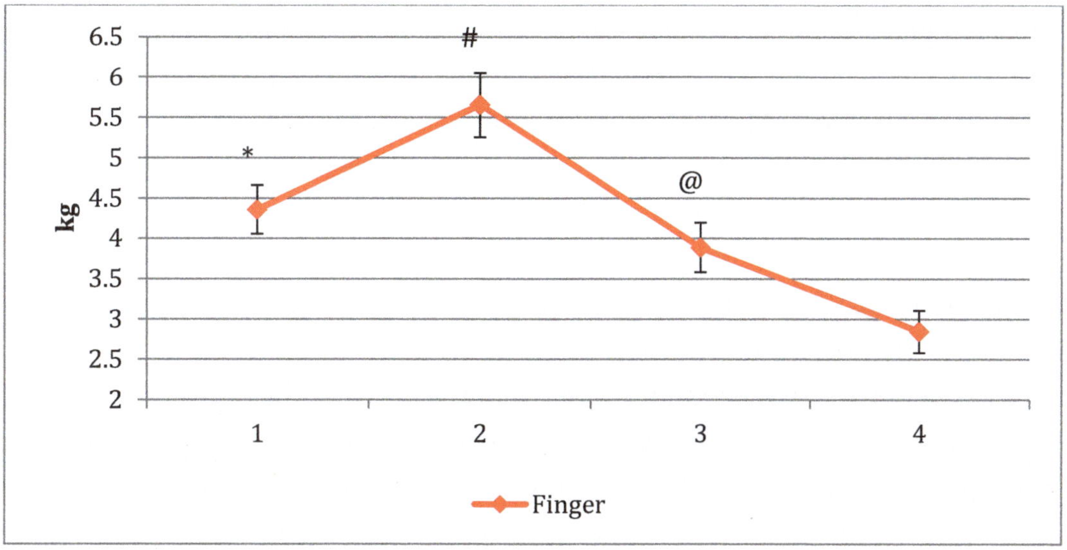

Figure 1. Mean ± SD of absolute finger strength. 1 = index, 2 = middle. 3 = ring and 4 = little. * Significantly ($P = 0.00$) greater than fingers 3 and 4; # Significantly ($P = 0.00$) greater than fingers 1,3 and 4; @ Significantly ($P = 0.00$) greater than finger 4.

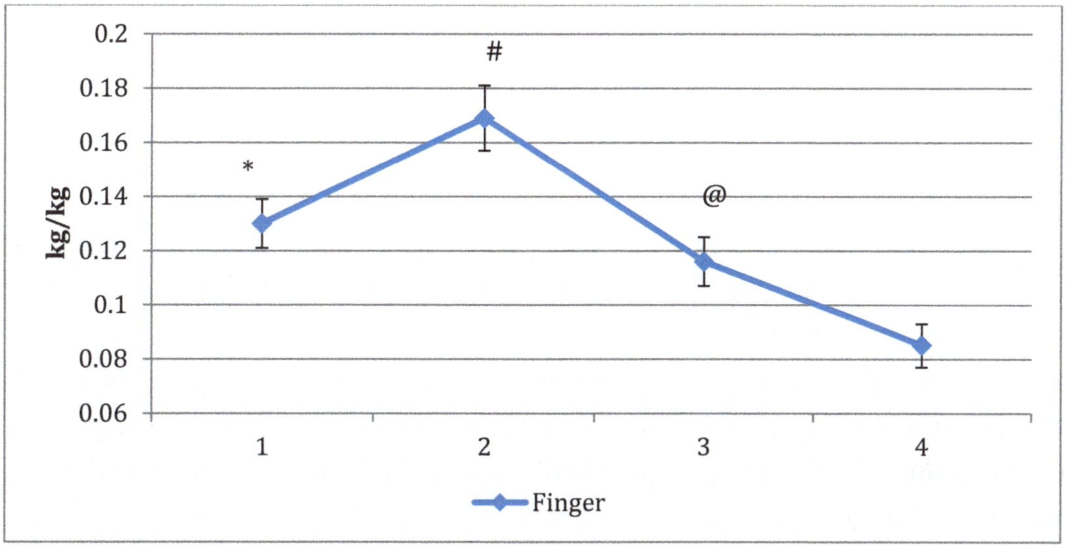

Figure 2. Mean ± SD of relative finger strength. 1 = index, 2 = middle. 3 = ring and 4 = little. * Significantly ($P = 0.00$) greater than fingers 3 and 4; # Significantly ($P = 0.00$) greater than fingers 1,3 and 4; @ Significantly ($P = 0.00$) greater than finger 4.

4. Discussion

The purpose of this study was to compare upper body strength between rock climbing and resistance trained men. The main findings were that rock climbers performed a significantly ($P = 0.03$) greater number of pull-ups, and had significantly greater relative grip ($P = 0.01$) and relative pinch ($P = 0.00$) strength than resistance trained men. This may be due to the physical demands required of rock climbing men to negotiate challenging routes successfully. These demands include lifting their body mass by pulling with their upper body musculature and supporting their body weight by many different handholds and grips [7,8]. Requirements for these demands include low body mass, strong pulling, pinching, and gripping strength to support body weight movements, and a large climbing volume in order to see increased relative strength and climbing ability [4,9,17]. In contrast, resistance trained men perform traditional weight room exercises and generally demonstrate greater absolute upper body strength but less relative strength than climbers. Grip strength of resistance trained men is developed through upper, and lower body exercises [18,19]. Climbers strengthen their upper body by lifting their own body mass and by directly working the grip via pinching and gripping [1,4,17]. Resistance trained men utilize exercises that indirectly strengthen their grip (*i.e.*, push-ups, squats, leg press, *etc.*) [18,19]. Therefore, it appears that both activities may be utilized to improve upper body strength.

In this study, we found that although groups were similar in height, climbers had significantly less body mass when compared to resistance trained men. This is probably due to the specific demands of each respective activity. Schweizer [20] determined that climbers had low levels of body mass and that body weight and height were negatively correlated with climbing performance. The current study corroborates that climbers' lower body mass probably led to greater relative strength.

In a contrasting study, Grant [4] demonstrated that there were no significant differences between elite, recreational and non-climbers for body mass, height, height:body mass ratio, or body fat %. It is important to note that they compared climbers to other climbers, not resistance trained men. So it is not known whether the elite climbers would have been significantly different in mass and body fat when compared to the resistance trained men of the current study. It is clear that low body fat and mass are desirable to climbers, however, there are numerous other variables that are used to determine climbing level such as type of training, climbing volume, grip, pinch, and finger strength [1,4,9,17]. For resistance trained men, training leads to hypertrophy and increased body mass which results in greater strength. This may be why resistance trained men in our study had significantly greater body mass. Despite differences in training, each group's goals overlap to some degree. Both desire increased upper body strength, which improves grip strength.

Balas [1] concluded that the practice of rock climbing resulted in increased upper body strength. He had young climbers, with little or no experience, participate in an 8-week climbing program and saw a significant increase in upper body strength, specifically, relative grip strength. In a similar study [17], he demonstrated that climbing volume and experience can predict performance, with a notable relationship between number of meters climbed per week, body fat, grip and bent- arm hang. Our results correspondingly showed that rock climbers had significantly greater relative pinch and grip strength. These two different grip types were chosen to be tested for the purpose of variation and specificity. The pinch is more climbing specific and the grip is more resistance training specific. It seems reasonable that if climbers utilized resistance training, focusing on larger lifts, it would result in improved upper body strength. However, a significant increase in mass might decrease climbing performance.

Several studies have shown that elite or advanced climbers demonstrate significantly greater MVC in a grip or pinch test [4,9,17,21]. Green [21] saw that trained climbers (similar to those in this study) had a significantly greater MVC and intermittent exercise capacity than untrained climbers. The conclusion is that climbing directly increases grip strength, similar to the current study.

Resistance training is commonly used to increase upper body strength. Thomas [18] observed the effects of a resistance training program on handgrip strength in young adults. Their results indicated that even though none of the movements in the training program involved specifically strengthening grip, each exercise contributed to overall improvement of absolute grip strength of the right hand only.

Another study by Wilmore [19] supports resistance training as a way to improve handgrip strength. Subjects participated in a training program that consisted of basic strength exercises and increased their absolute grip strength even though none of the exercises specifically strengthened handgrip. We hypothesized in the current study that resistance trained men would exhibit significantly greater absolute grip strength because absolute strength is the primary outcome of resistance training. However, we observed no difference between groups but climbers had significantly greater relative grip and pinch strength. Once again, this is probably due to climbers having less body mass.

Another hypothesis was that climbers would exhibit superior performance in tests of relative strength, such as push-ups and pull-ups. This was partially confirmed as climbers performed significantly more pull-ups than resistance trained men. Again, probably a result of climbers having significantly less body mass. Additionally, pull-ups are a very common movement performed in climbing and could lead to greater muscular endurance in rock climbers. Grant [4] also observed that elite climbers were able to perform significantly more pull-ups than recreational and non-climbers. In contrast, push-ups demonstrated no significant difference between groups. Push-ups were one of the exercises Balas [1] utilized in the resistance training program that indirectly improved grip strength. This suggests that push-ups could be part of a rock climbers training routine to aid in strengthening the upper body while also working the anterior chain in addition to the posterior chain, which is most often utilized while climbing. Resistance trained men are also at a slight disadvantage during push-ups as they must support greater overall body mass [13].

We did not find a significant difference in finger strength between groups. In contrast, Grant [4] found a significant difference in finger strength between elite and recreational climbers, but only for a climbing specific grip. The sensor used in the current study was very thin, making it less specific to a climbing grip and may not be a valid indicator of climbing finger strength. In addition, the resistance trained men were not familiar with the finger strength position.

Finally, Grant [9] compared climbing specific finger endurance in intermediate rock climbers, rowers, and aerobically trained men. This is the most similar study to ours comparing rock climbers to resistance trained men. Since the rowers followed a resistance training program it was thought that they would perform similarly to climbers. However, climbers demonstrated significantly greater MVC of a climbing specific grip when compared to rowers and aerobically trained men, but there was no difference between groups in endurance. These results further support that climbing directly improves grip strength.

5. Conclusions

Climbers demonstrated significantly greater relative grip and pinch strength and were also able to perform significantly more pull-ups than resistance trained men, due to their significantly lower body mass. Therefore, training for rock climbing should promote increased upper body strength in the absence of increased mass as relative strength appears to be an important parameter in this population. Additionally, testing rock climbers should focus on relative upper body strength as a positive indicator of performance.

Author Contributions

Kristina Macias, Lee Brown, Jared Coburn and David Chen were involved in study design, data collection, data interpretation, and manuscript writing.

Conflicts of Interest

The authors declare no conflict of interest.

References

1. Balas, J.; Strejcova, B.; Maly, T.; Mala, L.; Martin, A.J. Changes in upper body strength and body composition after 8 weeks indoor climbing in youth. *Isok. Exer. Sci.* **2009**, *17*, 173–179.
2. Limonta, E.; Ce, E.; Veicsteinas, A.; Esposito, F. Force control during fatiguing contractions in elite rock climbers. *Sport Sci. Health.* **2008**, *4*, 37–42.
3. Fanchini, M.; Violette, F.; Impellizzerim, F.M.; Maffiuletti, N.A. Differences in climbing-specific strength between boulder and lead rock climbers. *J. Strength Cond. Res.* **2013**, *27*, 310–314.
4. Grant, S.; Hynes, V.; Whittaker, A.; Aitchison, T. Anthropometric, strength, endurance, flexibility characteristics of elite and recreational climbers. *J. Sport Sci.* **1996**, *14*, 301–309.
5. Grant, S.; Hasler, T.; Dvies, C.; Aitchison, T.C.; Wilson, J.; Whittaker, A. A comparison of anthropometric, strength, endurance and flexibility characteristics of female elite and recreational climbers and non-climbers. *J. Sport Sci.* **2001**, *19*, 499–505.
6. MacLeod, D.; Sutherland, D.L.; Buntin, L.; Whitaker, A.; Aitchison, T.; Watt, I.; Bradley, J.; Grant, S. Physiological determinants of climbing-specific finger endurance and sport rock climbing performance. *J. Sports Sci.* **2006**, *25*, 1433–1443.
7. Schweizer, A.; Schneider, A.; Geohner, K. Dynamic eccentric-concentric strength training of the finger flexors to improve rock-climbing performance. *Isok. Exer. Sci.* **2007**, *15*, 131–136.
8. Mermier, C.M.; Janot, J.M.; Parker, D.L.; Swan, J.G. Physiological and anthropometric determinants of sport climbing performance. *Brit. J. Sports Med.* **2000**, *34*, 359–366.
9. Grant, S.; Shields, C.; Fitzpatrick, V.; Ming Loh, W.; Whitaker, A.; Watt, I.; Kay, J.W. Climbing-specific finger endurance: A comparative study of intermediate rock climbers, rowers, and aerobically trained individuals. *J. Sports Sci.* **2003**, *21*, 621–630.
10. Simon, B.; Draper, N.; Hodgson, C.; Blackwell, G. Development of a performance assessment tool for rock climbers. *Eur. J. Sport Sci.* **2009**, *9*, 159–167.
11. Jackson, A.S.; Pollock, M.L. Generalized equations for predicting body density of men. *Br. J. Nutr.* **1978**, *40*, 497–504.
12. Chen, K.W.; Chiu, P.K.; Lin, I.; Xu, K.F.; Hsu, M.; Liang, M.T. Study of basic military training of the physical fitness and physical self-concept for cadets. *J. Phys. Ed. Rec.* **2007**, *13*, 6–12.
13. Invergo, J.J.; Ball, T.E.; Looney, M. Relationship of push-ups and absolute muscular endurance to bench press strength. *J. Appl. Sport Sci. Res.* **1991**, *5*, 121–125.
14. Plowman, S.A. *Fitnessgram/Activitygram Reference Guide, 4th ed.*; Plowman, S.A., Meredith, M.D., Eds.; The Cooper Institute: Dallas, TX, USA, 2013.

15. Lee, S.; Kong, Y.; Lowe, B.; Song, S. Handle grip span for optimizing finger-specific force capability as a function of hand size. *Ergonomics* **2009**, *52*, 601–608.
16. Bacon, N.T.; Wingo, J.E.; Richardson, M.T.; Ryan, G.A.; Pangallo, T.C.; Bishop, P.A. Effect of two recovery methods on repeated closed-handed and open-handed weight assisted pull-ups. *J. Strength Cond. Res.* **2012**, *26*, 1348–1352.
17. Balas, J.; Pecha, O.; Martin, A.J.; Cochrane, D. Hand-arm strength and endurance as predictors of climbing performance. *Europ. J. Sport Sci.* **2011**, *12*, 16–25.
18. Thomas, E.M.; Shalber, M.; Svantesson, U. The effect of resistance training on handgrip strength and young adults. *Isok. Exer. Sci.* **2008**, *16*, 125–131.
19. Wilmore, J.H. Alterations in strength, body composition and anthropometric measurements consequent to a 10-week weight-training program. *Med. Sci. Sports Exer.* **1974**, *1*, 133–138.
20. Schweizer, A.; Furrer, M. Correlation of forearm strength and sport climbing performance. *Isok. Exer. Sci.* **2007**, *15*, 211–216.
21. Green, J.; Stannard, S. Active recovery strategies and handgrip performance in trained *vs.* untrained climbers. *J. Strength Cond. Res.* **2010**, *24*, 494–501.

4

Effectiveness of Different Rest Intervals Following Whole-Body Vibration on Vertical Jump Performance between College Athletes and Recreationally Trained Females

Nicole C. Dabbs [1,*], Jon A. Lundahl [2,†] and John C. Garner [2,†]

[1] Biomechanics and Sport Performance Laboratory, Department of Kinesiology, California State University, San Bernardino, 5500 University Parkway, San Bernardino, CA 92407, USA

[2] Applied Biomechanics Laboratory, Health, Exercise Science, and Recreation Management Department; The University of Mississippi, P.O. Box 1848, Oxford, MS 38677, USA; E-Mails: jonludndahl@gmail.com (J.A.L.); jcgarner@olemiss.edu (J.C.G.)

† These authors contributed equally to this work.

* Author to whom correspondence should be addressed; E-Mail: ndabbs@csusb.edu

Academic Editor: Lee E. Brown

Abstract: The purpose of this study was to evaluate the effect of different rest intervals following whole-body vibration on counter-movement vertical jump performance. Sixteen females, eight recreationally trained and eight varsity athletes volunteered to participate in four testing visits separated by 24 h. Visit one acted as a familiarization visit where subjects were introduced to the counter-movement vertical jump and whole-body vibration protocols. Visits 2–4 contained 2 randomized conditions. Whole-body vibration was administered in four bouts of 30 s with 30 s rest between bouts. During whole-body vibration subjects performed a quarter squat every 5 s, simulating a counter-movement vertical jump. Whole-body vibration was followed by three counter-movement vertical jumps with five different rest intervals between the vibration exposure and jumping. For a control condition, subjects performed squats with no whole-body vibration. There was a significant ($p < 0.05$) main effect for time for vertical jump height, peak power output, and relative ground reaction forces, where a majority of individuals max jump from all whole-body vibration conditions was greater than the control condition. There were significant ($p < 0.05$) group differences, showing that varsity athletes had a greater vertical jump height and peak power output compared to recreationally trained females. There were no significant ($p > 0.05$) group differences for relative ground reaction forces. Practitioners and/or strength and conditioning coaches may utilize whole-body vibration to enhance acute counter-movement vertical jump performance after identifying individuals optimal rest time in order to maximize the potentiating effects.

Keywords: rest time; counter-movement; warm-up; athletic women

1. Introduction

Identifying key variables in an athlete's performance is essential to improving athletic performance. It is common to use traditional training techniques, such as strength training, plyometrics, and weightlifting and it may be beneficial to incorporate non-traditional techniques to further enhance performance [1–3]. It has become increasingly popular to incorporate non-traditional training modalities such as, whole-body vibration (WBV) [4–8] to achieve performance enhancement.

Whole-body vibration uses a platform that oscillates, sending vibration to the whole body while standing on the platform. It has been shown to improve upper and lower body muscular activity in both trained and untrained individuals [7,9–16]. Previous research indicates WBV exposure at a moderate intensity is safe and effective in stimulating the neuromuscular system [4] and has been shown to induce non-voluntary muscle contractions [17]. Power output is a key variable for sports performance and previous research have shown an increase in power production by facilitation of an explosive strength effort [9,18,19] leading to augmentation of performance via muscular strength and motor function [20,21]. Bouts of WBV exposure have also been seen to improve sprinting and jumping performance [5,8,10,22,23], with little or no effort by the individuals [24]. Although many studies has shown positive effects, there are several studies have shown no performance enhancements following WBV [5,7,12,25–27], resulting in inconsistency in previous literature.

Warming up prior to any physical performance is highly recommended and a widely accepted and acknowledged practice. WBV is increasingly being utilized as a warm-up for its potentiating effects prior to performance [5,8,13,16,24,28,29], to prepare the body for active performance instead of traditional warm-up techniques [30–32]. Further, WBV has been used passively and/or combined with active movements due to its reported acute performance enhancing effects [5,8]. The acute lower body neuromuscular activation from WBV [22,33] may be beneficial in many power sports.

Numerous variables during WBV exposure can affect optimal performance outcomes such as frequency, amplitude, duration, rest intervals, platform type, and population tested [8,22,23,34]. Several combinations of these variables have been manipulated in previous research, attempting to identify optimal performance. Rest intervals, specifically, have been shown to effect performance outcomes, varying from too short of rest with possible over stimulation of the neuromuscular system or too long of rest with possible dissipating effects [8,22]. Therefore, to increase performance variables, optimal rest intervals are critical when utilizing whole-body vibration. Previous research have shown conflicting results using varying rest intervals following acute bouts of WBV, from immediately post to

10 min [5,8,10,12,22,23,35,36]. To our knowledge there is no current literature that has investigated this vibration protocol with these specific rest times comparing athletes *versus* non-athletes.

Therefore, the purpose of this study was to investigate the effect of different rest intervals following WBV on vertical jump (VJ) performance in female recreationally trained and varsity athletes. Identifying optimal rest intervals following WBV exposure is critical to maximize vertical jump performance in trained individuals. Additionally, identifying differences between female varsity athletes and recreationally trained females will allow conclusions to be made on the applications of WBV exposure to different trained populations.

2. Material and Methods

2.1. Subjects

Sixteen females, recreationally trained ($n = 8$, age: 22 ± 1 year, height: 162.87 ± 2.6 cm, body mass: 64.35 ± 4.64 kg) and varsity athletes ($n = 8$, age: 20 ± 1 year, height: 168.19 ± 7.73 cm, body mass: 61.35 ± 9.68 kg) volunteered to participate in four testing visits. The participants were selected randomly from responders to fliers distributed over the university campus, and by word-of mouth.

Participants who were recreationally trained were defined as individuals who within the last year participated in lower body strength and power activities about three times a week. Varsity athletes were defined as highly trained athletes currently on a Division I athletic team. Participants were asked to refrain from any physical activity 24 h prior to testing and were excluded if they reported any lower body orthopedic injury or musculoskeletal injury within the past year. Each visit was within plus or minus one hour from initial to all proceeding visits, separated by at least 24 h. Participants were asked to wear comfortable clothing and the same shoes for each visit. Diet and hydration were not recorded but participants were asked to keep fluid and food consistent throughout the duration of the study. Each subject read and signed a university Institutional Review Board approved informed consent form prior to participation.

2.2. Study Design

The purpose of the study was to investigate acute performance potentiation following WBV exposure as it might be used in a potentiation warm-up procedure. Therefore, this study used a mixed factor-repeated measures design by having subjects perform five different rest interval conditions and comparing VJ performance to a control condition without WBV in recreationally trained and varsity athletes. Rest intervals ranged from immediate post to four minutes post.

2.3. Procedures

Visit one served as a familiarization session, which included completing the informed consent, anthropometric measurements, familiarization with the countermovement vertical jump (CMVJ) and WBV protocol. During the familiarization session, each subject completed three CMVJ's to assess variability; if the three CMVJ's exceeded 5% difference in jump height, they were asked to return to the lab on a subsequent day to complete another three jumps until the criterion was met. Participants then performed six experimental conditions in three days with two conditions per day [23] separated by a

10 min rest period. This rest period was deemed sufficient since previous literature has shown that WBV is ineffective after 10 min of exposure [22]. The order in which the conditions were performed was randomized and days were separated by at least 24 h.

WBV was performed on an AIRadaptive (Power Plate, Inc.) vibration platform, which administered a tri-axial vibration frequency at 30 Hz [5,22] and an amplitude setting low (2–4 mm). WBV sessions entailed four bouts of 30 s [23] for a total of two minutes of vibration exposure with 30 s rest between bouts. During WBV, subjects performed quarter squats [23,37] every 5 s while also simulating the arm swing used in a CMJ's. Participants were instructed to step off the plate during the bouts of rest. Following WBV exposure subjects were instructed to walk quickly to the force plate (~15 feet) to complete their rest interval for that condition followed by the three CMVJ's.

One condition served as a control during which participants stood on the vibration platform with no vibration, completed the squatting protocol then immediately performed three CMVJ's. The other five conditions used rest intervals of either immediately post, 0.5 min, 1 min, 2 min, or 4 min followed by three CMVJ's [22]. In addition, each subjects max value during experimental conditions for each variable (vertical jump height, peak power output, relative ground reaction forces), regardless of rest interval, was analyzed as another condition, thereby making seven conditions overall.

During all conditions participants were instructed to begin with their arms at a 90-degree angle then perform a CMVJ to a self-selected depth with arm swing and jump as high and as explosively as possible. Fifteen seconds of rest separated each jump and all jumps were performed on an AMTI force plate (Advanced Mechanical Technology, Inc., Watertown, MA, USA). A Vertec® (Columbus, OH, USA) was used as a visual target and to measure jump height to the nearest half-inch and was positioned next to the force plate. Vertical jump height (VJH) was measured and peak power output (PPO) was calculated using the Sayers equation [38]. Peak relative ground reaction force (rGRF) was sampled at 1000 Hz and maximum values from the highest jump from each condition were used for analysis. After completing one condition subjects sat in a chair with no active movement for 10 min then completed the second condition for that visit.

2.4. Statistical Analyses

All statistical procedures were conducted using the Statistical Package for the Social Sciences (PASW 20.0 for Windows, SPSS, Inc., Chicago, IL, USA). An a-priori alpha was set at 0.05 to determine significance. Differences between groups for height, weight, and age were analyzed with a one-way ANOVA. Differences in VJH, Peak Power, and rGRF between conditions were analyzed with a 2 × 7 (training status by condition) mixed factor ANOVA.

3. Results

There were no significant differences between recreationally trained and athletes in height ($p = 0.08$), weight ($p = 0.44$), and age ($p = 0.07$). There was no significant interaction for training status and time for VJH ($p = 0.18$), PPO ($p = 0.18$), and rGRF ($p = 0.97$). There was a significant main effect for time for VJH ($p < 0.001$), PPO ($p < 0.001$), and rGRF ($p = 0.01$), where each individuals max jump from all WBV conditions was greater than the control condition (Figure 1), however no significant ($p > 0.05$) differences were found between all other conditions (Table 1). There was a significant group differences, showing that varsity athletes had a greater VJH (p < 0.001) and PPO (p < 0.001) compared to recreationally trained females. There were no significant (p = 0.96) group differences for rGRF (Figure 2). Additionally, where each participant reached their max jump during the experimental conditions is list here: IM = 4, 0.5 min = 2, 1 min = 3, 2 min = 6, and 4 min = 1.

Table 1. Vertical Jump Height (VJH), Peak Power Output (PPO), and relative ground reaction force (rGFR) maximum values and values for each condition (mean ± SD) for varsity athletes and recreationally trained.

Conditions	VJH (cm)		PPO (W)		rGRF (N)	
	Varsity	Rec	Varsity	Rec	Varsity	Rec
Control	50.48 ± 6.78	42.06 ± 5.74 *	4062.50 ± 411.54	3551.79 ± 348.27 *	1608.91 ± 510.74	1613.90 ± 356.66
0 min	50.95 ± 7.0	41.91 ± 4.55 *	4091.41 ± 425.11	3542.15 ± 276.42 *	1616.72 ± 502.40	1599.02 ± 363.28
5 min	51.91 ± 6.84	39.84 ± 5.72 *	4149.23 ± 415.01	3416.88 ± 347.05 *	1629.38 ± 561.86	1645.71 ± 327.41
1 min	48.89 ± 9.77	40.95 ± 6.29 *	3966.14 ± 592.85	3484.34 ± 381.57 *	1626.78 ± 468.27	1628.41 ± 289.14
2 min	50.16 ± 6.18	43.33 ± 2.29 *	4043.23 ± 375.40	3628.88 ± 145.32 *	1629.38 ± 525.42	1600.58 ± 384.68
4 min	50.80 ± 8.56	40.64 ± 6.40 *	4081.78 ± 519.59	3465.06 ± 388.73 *	1662.43 ± 634.03	1643.70 ± 387.99
Max	53.34 ± 7.25 #	44.45 ± 3.84 *#	4235.95 ± 439.96 #	3696.33 ± 233.10 *#	1727.36 ± 387.99 #	1692.04 ± 355.47 #

* indicates significant (p < 0.05) differences between varsity and recreational athletes; # indicates significant (p < 0.05) differences greater than control.

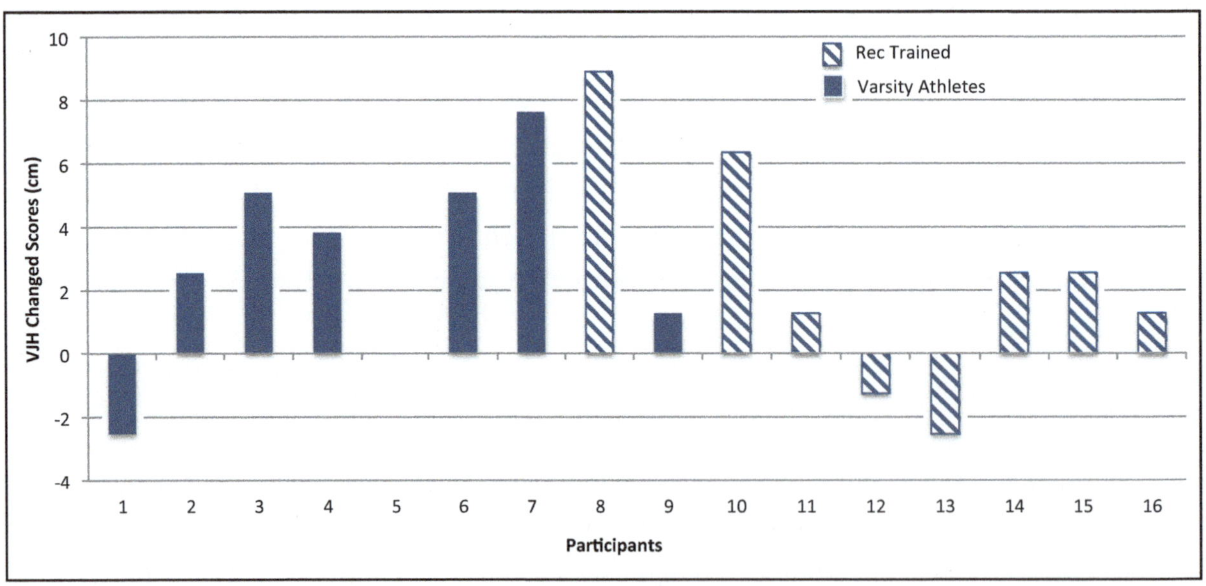

Figure 1. Individual differences between control and maximal VJ height (cm).

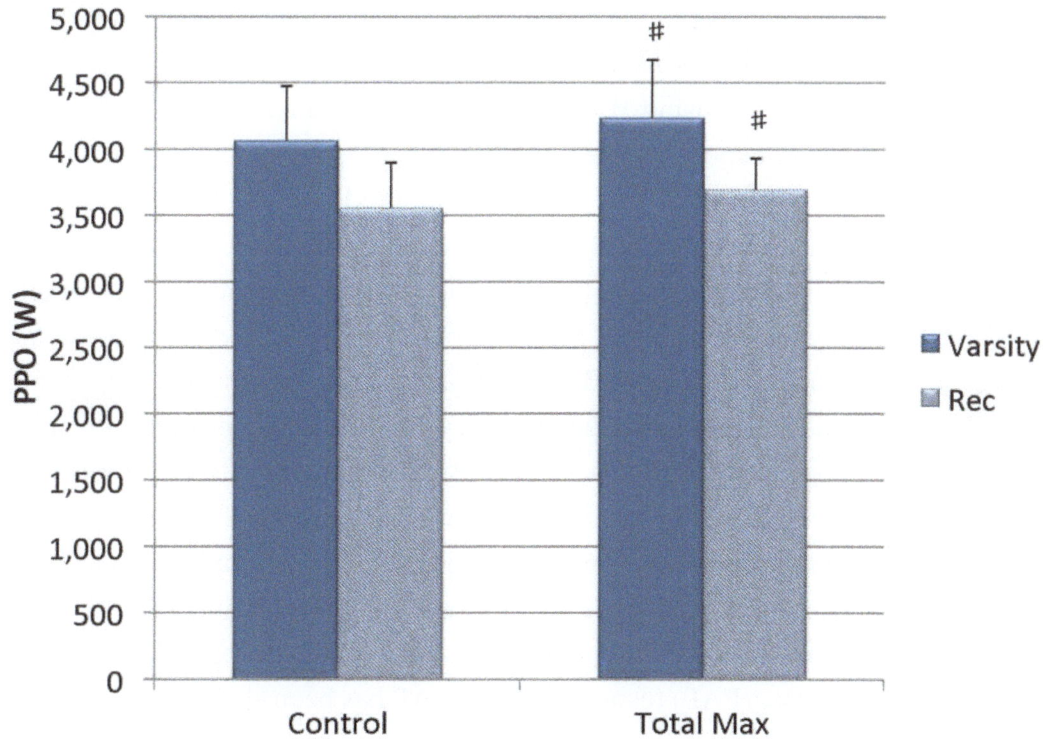

Figure 2. Differences between control condition and max condition for Peak Power Output (PPO) for varsity and recreationally trained females. # indicates significant ($p < 0.05$) differences between conditions; * indicates significant ($p < 0.05$) differences between groups.

4. Discussion

The aim of the current investigation was to determine the optimal rest interval following bouts of WBV on vertical jump performance variables. The main findings were that following WBV; VJH, PPO, and rGRF showed individual increases during one of the rest interval conditions with WBV exposure compared to the control condition (no WBV). Indicating that individuals respond differently to the WBV exposure, resulting in individual optimal rest times following WBV exposure. Another finding in this investigation was that for all conditions varsity female athletes had a greater VJH and PPO compared to the recreationally trained females.

In a previous study, the researchers found individual optimal rest intervals between WBV exposure and vertical jumping performance, similar to the current investigation using similar protocols but comparing recreationally trained males and females only [8] instead of an athletic population. These similarities indicate that regardless of training status or sex, a majority of individuals responded to the WBV exposure and had an increased vertical jump performance. The only other methodical difference from this particular previous research was that the current study used a tri-axial WBV platform, while the previous study used a pivotal vibration platform. Therefore, similar results in both studies indicate that the type of vibration platform exposure has similar benefits on vertical jump performance as well. This is a positive finding, since most research studies using WBV are done on a variety of platforms, it is often uncertain if researchers can make comparisons. Previous studies have examined the differences using different types of WBV platforms [34,39], since different platforms have different oscillatory motions. A recent study examined the differences in three platform types and found no differences on their acute vertical jump performance [34]. The researcher concluded that different devices could be used similarly for acute vertical jump performance bouts.

Other key variables are critical when using WBV for performance enhancement such as frequency, amplitude, rest times, and vibration exposure time. Frequency can easily be changed on most devices and can be described as the intensity of the vibration where amplitude can be described as the volume. Previous research has shown that 1 min rest post vibration exposure and a frequency of 30 Hz were optimal for vertical jump performance increases [22,23]. The frequency exposure was similar to the current study, however our study did differ in the time exposure of WBV. Bedient and Adams [22,23] exposed participants to one bout of 30 s of WBV and found an increase in CMVJ, resulting in a homogenous optimal rest interval of 1 min post when compared to immediate post, 5 min, or 10 min. In contrast, our study exposed subjects to four bouts of 30 s of vibration with a 1:1 rest ratio, and found individual optimal rest intervals for an increase in vertical jump performance. In contrast, another study examined varied frequencies and durations of vibration exposures and found no differences in vertical jump performance, indicating no conclusive frequency or vibration exposure time [34].

There are some research studies that conclude that using WBV prior to vertical jump performance induces a post-activation potentiation (PAP) response [5,35]. PAP has been shown to increase voluntary force development during muscle actions [40] but can induce fatigue if the intensity is too high or there is not sufficient rest periods before performance [41]. PAP has been shown to vary on an individual basis [42], some individuals have different optimal rest times and fatigue effects, which should be considered when inducing PAP [41]. Previous research that uses WBV for PAP to enhance vertical jump performance have seen positive effects at enhancing acute performance [5,8,35]. In the current investigation, no differences between rest intervals were found, however when taking individual max vertical jump values with WBV and comparing it to the control group, individuals showed an increase in vertical jump performance. Thus, the increases in vertical jump performance induced by WBV may have been sufficient enough to induce PAP but limited enough not to induce fatigue.

The current study compared female college athletes to recreationally trained females. As we expected, the college athletes performed at a higher level with greater vertical jump performance compared to the recreationally trained individuals. These results are most likely contributed to college athletes having a higher level of training, increasing their potential to develop a higher force generating capacity [42], resulting in a higher VJH. Additionally, the athletic population may have more experience with vertical jumping allowing them to have greater vertical jumping performance accompanied with a higher level of strength and conditioning periodized programs required by their college sport. However, there have been conflicting results in a variety of studies with athletic and recreationally trained individuals with WBV and jumping performance [7,8,43,44]. In the current study, there were no group differences in the rGRF but there was a difference for VJH and PPO. This may be due to the use of the Vertec® device to measure VJH instead of estimating flight time from the force plate. The use of the Vertec® doesn't account for changes in arm reach or trunk twist during the jumps, which may modify scores [45]. On the other hand, VJH estimation could be altered with landing mechanics when using the force plate [45].

Our study has a few potential limitations that may have influenced the results of our study. One may have been our testing protocol, there were two conditions performed in one testing day with a 10 min washout period between conditions. This was randomized to control for any learning effects however, it is possible that one condition influenced the other. Research suggests that after 10 min, WBV has no effect on vertical jump performance [22], therefore we do not suspect a learning effect occurred. Another limitation may have been that since our data reflects the maximum VJH for each condition, it is possible that it may have affected subsequent VJ performance. However, previous research shows that when analyzing kinetics during VJ performance there were no subsequent effects shown [46]. It is important to note that three of the participants actually perform better in the control condition compared to the experimental condition. This has been shown in other studies and has been suggested that there are responder and non-responders to WBV treatment [8]. Another important limitation to mention is the small power due to the sample size. A critical factor is the type of WBV platform utilized. The present study utilized a tri-axial platform where others [8,22,23,35] have utilized similar and other types (e.g., vertical, sliding horizontal, and pivotal), which may affect the outcome of the study.

5. Conclusions

Post activation potentiation was induced using whole-body vibration exposure on vertical jump performance on eight female college athletes and eight recreationally trained females. Four sets of 30 s bouts of WBV prior to vertical jump performance showed statistically significant differences between individual maximum jumps at different rest times with WBV compared to the control (no WBV). Therefore, it is recommended that practitioners determine individual optimal rest times following WBV prior to high level performance to obtain greatest potentiating effects. Acquiring individual optimal rest times prior to performance would allow individuals to maximum their potentiating acute effects in a single explosive movement. Therefore, this study specifically applies to female athletes that perform single bouts of explosive movements such as, high jumpers and long jumpers. Once optimal rest time is determined, it will allow for optimal performance during competition. This investigation has shown these effects to be applied to female athletic and recreationally trained individuals.

Author Contributions

Nicole Dabbs, Jon Lundahl, and John Garner were involved in study design, data collection, data interpretation, and manuscript writing.

Conflicts of Interest

The authors declare no conflict of interest.

References

1. Kraemer, W.J.; Ratamess, N.A. Fundamentals of resistance training: Progression and exercise prescription. *Med. Sci. Sports Exerc.* **2004**, *36*, 674–688.
2. Newton, R.U.; Gerber, A.; Nimphius, S.; Shim, J.K.; Doan, B.K.; Robertson, M.; Pearson, D.R.; Craig, B.W.; Häkkinen, K.; Kraemer, W.J. Determination of functional strength imbalance of the lower extremities. *J. Strength Cond. Res.* **2006**, *20*, 971–977.
3. Newton, R.U.; Kraemer, W.J.; Hakkinen, K. Effects of ballistic training on preseason preparation of elite volleyball players. *Med. Sci. Sports Exerc.* **1999**, *31*, 323–330.

4. Cardinale, M.; Bosco, C. The use of vibration as an exercise intervention. *Exerc. Sport Sci. Rev.* **2003**, *31*, 3–7.
5. Cormie, P.; Deane, R.S.; Triplett, N.T.; McBride, J.M. Acute effects of whole-body vibration on muscle activity, strength, and power. *J. Strength Cond. Res.* **2006**, *20*, 257–261.
6. Da Silva, M.E.; Fernandez, J.M.; Castillo, E.; Nuñez, V.M.; Vaamonde, D.M.; Poblador, M.S.; Lancho, J.L. Influence of vibration training on energy expenditure in active men. *J. Strength Cond. Res*. **2007**, *21*, 470–475.
7. Dabbs, N.C.; Brown, L.E.; Coburn, J.W.; Lynn, S.K.; Tran, T.T.; Biagini, M.S. Effect of Whole-body vibration warm-up on bat speed in women softball players. *J. Strength Cond. Res.* **2010**, *24*, 2296– 2299.
8. Dabbs, N.C.; Muñoz, C.X.; Tran, T.T.; Brown, L.E.; Bottaro, M. Effect of different rest intervals after whole-body vibration on vertical jump performance. *J. Strength Cond. Res.* **2011**, *25*, 662–667.
9. Bosco, C.; Cardinale, M.; Tsarpela, O. Influence of vibration on mechanical power and electromyogram activity in human arm flexor muscles. *Eur. J. Appl. Physiol. Occup. Physiol.* **1999**, *79*, 306–311
10. Bullock, N.; Martin, D.T.; Ross, A.; Rosemond, C.D.; Jordan, M.J.; Marino, F.E. Acute effect of whole-body vibration on sprint and jumping performance in elite skeleton athletes. *J. Strength Cond. Res.* **2008**, *22*, 1371–1374.
11. Cochrane, D.J.; Hawke, E.J. Effects of acute upper-body vibration on strength and power variables in climbers. *J. Strength Cond. Res.* **2007**, *21*, 527–531.
12. Cochrane, D.J.; Stannard, S.R. Acute whole body vibration training increases vertical jump and flexibility performance in elite female field hockey players. *Br. J. Sports Med.* **2005**, *39*, 860–865.
13. Dallas, G.; Kirialanis, P.; Mellos, V. The acute effect of whole body vibration training on flexibility and explosive strength of young gymnasts. *Biol. Sport* **2014**, *31*, 233–237.
14. Di Loreto, C.; Ranchelli, A.; Lucidi, P.; Murdolo, G.; Parlanti, N.; de Cicco, A.; Tsarpela, O.; Annino, G.; Bosco, C.; Santeusanio, F.; *et al.* Effects of whole-body vibration exercise on the endocrine system of healthy men. *J. Endocrinol. Investig.* **2004**, *27*, 323–327.
15. Jacobs, P.L.; Burns, P. Acute enhancement of lower-extremity dynamic strength and flexibility with whole-body vibration. *J. Strength Cond. Res.* **2009**, *23*, 51–57.
16. Despina, T.; George, D.; George, T.; Sotiris, P.; Alessandra, D.C.; George, K.; Maria, R.; Stavros, K. Short-term effects of whole-body vibration training on balance, flexibility and lower limb explosive strength in elite rhythmic gymnasts. *Hum. Mov. Sci.* **2014**, *33*, 149–158.
17. Issurin, V.B. Vibrationss and their applications in sport: A review. *J. Sports Med. Phys. Fit.* **2005**, *45*, 424–436.
18. Issurin, V.B.; Tenenbaum, G. Acute and residual effects of vibratory stimulation on explosive strength in elite and amateur athletes. *J. Sports Sci.* **1999**, *17*, 177–182.
19. Poston, B.; Holcomb, W.R.; Guadagnoli, M.A.; Linn, L.L. The acute effects of mechanical vibration on power output in the bench press. *J. Strength Cond. Res*. **2007**, *21*, 199–203.
20. Bosco, C.; Cardinale, M.; Tsarpela, O.; Colli, R.; Tihanyi, J.; von Duvillard, S.P.; Viru, A. The influence of whole body vibration on jumping performance. *Biol. Sports*. **1998**, *15*, 157–614.
21. Bosco, C.; Colli, R.; Introini, E.; Cardinale, M.; Tsarpela, O.; Madella, A.; Tihanyi, J.; Viru, A. Adaptive responses of human skeletal muscle to vibration exposure. *Clin. Physiol.* **1999**, *19*, 183–187.

22. Adams, J.B.; Edwards, D.; Serravite, D.H.; Bedient, A.M.; Huntsman, E.; Jacobs, K.A.; del Rossi, G.; Roos, B.A.; Signorile, J.F. Optimal frequency, displacement, duration, and recovery patterns to maximize power output following acute whole-body vibration. *J. Strength Cond. Res.* **2009**, *23*, 237–245.
23. Bedient, A.M.; Adams, J.B.; Edwards, D.A.; Serravite, D.H.; Huntsman, E.; Mow, S.E.; Roos, B.A.; Signorile, J.F. Displacement and frequency for maximizing power output resulting from a bout of whole-body vibration. *J. Strength Cond. Res.* **2009**, *23*, 1683–1687.
24. Rittweger, J.; Beller, G.; Felsenberg, D. Acute physiological effects of exhaustive whole-body vibration exercise in man. *Clin Physiol.* **2000**, *20*, 134–142.
25. De Ruiter, C.J.; van der Linden, R.M.; van der Zijden, M.J.; Hollander, A.P.; de Haan, A. Short-term effects of whole-body vibration on maximal voluntary isometric knee extensor force and rate of force rise. *Eur. J. Appl. Physiol.* **2003**, *88*, 472–475.
26. Kelly, S.B.; Alvar, B.A.; Black, L.E.; Dodd, D.J.; Carothers, K.F.; Brown, L.E. The effect of warm-up with whole-body vibration *vs.* cycle ergometry on isokinetic dynamometry. *J. Strength Cond. Res.* **2010**, *24*, 3140–3143.
27. Menefee, K.; Switzler, C.; Podlog, L.; Hickes-Little, C. The acute effects of two different foot positions during whole body vibration on vertical jump performance in females. *J. Athl. Med.* **2014**, *2*, 66–74.
28. Cochrane, D.J.; Stannard, S.R.; Sargeant, A.J.; Rittweger, J. The rate of muscle temperature increase during acute whole-body vibration exercise. *Eur. J. Appl. Physiol.* **2008**, *103*, 441–448.
29. Dallas, G.; Kirialanis, P. The effects of two different conditions of whole-body vibration on flexibility and jumping performance on artistic gymnasts. *Sci. Gymnast. J.* **2013**, *5*, 41–52.
30. Burkett, L.N.; Phillips, W.T.; Ziuraitis, J. The best warm-up for the vertical jump in college-age athletic men. *J. Strength Cond. Res.* **2005**, *19*, 673–676.
31. Chaouachi, A.; Castagna, C.; Chtara, M.; Brughelli, M.; Turki, O.; Galy, O.; Chamari, K.; Behm, D.G. Effect of warm-ups involving static or dynamic stretching on agility, sprinting, and jumping performance in trained individuals. *J. Strength Cond. Res.* **2010**, *24*, 2001–2011.
32. Gourgoulis, V.; Aggeloussis, N.; Kasimatis, P.; Mavromatis, G.; Garas, A. Effect of a submaximal half-squats warm-up program on vertical jumping ability. *J. Strength Cond. Res.* **2003**, *17*, 342–344.
33. Abercromby, A.F.; Amonette, W.E.; Layne, C.S.; McFarlin, B.K.; Hinman, M.R.; Paloski, W.H. Variation in neuromuscular responses during acute whole-body vibration exercise. *Med. Sci. Sports Exerc.* **2007**, *39*, 1642–1650.
34. Bagheri, J.; van den Berg-Emons, R.J.; Pel, J.J.; Horemans, H.L.; Stam, H.J. Acute effects of whole-body vibration on jump force and jump rate of force development: A comparative study of different devices. *J. Strength Cond. Res.* **2012**, *26*, 691–696.
35. McBride, J.M.; Nuzzo, J.L.; Dayne, A.M.; Israetel, M.A.; Nieman, D.C.; Triplett, N.T. Effect of an acute bout of whole body vibration exercise on muscle force output and motor neuron excitability. *J. Strength Cond. Res.* **2010**, *24*, 184–189.
36. Ronnestad, B.R. Acute effects of various whole-body vibration frequencies on lower-body power in trained and untrained subjects. *J. Strength Cond. Res.* **2009**, *23*, 1309–1315.
37. Cochrane, D.J.; Legg, S.J.; Hooker, M.J. The short-term effects of whole-body vibration training on vertical jump, sprint, and agility performance. *J. Strength Cond. Res.* **2004**, *18*, 828–832.

38. Sayers, S.P.; Harackiewicz, D.V.; Harman, E.A.; Frykman, P.N.; Rosenstein, M.T. Cross-validation of three jump power equations. *Med. Sci. Sports Exerc.* **1999**, *31*, 572–577.
39. Pel, J.J.; Bagheri, J.; van Dam, L.M.; van den Berg-Emons, H.J.; Horemans, H.L.; Stam, H.J.; van der Steen, J. Platform accelerations of three different whole-body vibration devices and the transmission of vertical vibrations to the lower limbs. *Med. Eng. Phys.* **2009**, *31*, 937–944.
40. Tillin, N.; Bishop, D. Factors modulating post-activation potentiation and its effect on performance of subsequent explosive ativities. *Sports Med.* **2009**, *39*, 147–166.
41. McCann, M.R.; Flanagan, S.P. The effects of exercise selection and rest interval on postactivation potentiation of vertical jump performance. *J. Strength Cond. Res.* **2010**, *24*, 1285–1291.
42. Chiu, L.Z.; Fry, A.C.; Weiss, L.W.; Schilling, B.K.; Brown, L.E.; Smith, S.L. Postactivation potentiation response in athletic and recreationally trained individuals. *J. Strength Cond. Res.* **2003**, *17*, 671–677.
43. Burns, J.D.; Miller, P.C.; Hall, E.E. *Acute Effects of Whole Body Vibration on Functional Capabilities of Skeletal Muscle*; Federación Española de Asociaciones de Docentes de Educación Física: Elon, NC, USA, 2015; pp. 180–183.
44. Naclerio, F.; Faigenbaum, A.D.; Larumbe-Zabala, E.; Ratamess, N.A.; Kang, J.; Friedman, P.; Ross, R.E. Effectiveness of different postactivation potentiation protocols with and without whole body vibration on jumping performance in college athletes. *J. Strength Cond. Res.* **2014**, *28*, 232–239.
45. Ferreira, L.C.; Schilling, B.K.; Weiss, L.W.; Fry, A.C.; Chiu, L.Z. Reach height and jump displacement: Implications for standardization of reach determination. *J. Strength Cond. Res.* **2010**, *24*, 1596–1601.
46. Jensen, R.L.; Ebben, W.P. Kinetic analysis of complex training rest interval effect on vertical jump performance. *J. Strength Cond. Res.* **2003**, *17*, 345–349.

5

The Effect of Kettlebell Swing Load and Cadence on Physiological, Perceptual and Mechanical Variables

Michael J. Duncan *, Rosanna Gibbard, Leanne M. Raymond and Peter Mundy

Centre for Applied Biological and Exercise Sciences, Coventry University, Coventry CV11 5FB, UK; E-Mails: gibbardr@uni.coventry.ac.uk (R.G.); raymondl@uni.coventry.ac.uk (L.M.R.); ab9674@coventry.ac.uk (P.M.)

* Author to whom correspondence should be addressed; E-Mail: michael.duncan@coventry.ac.uk

Academic Editor: Lee E. Brown

Abstract: This study compared the physiological, perceptual and mechanical responses to kettlebell swings at different loads and swing speeds. Following familiarization 16 strength trained participants (10 males, six females, mean age ± SD = 23 ± 2.9) performed four trials: 2 min kettlebell swings with an 8 kg kettlebell at a fast cadence; 2 min kettlebell swings with an 8 kg kettlebell at a slow cadence; 4 min kettlebell swings with a 4 kg kettlebell at a fast cadence; 4 min kettlebell swings with a 4 kg kettlebell at a slow cadence. Repeated measured analysis of variance indicated no significant differences in peak blood lactate or peak net vertical force across loads and cadences ($P > 0.05$). Significant main effect for time for heart rate indicated that heart rate was higher at the end of each bout than at mid-point ($P = 0.001$). A significant Load X cadence interaction for rating of perceived exertion (RPE) ($P = 0.030$) revealed that RPE values were significantly higher in the 8 kg slow cadence condition compared to the 4 kg slow ($P = 0.002$) and 4 kg fast ($P = 0.016$) conditions. In summary, this study indicates that the physiological and mechanical responses to kettlebell swings at 4 kg and 8 kg loads and at fast and slow cadence were similar, whereas the perceptual response is greater when swinging an 8 kg kettlebell at slow cadence.

Keywords: force; swing; nontraditional training; resistance exercise

---

1. Introduction

Kettlebells comprise a cast iron/steel weight, resembling a cannonball with a handle and are popular and widely used for resistance training. Their use has been advocated as a means to enhance muscular strength and endurance, and aerobic endurance whilst also reducing body fatness [1]. Unlike dumbbells, kettlebell training tends to comprise ballistic and swing movements where the centre of mass of the kettlebell is extended beyond the hand. Kettlebell training has also been recommended to condition occupation groups including the armed services [2] as well as being an efficacious rehabilitation tool [3,4]. While the use of the kettlebell dates back to circa 1700 s [1], scientific analysis of kettlebell training and individual movements with a kettlebell has only recently gathered momentum. Consequently, there are still significant gaps in the literature relating to the best use of kettlebells for strength and conditioning.

To date, studies examining kettlebell science have tended to focus on either physiological variables [5–7] or biomechanical variables [8,9]. A number of studies have also compared kettlebell exercise to treadmill running [7,10]. For example, Hulsey *et al.* [10] reported higher caloric expenditure, oxygen uptake (VO_2), metabolic equivalents and pulmonary ventilation during treadmill exercise, compared to 10 min kettlebell swinging. More recent work by Thomas *et al.* [7] compared a moderate-intensity kettlebell protocol with brisk walking performed on a treadmill. Ten novice participants performed a 30 min kettlebell protocol, comprising three continuous sets of 10 kettlebell swings followed by 10 sumo deadlifts (16 kg for males, 12 kg for females) with a 3 min rest between sets. This was compared to a 30 min treadmill walk (3,10 min bouts separated by 3 min rest) where VO_2 was matched from the kettlebell session. Their data indicated similar blood pressure, energy expenditure and respiratory exchange ratios between conditions but higher rating of perceived exertion (RPE) and heart rate during kettlebell exercise. Thomas *et al.* concluded that kettlebell training may therefore be used to enhance aerobic capacity to the same extent as brisk walking. Mechanically focused studies of kettlebell exercise have reported that kettlebell exercise results in a hip-hinge squat pattern, eliciting rapid muscle activation-relaxation cycles, opposite in polarity to that of traditional Olympic weightlifting techniques [9]. Other work [8] has reported on the mechanical demands of the kettlebell swing specifically. In their study, 16 males performed two sets of 10 kettlebell swings with 16, 24, and 32 kg kettlebells. Lake and Lauder [8] reported that swing mean and peak power was greater than power recorded during a back squat and comparable with power recorded from a jump squat.

A recent review of kettlebell research suggested a need to examine the effects of different kettlebell loads, as research has not fully examined responses across the range of kettlebell loads available [11]. Understanding the optimal loads for kettlebell training is an important consideration for coaches and athletes, yet without this initial comparison type research, this aspiration will not be elucidated. Moreover, in by far the majority of research using kettlebell training, participants have used different loads. For example, in Thomas *et al.* [7] kettlebell load differed between males and females, whereas in Lake and Lauder [8] participants performed two sets of 10 kettlebell swings across a standardised spectrum of kettlebell loads. As such, it is difficult to compare across kettlebell loads as the total volume of work will differ and therefore making inferences about the effect of load alone may be open to debate. Further, in research studies employing the kettlebell swing, there has seemingly been no standardisation of swing speed or cadence. Modification of swing cadence may result in different intensities of exercise, particularly if swing volume is set as a product of a set duration. The current study seeks to address this issue by comparing the physiological and mechanical responses to kettlebell swings at different loads and swing speeds. We hypothesized that heavier kettlebell load and faster swing speeds would elicit greater physiological and mechanical responses compared to lighter kettlebell load and slower swing speed.

2. Method, Results, Discussion

2.1. Method

2.1.1. Participants

Following institutional ethics approval, briefing regarding the study and provision of written informed consent, 16 strength trained participants (10 males, six females; mean age ± S.D. = 23 ± 2.9 years, height = 176.2 ± 9.2 cm, body mass = 76.3 ± 14.7 kg) volunteered to participate. Participants were recruited from the pool of MSc Strength and Conditioning Students at the institution where the testing took place. All participants had experience performing resistance exercise, including work with kettlebells, and were free of any musculoskeletal pain or disorders. Inclusion criteria included currently participating in > 10 h week^{-1} programmed physical activity including strength and endurance based activities and prior experience using kettlebells. Exclusion criteria included any musculoskeletal injury that would have prevented engagement in the experimental protocol. Mean ± S.D. of years training experience was 4.5 ± 1.5 years.

2.1.2. Procedures

This study used a within groups, repeated measures design, where participants undertook five visits to the human performance laboratory. The first visit was for familiarisation, and the subsequent four visits were counterbalanced experimental trials, which were all performed at the same time of day to minimise circadian variation. Participants were asked to refrain from strenuous exercise in the 24 h before exercise and to attend the laboratory in a hydrated state (e.g., minimum water consumption of 500 mL in the 3 h before testing). Participants engaged in the following four trials: 2 min kettlebell swings with an 8 kg kettlebell at a fast cadence; 2 min kettlebell swings with an 8 kg kettlebell at a slow cadence; 4 min kettlebell swings with a 4 kg kettlebell at a fast cadence; 4 min kettlebell swings with a 4 kg kettlebell at a slow cadence. Heart Rate (HR) and RPE were assessed at mid and end points of each bouts of swings. Blood lactate (BLa) was determined following each swing bout using a 5 μL capillary blood sample taken from the fingertip (Lactate Pro, Arkray Instruments, Kyoto, Japan). Peak net vertical force was also calculated from force platform data (AMTI AccuGait, Watertown, MA, USA), collected throughout each bout of kettlebell swings. Slow and fast cadence was determined via pilot work where different swing speeds were performed by an experienced strength and conditioning professional with 4 and 8 kg kettlebells. From this the two cadences chosen to represent slow (40 BPM) and fast (80 BPM) were selected as being ecologically sound in terms of use within fitness and strength and conditioning programmes. Throughout all trials a metronome (Seiko SQ44, Tokyo, Japan) was used to regulate cadence with a full swing (upwards and downwards phase) being completed in 2 BPM. This resulted in 20 full swings being completed per minute in the slow conditions and 40 full swings being completed in the fast conditions. In this manner, the total work completed in the slow and fast swing speed condition was the same when comparing across 4 kg and 8 kg kettlebell loads. All swings were performed in accordance with the technique reported by Tsatsouline [1] and as used in prior studies examining kettlebell swing performance [8]. Participants were positioned with feet shoulder width apart and standing on the force platform for each trial. Prior to each trial, all participants completed a 5 min warm up protocol at 25 W on a cycle ergometer (Monark, Vansbro, Sweden). They then began each trial 2 min after completion of the warm-up.

2.1.3. Statistical Analysis

In order to examine any changes in Heart Rate, Rating of Perceived Exertion and peak force, a series of 2 (4 kg *vs.* 2 kg kettlebell load) × 2 (slow *vs.* fast swing speed) × 2 (time, mid point *vs.* end point) ways repeated measures analysis of variance (ANOVA) were used. Any differences in post exercise blood lactate were examined using repeated measures ANOVA. Where any statistical differences were found, Bonferroni post-hoc multiple comparisons were used to determine where the differences lay. Partial η^2 ($P\eta^2$) was used as a measure of effect size. The statistical package for social sciences (SPSS, version 22, IBM Inc, New York, NY, USA) was used for all analysis and statistical significance was set as $P = 0.05$ *a priori.*

2.2. Results

In regard to heart rate, results indicated no significant higher order interaction or main effects due to load or cadence (all $P => 0.05$). However, there was a significant main effect for time ($P = 0.001$, $P\eta^2 = 0.621$), whereby heart rate at mid-point in each trial was significantly lower than heart rate at the end point of each trial ($P = 0.001$). Mean ± SE of heart rate was 148.1 ± 4.1 BPM and 155.5 ± 3.8 BPM at mid and end points respectively. There was also no significant difference in peak Bla across conditions ($P = 0.377$). For RPE there was a significant Load X cadence interaction ($P = 0.030$, $P\eta^2 = 0.293$, see Figure 1) where RPE was higher during the 8kg slow cadence condition compared to the 4 kg fast cadence and 4 kg slow cadence condition. Post hoc analysis indicated that there was a significant difference between 8 kg load at a slow cadence and 4 kg load at a slow cadence ($P = 0.002$) and 8 kg load at a slow cadence and 4 kg load at a fast cadence ($P = 0.016$). When peak vertical force was examined there were no significant differences between loads, cadence or time points (all $P > 0.05$). Mean ± SE of heart rate, peak blood lactate concentration and peak vertical force across loads and cadences and at mid and end point in each trial are presented in Table 1.

2.3. Discussion

The current study compared physiological, perceptual and mechanical variables during the kettlebell swing at two different loads and two different cadences. This is the first study to date to examine this issue in a manner where total work can be equalised across loads and cadence. The results of this study demonstrate that when this is the case the physiological and mechanical responses are similar between 4 and 8 kg kettlebells. However, when the 8 kg kettlebell swings at a slow cadence produced significantly higher perception of exertion than any of the other conditions. For strength and conditioning coaches and athletes this has useful implications for the development of kettlebell training programmes in that a heavier load (8 kg) when swung more slowly results in higher RPEs when the physiological and mechanical response is the same. In such cases, adherence to training programmes might be more effective if using a 4 kg load on the basis that it will feel more comfortable but elicit the same physiological response as an 8 kg load.

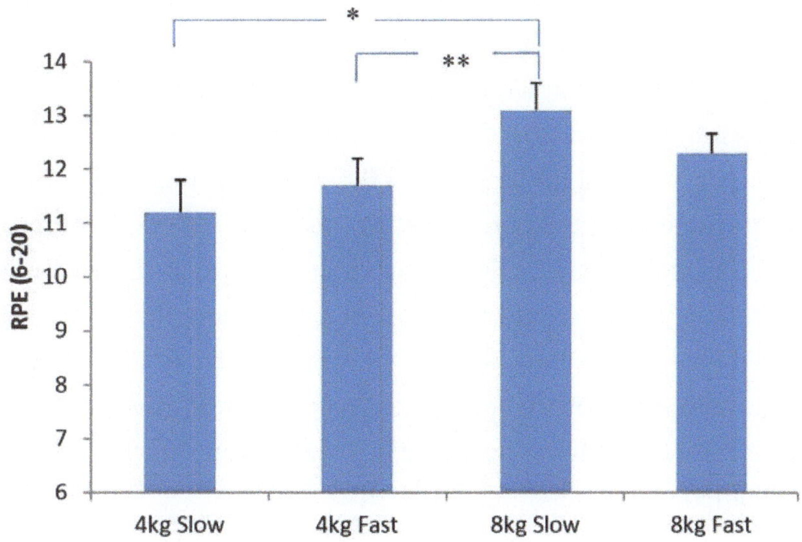

Figure 1. Mean ± SE of RPE values during kettlebell swings across loads and cadences (* $P = 0.002$, ** $P = 0.016$).

Table 1. Mean (SE) of heart rate, peak blood lactate concentration and peak vertical force at the mid point and end point of kettlebell swings at different loads and cadences.

	4 kg Slow		**4 kg Fast**		**8 kg Slow**		**8 kg Fast**	
	Mid Point	**End Point**	**Mid Point**	**End Point**	**Mid Point**	**End Point**	**Mid Point**	**End Point**
HR (BPM)	144 (4.8)	151 (4.4)	148 (3.9)	155 (3.7)	148 (7.1)	160 (4.3)	150 (3.7)	155 (4.2)
Bla (mmol/L)	-	5.8 (1.1)	-	4.9 (.55)	-	7.5 (1.6)	-	5.8 (1.1)
Peak Force (N)	562.5 (67.0)	551.2 (63.1)	516.2 (126.3)	462.9 (136.8)	623.1 (60.1)	585.4 (56.3)	557.6 (112.2)	539.3 (112.1)

In some respects it is difficult to compare the results of this study to prior work that has employed kettlebells as previous studies by Thomas *et al.* [7], Hulsey *et al.* [10], Lake and Lauder [10] have used discrete bouts of kettlebell exercise at different loads. Thus, the differences they report may be a consequence of greater work completed rather than a difference in the load employed. The results present in the current study build on this work by also examining different swing cadence. Prior research [7,8,10,12] has not tended to standardise or consider the effect of swing speed/cadence on responses to this type of exercise.

There are some limitations of the current study, due to lack of prior literature relating to optimum swing speed, cadence was determined via pilot study by strength and conditioning professionals. The two swing cadences employed may not however be "optimal" and additional research examining across the spectrum of possible swing speeds might be useful in determining whether there is an "optimum" kettlebell swing speed. Likewise, two relatively light loads (4 kg and 8 kg) were utilised in the present study. This was again based on pilot data in terms of what loads might conceivably be used for kettlebell swing durations over 2 min in duration. Research designs employed by previous authors have used kettlebell loads in excess of those used in the current study, and up to 32 kg e.g., [8]. They have also tended to use much longer durations of kettlebell swinging, which may lack ecological validity. For example, Hulsey *et al.* [10] employed a continuous 10 min period of kettlebell swings and Thomas *et al.* [7] employed three sets of 10 min kettlebell swings, each separated by a 3 min rest period. Such durations of kettlebell exercise seem in excess of what would realistically be engaged in within a gym setting, and particularly physically demanding. Hence the decision in the present to design to employ a smaller duration of swings, more akin to what might be used by the general exercising public. In addition only net peak net vertical force was assessed in the present study and future work that presents an analysis of overall mechanical demands, as well as asymmetry, may elucidate further information in relation to the biomechanics of the kettlebell swing. In regard to practical application, this study suggests that, when matched for work, 4 kg and 8 kg kettlebells when swung at fast or slow cadence, produce similar physiological and mechanical responses but the perceptual response was greater when the kettlebell was swung with an 8 kg load at a slow cadence. Thus, coaches and athletes may likely benefit to the same extent by swinging a 4 kg kettlebell than an 8 kg kettlebell.

3. Conclusion

The present study indicates that the physiological response to kettlebell swings at slow and fast cadences with 4 and 8 kg kettlebells is similar, as is the peak net vertical force. Perceived exertion values are higher when using an 8 kg kettlebell with a slow swing cadence. For coaches and athletes a 4 kg kettlebell swing protocol may be preferable as it results in similar physiological and mechanical response but lower RPE as compared to an 8 kg protocol.

Author Contributions

Michael J. Duncan, Rosanna Gibbard, Leanne M. Raymond and Peter Mundy designed the study, Rosanna Gibbard and Leanne M. Raymond collected the data. Michael J. Duncan and Peter Mundy analysed and interpreted the data. Michael J. Duncan, Rosanna Gibbard, Leanne M. Raymond and Peter Mundy wrote the manuscript. All authors critically reviewed, contributed to and approved the manuscript.

Conflicts of Interest

The authors declare no conflict of interest

References

1. Tsatsouline, P. *Enter the Kettlebell*; Dragon Door Publications: St. Paul, MN, USA, 2006.
2. O'Hara, R.B.; Serres, J.; Traver, K.L.; Wright, B.; Vojta, C.; Eveland, E. The influence of non-traditional training modalities in physical performance: Review of the Literature. *Aviat Space Environ. Med.* **2012**, *83*, 985–990.
3. Brumitt, J.; En Gilpin, H.; Brunette, M.; Meira, E.P. Incorporating kettlebells into a lower extremity sports rehabilitation program. *North Am. J. Sports Phys. Ther.* **2010**, *5*, 257–265.

4. Zebis, M.K.; Skotte, J.; Andersen, C.H.; Mortensen, P.; Petersen, M.H.; Viskaer, T.C.; Jensen, T.L.; Bencke, J.; Andersen, L.L. Kettlebell swing targets semitendinosus and supine leg curl targets biceps femoris: An EMG study with rehabilitation implications. *Br. J. Sports Med.* **2013**, *47*, 1192–1198.
5. Jay, K.; Frisch, D.; Hansen, K.; Zebis, M.K.; Andersen, C.H.; Mortensen, O.S.; Andersen, L.L. Kettlebell training for musculoskeletal and cardiovascular health: A randomized controlled trial. *Scand. J. Work Environ. Health* **2011**, *37*, 196–203.
6. Farrar, R.E.; Mayhew, J.L.; Koch, A.J. Oxygen cost of kettlebell swings. *J. Strength Cond. Res.* **2010**, *24*, 1034–1036.
7. Thomas, J.F.; Larson, K.L.; Hollander, D.B.; Kraemer, R.R. Comparison of two-hand kettlebell exercise and graded treadmill walking: Effectiveness as a stimulus for cardiorespiratory fitness. *J. Strength Cond. Res.* **2014**, *28*, 998–1006.
8. Lake, J.P.; Lauder, M.A. Mechanical demands of kettlebell swing exercise. *J. Strength Cond. Res.* **2012**, *26*, 3209–3216.
9. McGill, S.M.; Marshall, L.W. Kettlebell swing, snatch, and bottoms-up carry: Back and hip muscle activation, motion, and low back loads. *J. Strength Cond. Res.* **2012**, *26*, 16–27.
10. Husley, C.R.; Soto, D.T.; Koch, A.J.; Mayhew, J.L. Comparison of kettlebell swings and treadmill running at equivalent RPE Values. *J. Strength Cond. Res.* **2012**, *26*, 1203–1207.
11. Beardsley, C.; Contreras, B. The role of kettlebells in strength and conditioning: A review of the Literature. *Strength Cond. J.* **2014**, *36*, 64–70.
12. Borg, G. Perceived exertion as an indicator of somatic stress. *Scand. J. Rehab. Med.* **1970**, *2*, 92–98.

6

The Progression of Male 100 m Sprinting with a Lower-Limb Amputation 1976–2012

Bryce Dyer

Faculty of Science & Technology, Bournemouth University, Fern Barrow, Poole BH12 5BB, UK; E-Mail: brdyer@bournemouth.ac.uk

Academic Editor: Eling Douwe de Bruin

Abstract: Sprinting with a lower-limb amputation over 100 m has taken place in the Paralympic Games for over three decades. The aim of this paper is to statistically evaluate the performances and participation levels of such athletes during this period. The level of performance improvement over a 36-year period was proposed to be significantly greater than the able-bodied equivalent. Coupled with this, a major spike in amputee running performance improvement was shown to occur from 1984–1988. This supports previously recorded accounts of a major technological change being made at this time. Finally, whilst the average performance of the medallists has increased consistently over the 36-year history, the overall participation in the event fell significantly after 1988 and did not recover until 2012.

Keywords: amputee; sprinting; Paralympic Games

---

1. Introduction

Whilst other competitions such as World Championships and the Paralympic World Cup both offer competitive opportunities for athletes with a disability, the longest recorded and best known event is the Paralympic Games.

The first Paralympic Games took place in 1960 [1] and a specific event for lower-limb amputee sprinting began in 1976. The sprint running distances of 100, 200 and 400 m for both male and female athletes all exist within the Paralympic programme. However, only the male 100 m has consistently taken place since 1976.

Generally speaking, whilst an amputation is a disability, the level and type of any limb amputation will affect the performance of an athlete differently [2]. As a result, such athletes are classified based upon their functionality [3]. The classification of any athletes' disability has been undertaken either as a specific designation of their disability, or more recently through actual functional assessment [3]. This process clusters athletes with a similar level of disability together. The classification designated code for an athlete with a below-knee amputation in sprint athletics has changed over the 1976–2012 timeframe and has been defined in each Paralympic Games as:

- *MC* (1976 and 1980)
- *A4* (1984 and 1988)
- *TS2* (1992)
- *T44* (1996-current)

The current T44 class sprinter is typically characterised by a single amputation performed below the knee joint. An athlete with a double below-knee amputation can also race in the same event despite actually receiving a different formal classification (T43). This is known as a combined class and is often as a result of low levels of participation in any one classification [3]. However, even in a combined classification, prizes are only awarded to the first three athletes across the finish line. This makes parity between such mixed groups essential.

Sprinting with an amputation typically requires the use of a prosthetic limb. With functional prostheses, their purpose is to help a user maintain a full and active lifestyle [4]. However, the nature of prostheses when used in competitive sport is to facilitate the act of running and contribute to the best possible performance from an athlete. Running with a disability is unique in that it fundamentally requires technology to help facilitate it [5].

Whilst attention has focused on the act of amputee running [2], the behaviour of its technology [6] or characteristics when such athletes race [7], no study to date has investigated the male 100 m lower-limb amputee sprinting results and participation over the course of its history at the Paralympic Games. This study will evaluate both performance data from the Paralympic Games over the 1976–2012 period and then compare this to the able-bodied equivalent. It will also evaluate the level and type of athletic participation that has taken place during this time period.

2. Methods

2.1. Performance Data

The results of the male 100 m below knee classification from 1976–2012 was used as the basis of this study. The data was obtained from the sport's governing body website (http://www.paralympic.org/Athletes/Results).

Two statistical methods were used to track the progression of this event. The first method uses the *Performance Improvement Index* [8]. The Performance Improvement Index (PII) primarily assesses sports performance change from one set of performance data to another using the results of an event. It ultimately identifies proportions that could also be attributed to sports technology and provides a metric which forms a direct comparison to other sports that rely on different metrics (such as speed, distance, or time). Considering the typical requirement of a prosthetic limb when running with a lower-limb amputation [2] and the publicised controversy surrounding their use [6], use of this method may add further value to any discussions in the future. The PII has also been used to explore the impact of World Wars 1 and 2 upon running short, middle and long distance world records [9], and on the impact of technological innovation in Olympic field jumping events [10]. The PII cannot currently identify the exact proportion of impact of sports technology change, but it has been shown to corroborate anecdotal evidence of change such as the inception of new materials used for the pole vault or a change in the aerodynamic design of bicycles [8]. As a result, it is a complementary tool to inform debate rather than to generate substantive findings. When considering timed events over fixed distances, Haake [8] defines the Performance Improvement Index as:

$$\text{Index} = \left[\left(\frac{t_1}{t_2}\right)^2 - 1\right] \times 100 \tag{1}$$

This formula was initially derived as part of a linear regression process [8]. This formula addresses work done by a body overcoming aerodynamic drag when moving and for a fixed air density. It comprises a first timed performance t_1 divided by a second performance t_2. The rest of the formula converts the change between two performances and expresses it as a percentage. This formula assumes events requiring motion to be dominated by aerodynamics. However, it should be noted that air resistance increases exponentially as speed increases [11]. The proportion attributed to the air resistance of a 100 m sprinter running at 36 km/h is going to be exponentially less than a cyclist performing a 4 km individual pursuit at 50 km/h. As a result, the magnitude of the PII index may be skewed if comparing events that result in different absolute and average speeds.

The second method was the percentage increase of a performance from one Paralympics Games to the next. This was expressed as:

$$\text{Index} = \left[\left(\frac{t_1}{t_2}\right) - t_1\right] \times 100 \tag{2}$$

Like the PII, t_1 is the first performance (race time) and t_2 the next performance (race time). The result of this change was also expressed as a percentage.

The mean average of the finishing time of the 3 medal podium runners from each successive Paralympic Games was calculated as a basis for methods one and two. By considering a group of runners (rather than outright world records or event winners), any individual outliers are reduced in impact to help prevent skew. Each events sample of three allows a normalised comparison of all results despite participation likely varying at each games.

Both amputee sprinting and its able-bodied equivalent could be considered the same in philosophical nature. As a result, to provide a base of reference to the amputee race analysis, both methods one and two were compared to able-bodied 100 m sprinting to the nearest able-bodied equivalent, the *Olympic Games*. The Olympic Games and Paralympic Games have both taken place every 4 years and (since 1992) at the same venue. To provide the basis for such comparison (and to also provide several methods of normalising the relative infancy of sprinting with a disability with those of the able-bodied equivalent), three 36-year data evaluations were compared. These are:

- Amputee sprinting (AS): The PII change from Paralympic Games to Paralympic Games over the 1976–2012 time period.
- Able-bodied Inception Period (IP): The change from Olympic Games to Olympic Games over the 1896–1932 time period.
- Able-bodied Modern Period (MP): The change from Olympic Games to Olympic Games over the 1976–2012 time period.

It should be noted that only legal competitive performances were used in this study. Any sprinting performance which were rejected in the official results due to illegal practises such as doping, were also excluded here.

2.2. Event Participation

Athlete participation data was used to track trends to ascertain any level of change over the 36 year time periods. These were drawn from the classifications inception in 1976 up to the 2012 games using those described in the introduction section of this paper. The athletes' total participation number and country of representation was recorded from the total entry of the event—not just those qualifying for the final.

The data of athlete participation was also derived from the official governing body's website (http://www.paralympic.org/Athletes/Results).

3. Results

3.1. Performance Improvement

3.1.1. Performance Improvement of AS

The data derived from the timed performance of lower-limb amputee sprinting from Paralympics to subsequent Paralympics over the 1976–2012 timeframe is shown in Table 1.

Table 1. Amputee sprinting (AS) performance improvement 1976–2012.

Paralympic Games	Mean podium time (s)	Percentage improvement from prior games (%)	PII improvement from prior games (%)	PII improvement from 1976 baseline (%)
1976	14.40	-	-	-
1980	14.01	2.7	6	6
1984	13.62	2.8	6	12
1988	12.37	9.2	21	36
1992	12.19	1.5	3	40
1996	11.78	3.4	7	49
2000	11.40	3.2	7	60
2004	11.12	2.5	5	68
2008	11.29	−1.5	−3	63
2012	11.00	2.6	5	71

Note: PII = performance improvement index.

It is evident in Table 1 that both the "games to games" percentage increase and the PII demonstrates substantial improvement in 1988 with an increase well in excess of other AS "games to games" scores. There is no evidence of a change in PII to the same magnitude as 1988—either prior to it or after this date. Improvements in performance can be demonstrated until 2008 when performance times generally decrease.

3.1.2. Performance Improvement of Able-Bodied IP

The data derived from the timed performance of able-bodied sprinting from their inception at the Olympics over the 1896–1932 timeframe is shown in Table 2.

Table 2. Inception Period (IP) performance improvement 1896–1932.

Olympic Games	Mean podium time (s)	Percentage improvement from prior games (%)	PII improvement from prior games (%)	PII improvement from 1896 baseline (%)
1896	12.27	-	-	0
1900	11.10	9.5	22	22
1904	11.13	−0.3	−1	21
1908	10.90	2.1	4	27
1912	10.87	0.3	1	27
1920	10.80	0.6	1	29
1924	10.70	0.9	2	31
1928	10.87	−1.6	−3	27
1932	10.42	4.29	9	39

Note: PII = performance improvement index.

Able bodied sprinting from its Olympic Games inception saw progressively low rates of improvement. However, there was a spike, (equal to that of the AS 1984–1988 Paralympic sprinting improvement) from 1896–1900. The specific reason for this (be it social, technological or other) is not known. It should also be noted that a gap in the data occurred in 1916 since the Olympic Games were cancelled that year due to World War 1.

3.1.3. Performance Improvement of Able-Bodied MP

The data derived from the timed performance of able-bodied sprinting from their inception at the Olympics over the 1976–2012 timeframe is shown in Table 3.

Table 3. Modern Period (MP) performance improvement 1976–2012.

Olympic Games	Mean podium time (s)	Percentage improvement from prior games (%)	PII improvement from prior games (%)	PII improvement from 1976 baseline (%)
1976	10.09	-	-	0
1980	10.31	−2.2	−4	−4
1984	10.13	1.7	3	−3
1988	9.96	1.7	4	3
1992	9.99	−0.3	−1	2
1996	9.88	1.1	2	4
2000	9.97	−0.9	−2	3
2004	9.86	1.1	2	5
2008	9.83	0.3	1	5
2012	9.72	1.1	2	8

Note: PII = performance improvement index.

The degree of improvement of able-bodied MP PII is very low and significantly lower than those illustrated in Tables 1 and 2. Any gains are typically around 1% which is less than half of the typical gain that AS see during the same time period.

The general trend progressions of the mean podium of IP, MP and AS are now illustrated for comparative purposes in Figure 1.

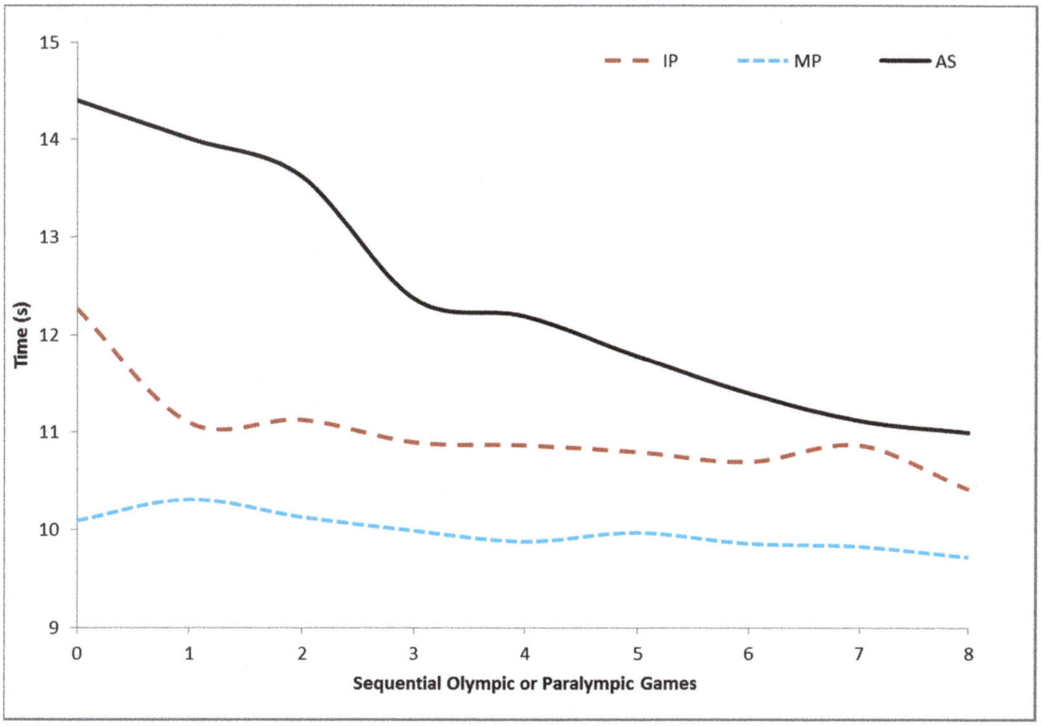

Figure 1. Performance improvement index (PII) of evaluated timeframes. IP = able-bodied inception period; MP = able-bodied modern period; AS = amputee sprinting.

Visual inspection of Figure 1 reveals that whilst it can be seen at the start of the evaluated time period that the three traces are wide apart, by the end of a 36-year duration they have narrowed considerably. Whilst the MP group has seen relatively little progression, AS has been subjected to a substantial reduction in the mean podium performances, illustrated with a far steeper gradient in its trace. Both IP and MP are also reducing but this is at a far more conservative rate. The three sub-groups decaying downward traces suggest that they are all likely to improve further in the future but that AS will likely be subjected to the greatest level of improvement.

The "games to games" PII changes of AS and able-bodied MP and IP over their 36 year periods can be compared together as shown in Figure 2.

It should be noted that the gap in IP's trace in Figure 2 was due to there being no Olympic Games held in 1916. The magnitude of the change in the AS event is shown by the steep peak in 1988 (games no. 3). After this point, the AS rate reduces until games no. 9. The IP timeframe too sees a slight increase at the end of its 36-year period, despite relative stability prior to it. The MP period seems to be in a state of relatively marginal improvement.

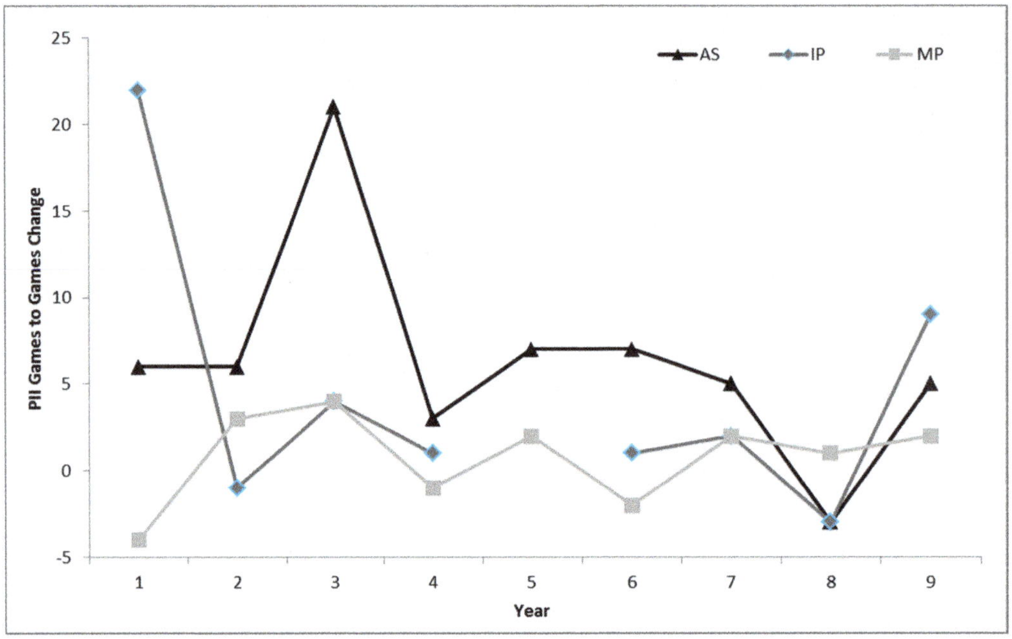

Figure 2. PII of timeframes. PII = performance improvement index; IP = able-bodied inception period; MP = able-bodied modern period; AS = amputee sprinting.

3.2. Event Participation

36 different countries sent athletes to the eight Paralympic games held between 1976 and 2012. The total number of eligible race "starts" by athletes was 159 (inclusive of those who did not finish). Figure 3 illustrates the number of nations participating and the total number of athletes competing in the lower-limb amputee 100 m sprint event at each games.

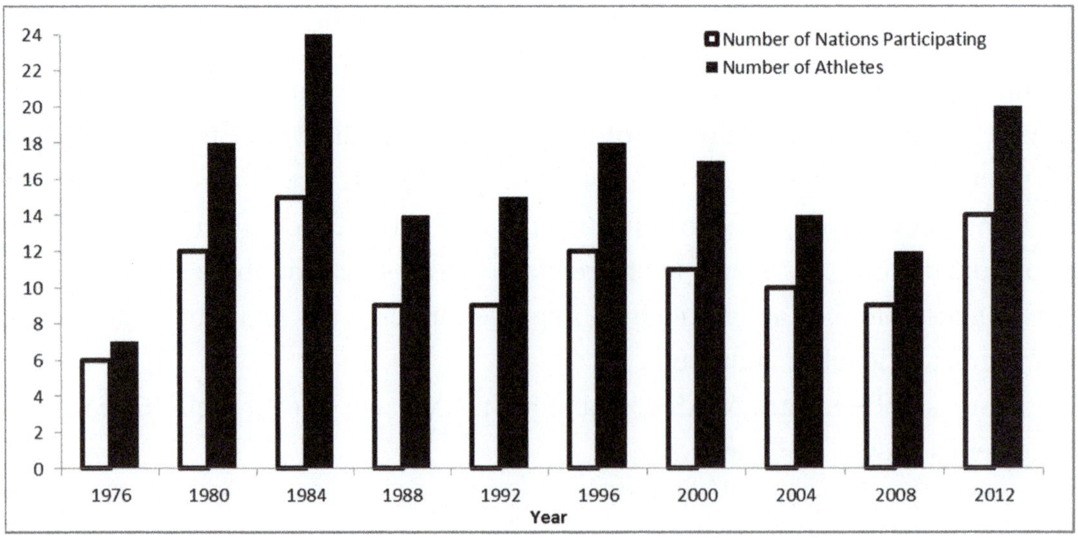

Figure 3. Amputee sprinting historical participation levels.

It can be seen that the number of competing athletes peaked in 1984 with a sharp decline in 1988. There is a gradual second (but smaller) peak at the 1996 games and then a gentle decline until the biggest increase seen since 1984 in 2012. This trend is also reflected by the total number of countries sending athletes to compete in this event. It is unclear what may have caused a positive increase in 2012, having suffered a gradual decline prior to it. It should be noted that (as mentioned in the introduction) the disability classification codes were changed 4 times over this full period. Crucially though, there was no such change in these between 1984 and 1988.

The relationship between the number of athletes and the number of nations taking part from 1976–2012 can be expressed as a ratio. This is illustrated in Figure 4.

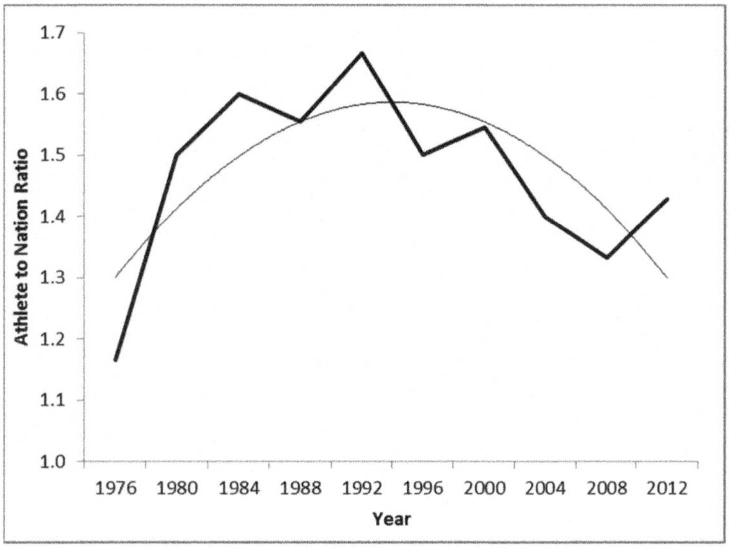

Figure 4. Athlete to nation ratio 1976–2012.

The ratio had its higher level from 1984–1992 but has been in decline since then. This demonstrates that the number of athletes a country could have is not increasing—despite the increase in AS illustrated in Figure 1. Secondly, Figure 3 has not indicated an increase in the number of nations competing. As a result, whilst the strength in competition is clear, its depth is not.

4. Discussion

Able-bodied sprinting has generally shown consistent, yet marginal improvements in performance. Amputee sprinting on the other hand has not directly followed the trends of able-bodied sprinting—either with their original inception into the Olympic Games nor over the same timeframe from 1976–2012. Amputee sprinting has seen a greater and faster rate of performance improvement compared to both of the able-bodied time period comparisons.

In addition, a noticeable peak in PII took place from 1984–1988. The specific reason for this peak can only be speculated. It has been demonstrated that of a typical historical performance improvement change, some of this can be attributed to clothing [8] or the social impact of war [10], but the able-bodied athlete's data over the same evaluated time period do not reflect similar sudden increases in PII that the amputee sprinting group demonstrated. Acknowledging that there were no changes in disability classification at the Paralympics between 1984 and 1988 (which may account for the sudden change in performance or participation), this suggests that there are other causative factors involved which are unique to disability sprinting. It has been proposed that a significant change in prosthetics technology took place from 1988 with the introduction of energy storage and return prostheses [8]. The PII magnitude of this peak (21%) is extremely large compared to any other Paralympic Games to Games increase over the evaluated period. This PII peak value is not as high as other values reported [8] such as javelin technology (95%), pole vault design (86%) or the cycling individual pursuit (35%). However, those examples were all calculated over much greater timeframes of at least 80 years. Considering that the maximum change in able-bodied sprinting would be 24% over a 100 year period [8], the level of progression shown by AS of 21% over just a 4 year period could be regarded as somewhat unusual and supportive of the notion that the technological change occurring in 1988 reported by Nolan [2], has positively contributed to the running ability of a lower-limb amputee. It has been suggested that to break plateaus in sporting performance, greater athletic improvements will be driven by revolutions in sports technology [10]. If this is true (and if a technological change was the sole cause of the large increase in PII), the use and role of prosthetics technology requires clarification by the sports stakeholders.

The general rate of performance improvement progression, whilst remaining positive, has generally decayed over the 36 year history. Such decay is typical in nature of sporting records and has also been recorded in the able-bodied 100 m world record generally [9]. This suggests that the sport will continue to develop for the foreseeable future but that the margins of improvement will become increasingly smaller in magnitude.

The evidence presented here also demonstrates a declining level of participation coupled with increasing levels of performance, even though overall athlete attendance at the Paralympic Games has been stated to continually increase [12]. In addition, the ratio of athlete to nation entering the 100 m at the Paralympic Games is also in decline—even as its performances are. If an increase in participation is desirable to the sport, any perceived barriers need to be identified to improve this. There are caveats to this proposal—it is not known what restrictions any nations might have applied to the number of athletes sent during this allotted time-period. The changes in participation levels could hypothetically be attributed to countries changing their attitude to athlete selection. It would be worthwhile to find out why smaller nations such as Poland, Israel or Myanmar (who sent several athletes prior to 1988) suddenly failed to do so from this point onwards. It is possible that their athletes simply were not replaced when they retired by younger ones of comparable standard but it would be a significant coincidence that several nations had this issue around the same time, who were all previously successful. It is of note that if a change in prosthetics technology took place from 1988 as discussed earlier, whether this impacted on athlete participation. The supply, demand or access to prostheses technology should be investigated to see if that was a contributory factor.

5. Conclusions

Amputee sprinting was evaluated from 1976–2012 and compared to able-bodied sprinting over the same duration and time period to its change in Paralympic Games event to event performance. The rate of improvement is significantly higher in amputee sprinting than an able-bodied equivalent. However, the performance trend of lower-limb amputee sprinting demonstrates a decaying rate of improvement which is typical of other sports. A large increase in amputee sprinting performance improvement was identified in 1988. This evidence supports previously reported anecdotes of a technological change made at this time. Finally, whilst the running performance has steadily improved, the level of participation has not. The nations sending athletes to the Paralympic Games changed significantly before and after 1988 but it is not clear if this is linked to the increase in performance improvement that occurred at the same time.

Acknowledgments

Both Philip Sewell and Siamak Noroozi of Bournemouth University are thanked for their feedback on the original data that contributed to this paper.

Conflicts of Interest

The author declares no conflict of interest.

References

1. Gold, J.; Gold, M. Access for all: The rise of the Paralympic Games. *J. R. Soc. Promot. Health* **2007**, *127*, 133–141.
2. Nolan, L. Carbon fibre prostheses and running in amputees: A review. *Foot Ankle Surg.* **2008**, *14*, 125–129.
3. Tweedy, S.; Vanlandewijck, Y. International Paralympic Committee position stand—Background and scientific principles of classification in Paralympic Sport. *Br. J. Sports Med.* **2011**, *45*, 259–269.
4. Gutfleisch, O. Peg legs and bionic limbs: The development of lower extremity prosthetics. *Interdiscip. Sci. Rev.* **2003**, *28*, 139–148.
5. Burkett, B. Technology in Paralympic sport: Performance enhancement or essential for performance? *Br. J. Sports Med.* **2010**, *44*, 215–220.
6. Bruggemann, G.; Arampatzis, A.; Emrich, F.; Potthast, W. Biomechanics of double transtibial amputee using dedicated sprinting prostheses. *Sports Technol.* **2008**, *1*, 220–227.
7. Dyer, B.; Noroozi, S.; Sewell, P. Sprinting with an amputation: Some race-based lower-limb step observations. *Prosthet. Orthot. Int.* **2014**, doi:10.1177/0309364614532863.
8. Haake, S. The impact of technology on sporting performance in Olympic Sports. *J. Sports Sci.* **2009**, *27*, 1421–1431.
9. Foster, L.; James, D.; Haake, S. Understanding the influence of population size on athletic performance. *Proced. Eng.* **2010**, *2*, 3183–3189.
10. Balmer, N.; Pleasence, P.; Nevill, A. Evolution and revolution: Gauging the impact of technological and technical innovation on Olympic performance. *J. Sports Sci.* **2012**, *30*, 1075–1083.
11. Kyle, C. Ergogenics for bicycling. *Perspect. Exercise Sci. Sports Med.* **1991**, *4*, 373–413.
12. Legg, D.; Steadward, R. The Paralympic Games and 60 years of change (1948–2008): Unification and restructuring from a disability and medical model to sport-based competition. *Sport Soc.* **2011**, *14*, 1099–1115.

7

Outcomes following Hip and Quadriceps Strengthening Exercises for Patellofemoral Syndrome: A Systematic Review and Meta-Analysis

Adebisi Bisi-Balogun * and Firdevs Torlak

Clinical Exercise Science, Faculty of Health Science, University of Potsdam Out-Patient Clinic, Potsdam 14469, Brandenburg, Germany; E-Mail: torlak@uni-potsdam.de

* Author to whom correspondence should be addressed; E-Mail: bisibalo@uni-potsdam.de

Academic Editor: Lee E. Brown

Abstract: There is growing evidence to support change in the rehabilitation strategy of patellofemoral pain syndrome (PFPS) from traditional quadriceps strengthening exercises to inclusion of hip musculature strengthening in individuals with PFPS. Several studies have evaluated effects of quadriceps and hip musculature strengthening on PFPS with varying outcomes on pain and function. This systematic review and meta-analysis aims to synthesize outcomes of pain and function post-intervention and at follow-up to determine whether outcomes vary depending on the exercise strategy in both the short and long term. Electronic databases including MEDLINE, EMBASE, CINAHL, Web of Science, PubMed, Pedro database, Proquest, Science direct, and EBscoHost databases were searched for randomized control trials published between 1st of January 2005 and 31st of June 2015, comparing the outcomes of pain and function following quadriceps strengthening and hip musculature strengthening exercises in patients with PFPS. Two independent reviewers assessed each paper for inclusion and quality. Means and SDs were extracted from each included study to allow effect size calculations and comparison of results. Six randomized control trials met the inclusion criteria. Limited to moderate evidence indicates that hip abductor strengthening was associated with significantly lower pain post-intervention (SMD −0.88, −1.28 to −0.47 95% CI), and at 12 months (SMD −3.10, −3.71 to −2.50 95% CI) with large effect sizes (greater than 0.80) compared to quadriceps strengthening. Our findings suggest that incorporating hip musculature strengthening in management of PFPS tailored to individual ability will improve short-term and long-term outcomes of rehabilitation. Further research evaluating the effects of quadriceps and hip abductors strengthening focusing on reduction in anterior knee pain and improvement in function in management of PFPS is needed.

Keywords: anterior knee pain; function; hip; muscle strengthening; muscle endurance

1. Introduction

Patello-femoral pain syndrome (PFPS) is one of the most diagnosed knee pain syndromes in paediatric physical therapy or orthopaedic outpatient clinics [1–3] and is thus implicated as the primary cause of knee pain in clinical settings in up to 40% of cases [4,5]. PFPS is prevalent in active young adults with a noticeable peak of prevalence in young, active adolescents between the ages of 12 and 17 years with double the annual incidence in women compared to men [1–3].

Diagnosis and treatment of PFPS poses a challenge in clinical practice, as its exact aetiology is unknown. However, PFPS describes anterior knee pain resulting from several intrinsic factors including increased Q-angle in the weight-bearing position, genu valgus, tibia internal rotation, patellar mal-alignment, muscular imbalance around the hip and knee joints, and over-activity [6]. Thus, diagnosis of PFPS requires exclusion of other conditions including intra-articular pathologic abnormality, plica syndromes, Osgood-Schlatter disease, neuromas, and other rare causes [6,7].

Conservative management options, which have been suggested for PFPS, include quadriceps strengthening, stretching, bracing, and patella taping although no specific intervention has been reported to be most effective in management of PFPS [8–10]. Quadriceps strengthening in the management of PFPS has been the focus of clinical interventions to correct patella tracking, alignment, and motion seen in PFPS thus reducing resultant increased patellar joint pressure and pain [8,10]. However, abnormal hip motion in both frontal and transverse planes due to weak hip muscles occurs in PFPS further influencing pain, knee kinematics, and function [9]. Poor eccentric hip abductors and external rotator muscle strength causes a resultant femoral adduction and medial rotation during weight-bearing activities, causing a lateral patellar tracking as the femur medially rotates beneath the patella, resulting in patellar mal-alignment [10,11].

Studies have reported that when compared to healthy controls, persons with PFPS show deficits in hip abductor, extensor, and external rotator muscle strength [12,13]. A deficit in hip abductor strength deficit compared with healthy controls of up to 14% has been reported in persons with PFP syndrome, resulting in impaired medial–lateral postural stability with diminished quantitative balance performance difference of up to 39%–45% [14]. This strength deficit plays huge biomechanical significance as seen in diminished single leg stance performance with following fatiguing of the hip abductor muscles [15] and also a reported correlation between balance performance and hip muscle abductor strength in adults [16]. The gluteus medius is an important muscle in controlling frontal-plane motion in a far reaching movement of the arm compared to ankle evertors and invertors, and as such play a significant role in maintaining normal posture in response to medial-lateral perturbations on the body [17].

The primary goals in management of PFPS, either surgical or conservative management, are the reduction in intensity of anterior knee pain, and restoration of patient optimal function (aspects of interaction between a person's health status and their contextual factors either environmental and personal factors) [8,13]. Evaluation of pain intensity and function pre and post intervention, provides a means of determining whether goals of conservative management of PFPS are achieved and serve as a means of assessing severity of patient symptoms at different time points during the course of management [8].

Although several studies have focused on the effects of both quadriceps strengthening and hip abductor strengthening on pain, hip muscle function and functional activities in PFPS reported mixed and inconclusive results.

Therefore, this meta-analysis was aimed to:

a. Determine differences in patient-reported anterior knee pain intensity in management of PFPS following quadriceps strengthening or hip abductor strengthening programs in management of PFPS.
b. Determine differences in function following quadriceps strengthening or hip abductor strengthening programs in management of PFPS.

2. Materials and Methods

2.1. Type of Participants

Studies were included if they reported having both male and female participants aged 15 to 40 years with a diagnosis of PFPS by medical and radiographic examination.

2.2. Types of Studies

Studies selection was limited to randomized control trial studies to reflect the highest level of clinical research quality. All studies reported pre and post intervention data of outcomes of anterior knee pain intensity and function following quadriceps strengthening and hip abductor strengthening programs in management of PFPS.

2.3. Type of Interventions

The interventions under consideration were quadriceps strengthening alone or hip abductor and external rotator strengthening programme in management of PFPS.

2.4. Outcome Measurements

Outcome measures used in selected studies in this review to evaluate pain and function included:

- Function—Evaluated with outcome measures including lower extremity function score (LEFS), Western Ontario and McMaster Universities Arthritis Index (WOMAC), or anterior knee pain score (AKPS), which have all been consistently used in research to assess function of the lower extremity pre and post intervention in management of PFPS [8].
- Pain as measured with outcome measures including the visual analogue scale or numerical pain rating scale (0/10) which have both been consistently used in research to assess anterior knee pain intensity pre and post intervention, in management of PFPS [3,8].

Validity and Reliability of Outcome Measures

Reliability for the LEFS and AKPS has been reported to be $R = 0.98$ and $R = 0.95$ in subjects with PFPS [18]. Reliability and validity of outcome measures of pain selected for this study, including the visual analogue scale (VAS) and numerical pain rating scale (NPRS) have been described in literature.

The VAS and the NPRS compared to other pain rating tools has a better responsiveness compared to other rating tools with an inter-rater reliability of ICC = 0.76 and 0.84 respectively [3,8].

2.5. Electronic Search

An electronic online search was conducted using a systematic search strategy to identify relevant articles in electronic databases including MEDLINE, EMBASE, CINAHL, Web of Science, PubMed, Pedro database, Proquest, Science direct, and EBscoHost for studies published in English between 2008 and May 2015 to reflect current research knowledge. Key word combinations used included: patellofemoral pain syndrome, anterior knee pain, function, hip, muscle strengthening, and muscle endurance. The electronic data search was limited to randomized control trial studies only to reflect the highest level of clinical research quality included in this review. In addition, a manual searching of the references of all articles selected for the review and bibliographies of relevant texts and journals was conducted. Depositories of unpublished research were not perused and although the authors agree this may potentially lead to publication bias [19], it is impossible to exhaustively peruse all unpublished work on effects of strength training interventions associated with PFPS from all authors and institutions around the world related to this research area.

2.6. Inclusion and Exclusion Criteria

Inclusion Criteria—Studies with

- Participants aged 15–40 years.
- Comparison of pre and post intervention outcomes following quadriceps strengthening or hip abductor strengthening programs in management of PFPS including anterior knee pain and patient reported function.
- Incidence of PFPS of at-least four weeks onset. Participants had to report anterior, retro, or peri-patellar pain during at least two or three of the following provocative activities: squatting, kneeling, prolonged sitting, ascending or descending stairs, running, hopping, jumping, palpation or compression of medial or lateral patella facet, and isometric quadriceps contraction.
- Studies published between 1st of January 2005 and 31st of June 2015.

Exclusion criteria

- o Studies were excluded if they reported inclusion of participants with a previous history of knee surgeries, lower limb pathology, or dysfunctions including knee/patellar osteoarthritis, bursitis, meniscal injuries and knee collateral or cruciate ligament injuries, or other pathological diseases of the knee joint.

2.7. Study Selection

Two reviewers independently performed the process of study selection based on the title and the abstract. Articles not excluded by both reviewers were assessed in full-text and disagreement regarding inclusion was resolved by consensus.

Quality Rating of Selected Studies

For studies meeting inclusion criteria, the PEDRO scale was used to appraise their methodological quality. It has a fair inter-rater agreement for individual domains and substantial agreement for the final grade in contrast to similar rating tools (ICC = 0.56–0.68) [19]. This was independently applied by two reviewers, with discrepancies resolved during a consensus meeting.

2.8. Data Abstraction

Data relating to study design, participants, PFPS definitions, and protocol for exercise intervention (frequency, intensity, type, and time) were extracted from all studies. The mean differences of pre and post intervention for anterior knee pain using the Visual Analogue Scale/Numerical Pain rating Scale were determined. Similarly, pre and post intervention mean differences of outcome measures of function of the lower extremity using the Anterior Knee Pain Scale (AKPS), Lower Extremity Function Scale (LEFS) and WOMAC (The Western Ontario and McMaster Universities Arthritis Index) questionnaires between subjects with PFPS in both quadriceps strengthening group and hip abductor and external rotator groups were extracted. If data were missing, information was requested from the authors to allow effect size (ES) calculations.

2.9. Data Analysis

The Cochrane review statistical program Revman 5.3 was used for statistical data analysis of effect size, heterogeneity, and Standard Error of Effect size estimate. Data were pooled for pain with the VAS and where studies evaluated lower extremity function, results were pooled using functional outcome measures for the lower extremity function variable. Calculated individual or pooled ES were categorised as small (=0.59), medium (0.60–1.19) or large (=1.20). The level of statistical heterogeneity for pooled data was established using the Chi^2 and I^2 statistics (with heterogeneity defined as $p < 0.05$). Thus, the summary measure of treatment effect was the between-groups difference in mean levels of post intervention pain reduction and increase in function, expressed as a standardised mean difference (SMD) using Hedges' (adjusted) g, which includes a correction term for sample size bias [20] Statistical heterogeneity was assessed by the I^2 test, which describes the percentage of variability among effect estimates beyond that expected by chance. Heterogeneity can be considered as unlikely to be important for I^2 values up to 40%. In the absence of statistical heterogeneity (I^2 less than or equal to 40%), individual effect sizes were combined statistically using the inverse variance random-effects method, which assumes that true effects are normally distributed [21]. Levels of evidence definitions employed in this study were as recommended by van Tulder *et al.* [22].

3. Results

The literature search produced a total of 402 studies. Six randomized control trials met the inclusion and exclusion criteria for this review. Manual search of literature sources did not produce any additional study. The search strategy is itemized in Figure 1 below.

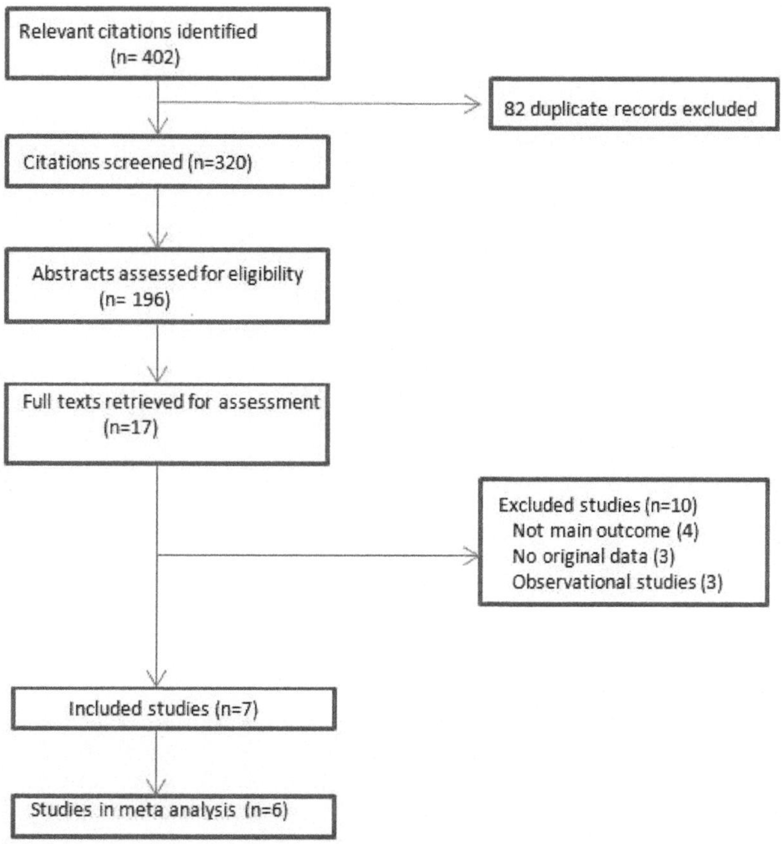

Figure 1. Flow chart showing search strategy.

3.1. Study Characteristics

A total of six randomized controlled trials met the inclusion and exclusion criteria and were included in the review. All six studies [23–28] evaluated anterior knee pain intensity (VAS/NPRS 0/10) as a pre and post intervention outcome measure. A total of four studies examined function using the functional assessment tools AKPS [25,26], LEFS [25,26,28] and WOMAC [27]. All six studies randomized a total of 214 participants (89.7% female), with sample size ranging from 14 to 54 subjects. The mean age of studies populations ranged from 16 to over 40 years. Participant eligibility was determined by clinician diagnosis of PFPS of at least four weeks onset, and a fulfilment of an inclusion and exclusion criteria as itemized in Table 1. Interventions typically involved exercising for three 30-45 min sessions per week for 4-8 weeks, a range of 12–24 sessions per trial [23–28].

Table 1. Description of Methods and characteristics of included studies with quality ratings score.

Author	Study Population/ Group Allocation	Inclusion/Exclusion Criteria	Follow up/ Monitoring	Intervention Description	Pre and Post-Operative Measurements	Randomisation Process	Pedro Score (0/10)
Nagakawa *et al.* 2008 [23] RCT	14 subjects (4 male; 10 females); QUADSG (7) HABLG (7)	Inclusion—Clinically diagnosed with PFP; anterior knee pain; insidious onset of pain unrelated to a traumatic incident and persistent for at least four weeks; presence of pain on palpation of the patellar facets. Exclusion—Intra-articular pathologic conditions; cruciate or collateral ligament involvement; tenderness over patellar tendon, iliotibial band, or pes anserinus tendon; patellar apprehension; Osgood-Schlatter or Sinding-Larsen-Johansson syndromes; hip or lumbar referred pain; a history of patellar dislocation; knee effusion; or previous patellofemoral joint surgery.	No follow-up period	Duration—5 sessions/week for 6 weeks, 1 supervised and 4 unsupervised weekly session. QUADSG— 1. Open and closed kinetic chain exercises for quadriceps strengthening, 2. Sitting hamstring stretch, 3 repetitions/30-s hold; patellar mobilization, Standing quadriceps, calf and iliotibial band stretch. 3. Isometric quadriceps contractions while sitting with 90° of knee flexion 2 sets of 10 repetitions/10-s hold 4. Straight-leg raise in supine position 3 sets of 10 repetitions 5. Mini squats to 40° of knee flexion 4 sets of 10 repetitions Balance training 3 sets. HABSG—Same as QUADSG with addition of 1. Transversus abdominis muscle contraction in the quadruped position 2 sets of 15 repetitions/10-s hold. 2. Isometric combined hip abduction-lateral rotation in side-lying and then quadruped position with the hips using elastic resistance 2 sets of 15 repetitions/10-s hold for each position. 3. Side-lying isometric hip abduction with extended knee 2 sets of 15 repetitions/10-s hold. 4. Additional elastic resistance around the affected leg in the forward lunges to encourage lateral rotation and abduction of the hip. All subjects performed the rehabilitation exercises once a week under the supervision of the principal investigator and four times a week at home, for a total of five sessions a week for six weeks.	Pain—Worst and usual pain; Pain during stair ascending and descending (VAS)	Sealed envelope, blinded assessors, single blinded	9

Table 1. *Cont.*

Author	Study Population/ Group Allocation	Inclusion/Exclusion Criteria	Follow up/ Monitoring	Intervention Description	Pre and Post-Operative Measurements	Randomisation Process	Pedro Score (0/10)
Razeghi *et al.* 2010 [24] RCT	32 females; mean age 22.62 ± 2.67 years (18–30); QUADSG (16) HABLG (16)	Inclusion—Clinically diagnosed with PFP; anterior knee pain; insidious onset of pain unrelated to a traumatic incident of at least four weeks onset; pain during patellar orthopaedic test or facet tenderness. Exclusion—Intra-articular pathologic conditions; cruciate or collateral ligament involvement; tenderness over iliotibial band, patella or pes anserinus tendon; patellar apprehension; Osgood-Schlatter or Sinding-Larsen-Johansson syndromes; hip or lumbar referred pain; a history of patellar dislocation; Pregnancy; history of being on a steroidal or nonsteroidal medication in last 6 months	No follow-up	Duration—4-week treatment program, supervised. QUADSG—Strengthening exercise in the control group focused only on the quadriceps muscle. The treatment program consisted of progressive resistive exercises for the hip muscles and terminal and 90° to 50° resistive knee extension and mini squat for the quadriceps. The Mc Queen progressive resistive technique was applied to increase exercise resistance. HABSG—Exercise intervention not properly described.	Usual pain measured with VAS	Random allocation	5

Table 1. *Cont.*

Author	Study Population/ Group Allocation	Inclusion/Exclusion Criteria	Follow up/ Monitoring	Intervention Description	Pre and Post-Operative Measurements	Randomisation Process	Pedro Score (0/10)
Fukuda *et al.* 2010 [25] RCT	70 females; mean age 25 years (20–40); QUADSG (22); HABSG (23) Control group (25)	Inclusion—History of anterior knee pain of more than 3 months onset; reported pain in 2 or more daily activities; sedentary for at least the past 6 months. Exclusion—Pregnant or had any neurological disorders; hip, knee, or ankle injuries; low back or sacroiliac joint pain; rheumatoid arthritis; used corticosteroids or anti-inflammatory drugs; a heart condition that prohibited performing the exercises; or previous surgery involving the lower extremities.	No follow up	Duration—3 sessions per week for 4 weeks, totalling 12 sessions, supervised. QUADSG— 1. Stretching and strengthening of knee musculature. Stretching (HM, PF, quadriceps, and ITB), 3 sets/30 s 2. Iliopsoas strengthening in non-weight bearing, 3 sets/10 repetitions. 3. Seated knee extension 90°–45°, 3 sets/10 repetitions. 4. Leg press 0°–45°, 3 sets/10 repetitions 5. Squatting 0°–45°, 3 sets/10 repetitions. HABSG—Same protocol as QUADSG, with the addition of exercises to strengthen the hip abductor and lateral rotator muscles. Standardized to 70% of the 1-repetition maximum. 1. Hip abduction against elastic band (standing), 3 sets/10 repetitions 2. Hip abduction with weights (side-lying), 3 sets/10 repetitions 3. Hip external rotation against elastic band (sitting), 3 sets/10 repetitions. 4. Side-stepping against elastic band, 3 reps/1 min.	Pain during stair ascending and descending (NPRS); Lower extremity function with LEFS and AKPS	Random allocation using opaque and sealed envelopes containing the names of the groups	8

Table 1. *Cont.*

Author	Study Population/ Group Allocation	Inclusion/Exclusion Criteria	Follow up/ Monitoring	Intervention Description	Pre and Post-Operative Measurements	Randomisation Process	Pedro Score (0/10)
Fukuda *et al.* 2012 [26] RCT	54 females; mean age 23 years QUADSG (26); HABSG (28)	Inclusion—History of anterior knee pain of more than 3 months onset; reported pain in 2 or more daily activities; sedentary for at least the past 6 months. Exclusion—Pregnant or had any neurological disorders; hip, knee, or ankle injuries; low back or sacroiliac joint pain; rheumatoid arthritis; used corticosteroids or anti-inflammatory drugs; a heart condition that prohibited performing the exercises; or previous surgery involving the lower extremities.	1 year	Duration—3 sessions per week for 4 weeks, totalling 12 sessions, supervised exercise sessions QUADSG— 1. Stretching and strengthening of the knee musculature. Stretching (HM, PF, quadriceps, and ITB), 3 sets/30 s 2. Iliopsoas strengthening in non-weight bearing, 3 sets/10 repetitions. 3. Seated knee extension 90°–45°, 3 sets/10 repetitions. 4. Leg press 0°–45°, 3 sets/10 repetitions 5. Squatting 0°–45°, 3 sets/10 repetitions. HABSG—Same protocol as QUADSG, with the addition of exercises to strengthen the hip abductor and lateral rotator muscles. Standardized to 70% of the 1-repetition maximum. 1. Hip abduction against elastic band (standing), 3 sets/10 repetitions 2. Hip abduction with weights (side-lying), 3 sets/10 repetitions 3. Hip external rotation against elastic band (sitting), 3 sets/10 repetitions. 4. Side-stepping against elastic band, 3 reps/1 min.	Pain during stair ascending and descending (NPRS); Lower extremity function with LEFS and AKPS	Random allocation using opaque and sealed envelopes containing the names of the groups	8

Table 1. *Cont.*

Author	Study Population/ Group Allocation	Inclusion/Exclusion Criteria	Follow up/ Monitoring	Intervention Description	Pre and Post-Operative Measurements	Randomisation Process	Pedro Score (0/10)
Khayambashis *et al.* 2014 [27] RCT	36 (18 male; 18 female); mean age 27.3 ± 7 years (19–35 years); QUADSG (18) HABSG (18)	Inclusion—Unilateral or bilateral PFP diagnosed by a physician. Exclusion—Ligamentous laxity; meniscal injury; pes anserine bursitis; iliotibial band syndrome; patella tendinitis; or a history of patella dislocation, patella fracture, knee surgery or symptoms that had been present for ≤6 months.	6 months	Duration—3 sessions/week for 8 weeks totalling 24 sessions; 3 sets, 20–25 reps/set, supervised exercise sessions. QUADSG— 1. Resisted knee extension using an elastic with subjects extending the knee from 30 of knee flexion to full knee extension. 2. Partial squat against resistance from the start position to full knee extension while squeezing a ball between both knees HABSG— 1. Hip abductor strengthening in side lying on a treatment table with elastic tubing providing resistance by abducting the hip from 0° to 30° 3 sets, 20–25 reps/set 2. Hip external rotator strengthening performed seated at the edge of a treatment table and the knee flexed to 90° with elastic tubing tied around the ankle providing resistance as subjects externally rotated the hip from 0° to 30°.	Usual pain (VAS); Lower extremity function (WOMAC).	Controlled clinical trial	5

Table 1. *Cont.*

Author	Study Population/ Group Allocation	Inclusion/Exclusion Criteria	Follow up/ Monitoring	Intervention Description	Pre and Post-Operative Measurements	Randomisation Process	Pedro Score (0/10)
Doldak *et al.* 2011 [28] RCT	33 females; aged 16–35 years; QUADSG (16) HABSG (17)	Inclusion—Clinically diagnosed with PFP; anterior knee pain; insidious onset of pain unrelated to a traumatic incident of at least four weeks onset; pain during patellar orthopaedic test or facet tenderness. Exclusion—Symptoms present for less than one month; self-reported other knee pathology; history of knee surgery within the last year; a self-reported history of patella dislocations or subluxations; and other concurrent significant injury affecting the lower extremity.	No follow up	Duration—8 weeks, 3 sessions per week. 1 supervised, 2 unsupervised at home (3 sets/10 reps). 1st rehabilitation phase—4 weeks HABSG— 1. Standing; side-lying hip abduction and external rotation with 3%–5% body weight 2. Side-lying hip abduction and external rotation with 5%–7% body weight and quadruped hydrant QUADSG— 1. Short arc quads with 3%–7% body weight; Straight leg raises with 3%–7% body weight. 2. Terminal knee extensions with 3%–7% body weight. 2nd Phase—Both groups performed similar flexibility exercises (5–8 weeks) 1. Single-leg balance with front pull or standing on Airpex pad, (3 sets/10 reps) 2. Lateral step-downs off a 10–20.3-cm step (3 sets of 10 repetitions) 3. Lunges to a 10–20.3-cm step; Single-leg calf raises alone or on Airex pad.	Usual pain (VAS), Lower extremity function with LEFS.	Participants were randomly assigned to a hip strengthening program (hip group) or a quadriceps strengthening program (quad group) for 4 weeks.	6

In three of the six studies, [23,25,26] the hip abductor strengthening group (HABSG) performed both hip abductor, external rotator, and quadriceps muscle strengthening exercises, while the quadriceps strengthening group (QUADSG) performed quadriceps muscle strengthening exercises alone. In the other three studies [24,27,28], the hip abductor strengthening group performed hip abductor and external rotator strengthening exercises alone, while subjects in the quadriceps strengthening group performed quadriceps strengthening exercises alone.

In four studies, all subjects performed stretching exercises as part of their exercise intervention sessions in both hip abductor strengthening groups and quadriceps strengthening groups [23–25,28], while stretching was not performed in the other two trials [26,27]. In two studies, all weekly exercise sessions were performed in a rehabilitation setting and supervised by the investigator [24–27] while in the other two of the studies [23,28], one out of five session weekly sessions [23] and one out of three weekly sessions [28] were supervised in the clinic by the investigator while all other sessions were performed by the subject at home unsupervised (Table 1). Only two of the six studies [26,27] reported a post-intervention follow-up period (6 and 12 months respectively).

3.2. Effect of Hip Abductor and Quadriceps Strengthening Exercise on Anterior Knee Pain

Post Intervention: The point estimate of effect size for each study indicated a greater reduction in PFPS amongst subjects in the hip abductor and external rotator muscle strengthening group compared with subjects in the quadriceps muscle strengthening groups post intervention (Figure 2). In four out of six trials [23,24,26,27] the post intervention difference in intensity of anterior knee pain was statistically significant between both groups ($p < 0.05$). One study reported non-statistically significant differences in post intervention usual pain [28] and in ascending pain post intervention [25]. In the presence of statistical heterogeneity (I^2 greater or equal to 40%), individual effect sizes could not be combined statistically using the inverse variance random-effects method, which assumes that true effects are not normally distributed. Synthesis of data showed evidence of high statistical heterogeneity ($I^2 = 78\%$, $p < 0.05$), and therefore effect size estimates from the three subgroups (usual pain, pain during ascending stairs, and descending stairs) could not be pooled (Figure 2).

However, from results of analysis of overall pain, focusing on usual pain as a subgroup of overall pain, analysis of estimates of effect sizes of usual pain intensity from four studies [23,24,27,28] indicated that there is moderate evidence showing that the hip abductor strengthening group compared to the quadriceps strengthening alone in management of PFPS resulted in more significant reduction in usual pain ($I^2 = 28\%$, $p = 0.24$) with a medium pooled ES (SMD −0.88, −1.28 to −0.47 95% CI) (Figure 2).

Six months follow up: In the presence of statistical heterogeneity ($I^2 = 67\%$), effect size estimates could not be pooled statistically. However, sub group analysis of inverse variance random effects showed an increase in effect size at six months follow-up from post-intervention levels between both groups in usual pain intensity (−0.87 to −1.43), during stair ascending (SMD −1.12 to −2.65 95% CI), and stair descending (SMD −1.09 to −2.50 95% CI) (Figure 3).

Twelve months follow up: In the absence of statistical heterogeneity ($I^2 = 0\%$, $p = 0.07$), synthesis of data at 12 months follow up from one high quality study [26] shows limited evidence for significant differences in pain reduction between both the hip abductor strengthening group and the quadriceps strengthening group at six months follow-up with no evidence of statistical heterogeneity among the pooled estimates and a large pooled effect size (SMD −3.10, −3.71 to −2.50 95% CI) (Figure 4). However, sub group analysis of inverse variance random effects showed a more significant increase in effect size estimates at 12 months follow-up between both groups in pain intensity during stair ascending (SMD −2.65 to −2.99 95% CI) and stair descending (SMD −2.50 to −3.22 95% CI) (Figure 4).

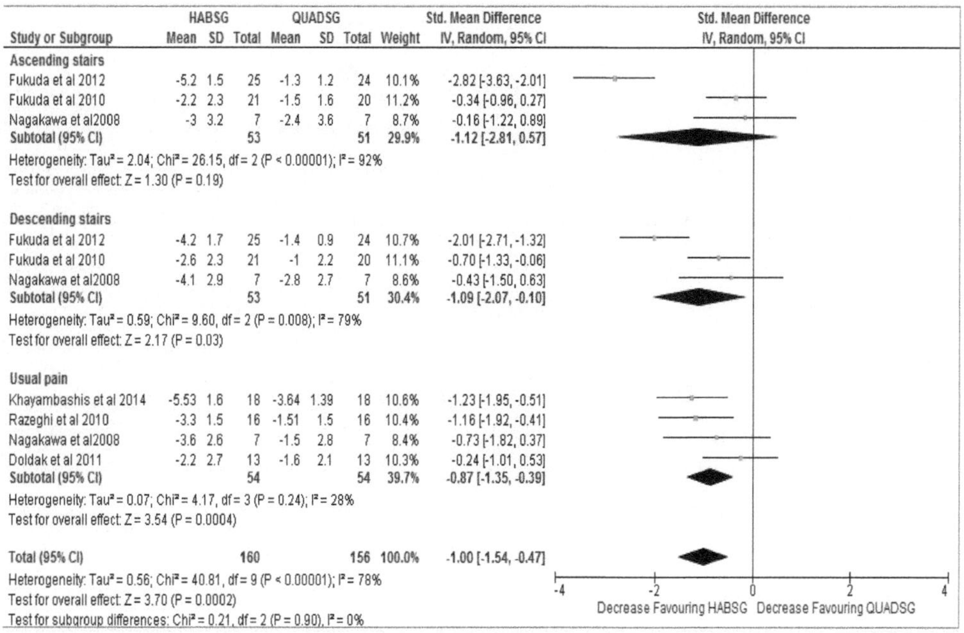

Figure 2. Post intervention: Effect size comparison and estimate of anterior knee pain intensity measured a 10 point visual analogue scale (VAS) and numerical pain rating scale (NPRS) (0/10) in both Hip abductor strengthening group (HABSG) and Quadriceps strengthening group (QUADSG).

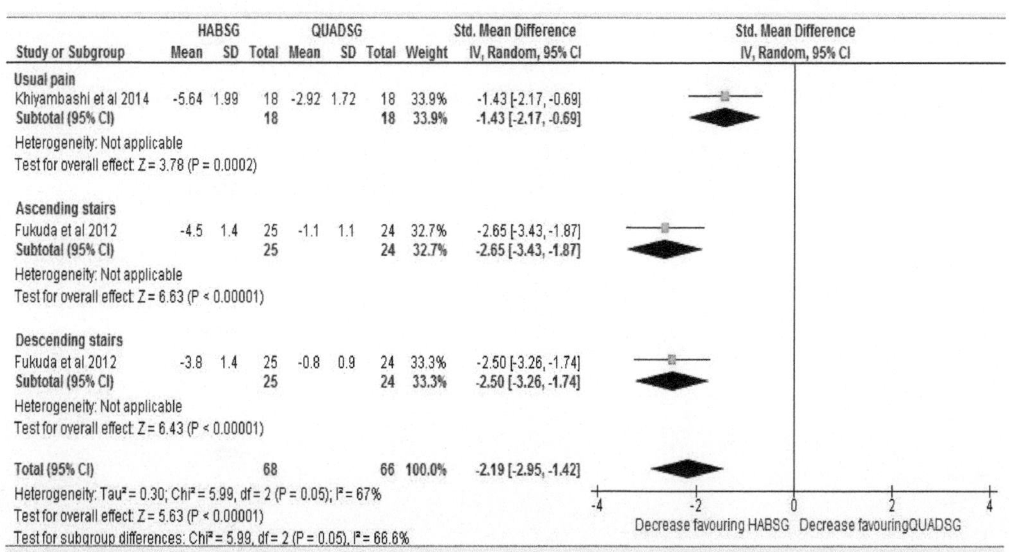

Figure 3. At six months follow-up: Effect size comparison and estimate of anterior knee pain intensity measured with a 10 point visual analogue scale/NPRS (0/10) in both Hip abductor strengthening group (HABSG) and Quadriceps strengthening group (QUADSG).

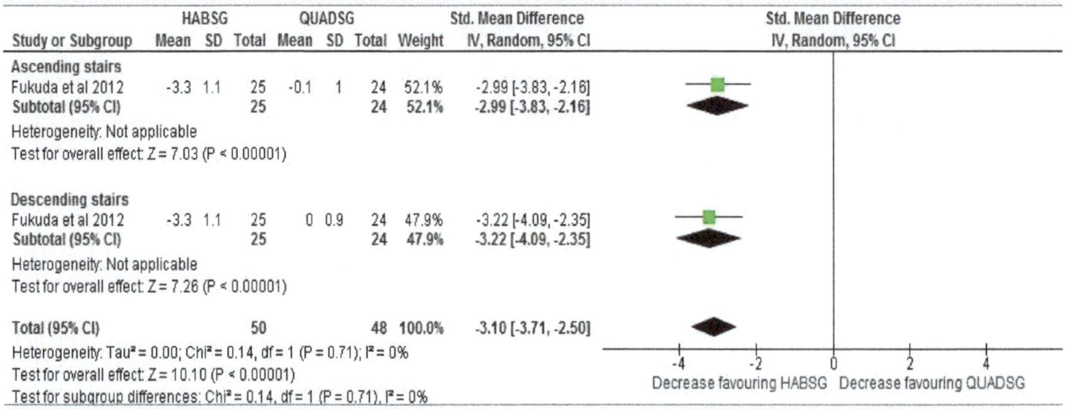

Figure 4. At 12 months follow-up: Effect size comparison and estimate of anterior knee pain intensity measured with a 10 point VAS/NPRS (0/10) in both Hip abductor strengthening group (HABSG) and Quadriceps strengthening group (QUADSG).

3.3. Effect of Hip Abductor and Quadriceps Strengthening Exercise on Function

Post intervention: Four trials evaluated function pre and post intervention. The point estimate of effect size of each study [25–27] excluding Doldak *et al.* [28] indicated a greater increase in function amongst subjects in the hip abductor strengthening group compared with subjects in the quadriceps muscle strengthening group. Contrastingly, Doldak *et al.* [28] showed a point estimate of effect size indicating a greater increase in function post-intervention in the quadriceps strengthening group compared to the hip abductor strengthening group (Figure 5). In two out of four studies [26,27] the post intervention differences in increased function between both groups were statistically significant and non-significant in the other two studies [25,28] ($p < 0.05$) (Figure 5). Synthesis of data showed evidence of high statistical heterogeneity ($I^2 = 87\%$, $p < 0.05$), and therefore effect sizes from the three subgroups (LEFS, AKPS and WOMAC) could not be pooled for further analysis.

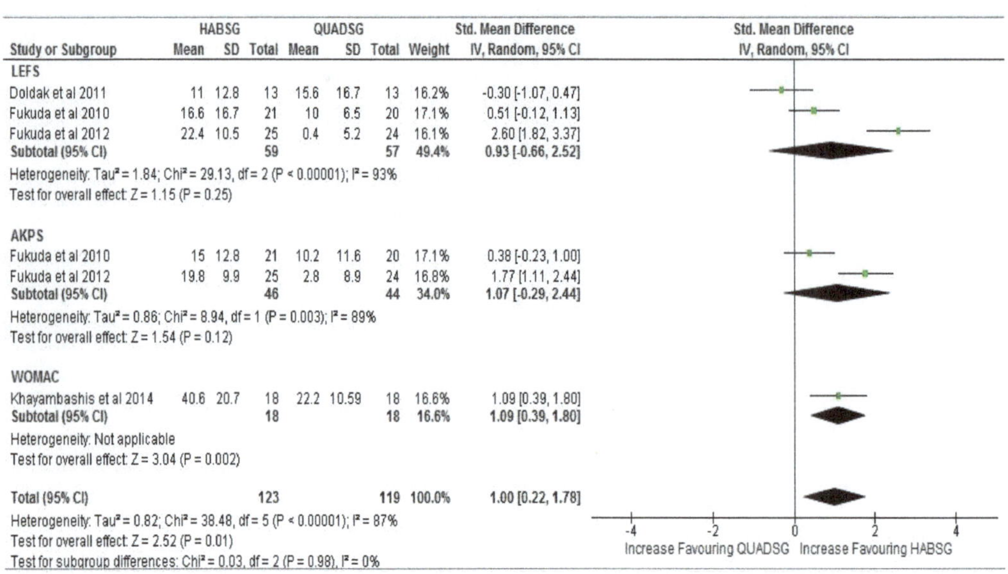

Figure 5. Post intervention: Effect size comparison of estimates of Function in subjects with Patellofemoral pain in both Hip abductor strengthening group (HABSG) and Quadriceps strengthening group (QUADSG).

Six months follow up: Due to high statistical heterogeneity ($I^2 = 66\%$, $p = 0.05$) individual effect sizes could not be combined statistically assuming that true effects are not normally distributed. Therefore, ES estimates from the three subgroups (LEFS, AKPS and WOMAC) could not be pooled (Figure 6). However, sub group analysis showed a more significant increase in effect size estimates (SMD) of function at six months follow-up from post-intervention levels between both groups in LEFS (SMD 0.99 to 2.49 95% CI); AKPS (SMD 1.07 to 1.86 95% CI); WOMAC (SMD 1.09 to 1.20 95% CI) (Figure 6).

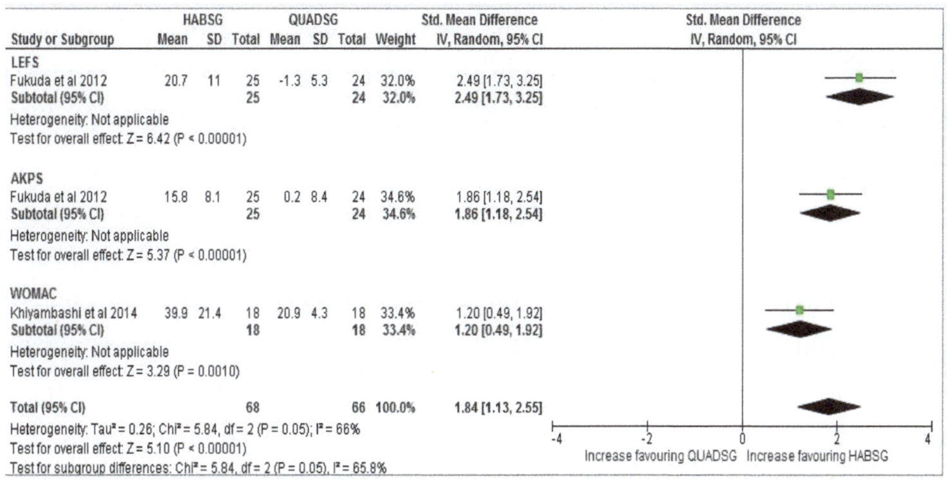

Figure 6. At six months follow-up: Effect size comparison of estimates of Function in subjects with patellofemoral pain in both Hip strengthening group (HABSG) and Quadriceps strengthening group (QUADSG).

Twelve months follow up: Due to high statistical heterogeneity ($I^2 = 65\%$, $p = 0.05$) individual effect sizes could not be combined, assuming that true effects are not normally distributed. Results from only one high quality study [26] showed a more significant increase in effect size estimates of function at from six to 12 months follow-up levels between both groups in LEFS (SMD 2.49 to 2.65 95% CI) and a slight decrease in AKPS (SMD 1.86 to 1.76 95% CI) (Figure 7).

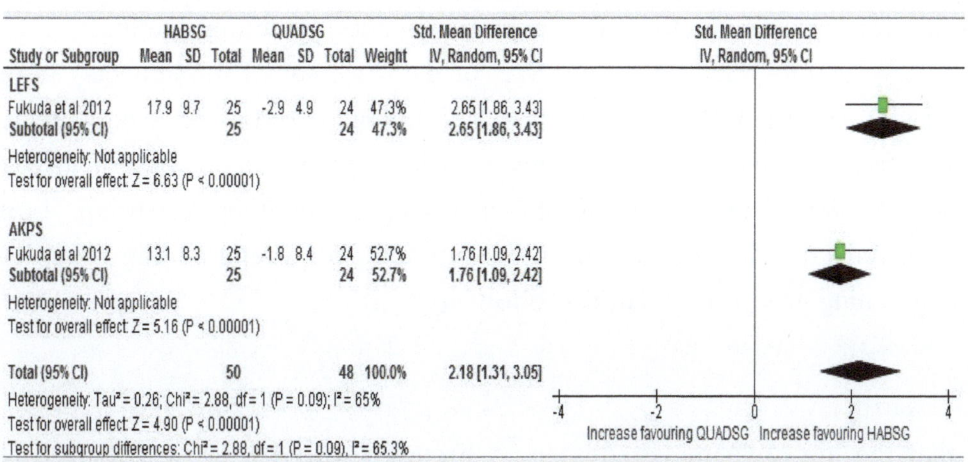

Figure 7. At 12 months follow-up: Effect size comparison and estimate of Function in subjects with patellofemoral pain in both Hip abductor strengthening group (HABSG) and Quadriceps strengthening group (QUADSG).

4. Discussion

The aim of this meta-analysis was to compare effects of hip abductor strengthening and quadriceps strengthening in management of PFPS. Results from individual studies indicated significant differences in usual pain intensity post intervention, and pain and function at six and 12 months follow-up with large effect sizes. However, these post intervention differences were not consistent in their level of statistical significances across all studies and tasks with high statistical heterogeneity of data during synthesis. While attempting to identify methodological differences to explain this disparate finding, one possible explanation could be because PFPS diagnosis is based on a group of symptoms and not a specific test. And although inclusion and exclusion criteria were similar, they differed between studies with some variability in terms of localization, onset of pain and pre-intervention level of function of subjects meeting eligibility criteria for inclusion across studies. In two studies [23,28] onset of PFPS as an inclusion criteria of participants was minimum of four weeks onset of PFPS while the four remaining studies [24–27] reported an inclusion criteria of a minimum of six months onset of PFPS (Table 1).

Due to high level of statistical heterogeneity, outcomes of overall pain post-intervention and at six months follow-up and function post intervention and at six months and 12 months follow-up were not pooled. Thus, individual effect sizes could not be combined statistically using the inverse variance random-effects method, assuming that true effects were not normally distributed across studies.

4.1. Anterior Knee Pain

Post intervention, effect sizes were medium-to-strong, indicating that the hip strengthening group demonstrated greater improvements in usual pain post intervention (Figure 2) and overall pain at 12 months follow-up (Figure 4) compared with the quadriceps strengthening group. Moderate evidence indicates that usual pain was significantly reduced in the hip abductor strengthening group compared to the quadriceps strengthening group with a moderate effect size (SMD −0.88, −1.28 to −0.47 95% CI) immediately post-intervention (analysis of a total of 108 subjects). While hip abductor strengthening exercises and quadriceps strengthening exercises reduced usual pain intensity post-intervention, there was a significant difference in the magnitude of this post-intervention usual pain reduction between both groups, with far greater pain reduction in the hip abductor strengthening groups.

At 12 months follow-up for overall pain, analysis of data (a total of 49 subjects) showed a large pooled effect size (SMD −3.10, −3.71 to −2.50 95% CI). This increased effect size estimate compared to post intervention effect sizes between both groups may be explained as a consequence of a gradual increase in overall pain post-intervention in the quadriceps strengthening group. Low evidence indicates an increased reduction in overall pain in the hip abductor strengthening group compared to the quadriceps strengthening group at 12 months follow up.

4.2. Function

Results show that the hip abductor strengthening groups showed a greater increase in function post-intervention and at six and 12 months follow-up compared to the quadriceps strengthening groups according to point estimates of effect sizes across subgroups for LEFS, AKPS [25,26,28] and WOMAC [27]. However, the magnitude of effect sizes of function between both groups became more significant at six and 12 months follow-up compared to post intervention estimates. This may be explained to be as a result of a noticeable steady decline in function in the quadriceps strengthening groups compared to the hip abductor strengthening group from post intervention levels, widening the point estimates of effect size between groups in the long term as seen from the results. Overall estimates of function could not be pooled due to heterogeneity of effect size estimates across studies. Although individual studies report increased function post intervention, no evidence exists due to statistical heterogeneity of outcomes reported.

A recently published study by Regelski *et al.* (2015) [29] reported similar outcomes post intervention and at follow-up by interpreting pooled effect sizes of individual studies post-intervention and at follow-up where applicable. However, they did not provide a clear interpretation of data as they did not perform further analysis with pooling and synthesis of data with recommendations made from effect sizes from individual studies.

4.3. Exercise Interventions

Changes in lower limb kinetics and kinematics occur in PFPS with weakness of hip muscles, a clinical finding in PFPS, associated with changes in hip and knee joint kinematics in PFPS [8–10]. Incorporating hip musculature strengthening (abductors and external rotator) into rehabilitation programs in management of PFPS may increase patient function and reduce severity of PFPS symptoms [23]. Amongst included trials, there were similarities in hip strengthening and quadriceps protocols with regards to exercise frequency: three sessions weekly for four weeks [24 26,28]. Two studies, Khayambashi *et al.* [27] and Nakagawa *et al.* [23] required patients to perform exercises three times per week for eight weeks and five times per week for six weeks, respectively. However, the types of exercises performed varied across studies. Apart from the study by Razeghi *et al.* [24] where exercise protocol was not properly described, five studies incorporated stretching of the hamstrings, quadriceps, and triceps surae as part of the PFPS protocols and used side-lying hip abduction in the hip strengthening protocol [23,25–28].

Standing hip abduction exercise was performed in three studies [25,26,28] while three studies [25–27] progressed hip abduction exercises in side-lying and standing by incorporating use of an elastic band. Four studies performed strengthening of the hip external rotation in sitting with or without the use of an elastic band [25–28]. Dolak *et al.* [28] and Nakagawa *et al.* [23] combined hip abduction and external rotation in side-lying to strengthen both abductors and external rotators. With reference to exercise types, Nakagawa *et al.* [23] used isometric exercises while the other five studies used isotonic exercises.

While there is no evidence of effects of different quadriceps strengthening and hip abductor strengthening exercise protocols influencing rehabilitation outcomes in management of PFPS, there is a possibility that this may have contributed to the high heterogeneity of pooled data across studies included in this review.

4.4. Strengths and Limitations and Recommendations

Strengths of this study include synthesis of homogenous data only where data are assumed to reflect similar effects across studies and are normally distributed. Therefore, this review not only provides data crucial to healthcare decision-making, such as uptake of hip strengthening exercise in rehabilitation strategies for PFPS, but data that are derived from trials conducted under conditions that most closely match the context of usual healthcare practice.

Limitations of this review include inclusion of a small number of studies as only the six included RCTs met the inclusion criteria. Additionally, as a result of the high heterogeneity of pooled data (I^2 greater or equal to 40%), further analysis of pooled data for overall pain post-intervention and function post-intervention and at follow-up could not be made. Future studies should systematically homogenize participant's eligibility criteria for selection of patients with PFPS to improve the quality research and consistency of outcomes in management of PFPS. While methodological quality across all studies was moderate to high with the Pedro scale, only one of the studies stated that the assessors responsible for collecting baseline and post-intervention outcomes were blinded to group assignment. Heterogeneity of reported outcomes in research on PFPS is too large to allow a clinically and scientifically sound meta-analysis of data. Better designed studies should be conducted considering limitations of currently existing studies.

In addition, valid and reliable scales, responsive to PFPS specifically, like the anterior knee pain scale (AKPS) (also known as the Kujula scale) was used by only two of the included studies [25,26]. The systematic use of the AKPS in studies on PFPS could allow optimal comparability between participants. PFPS is a multifactorial and complex condition and it is evident that the target population is often heterogeneous and thus could be separated in subgroups. Also, similarities and variances in exercise protocols provide a strong basis to incorporate a standardised exercise protocol and regimen for hip abductor or quadriceps strengthening exercises in conservative management of PFPS to aid future research into this condition.

5. Conclusions

Although results indicate that quadriceps strengthening may also reduce intensity of usual pain post-intervention, for greater significant post-intervention and clinically beneficial long-term outcomes, hip strengthening should be the preferred treatment approach for management of PFPS. However, there is currently low to moderate quality evidence to support this recommendation. Future studies should seek development of eligibility criteria/PFPS subject checklists for inclusion of subjects into studies on PFPS, and also take into consideration limitations of current studies so as to minimize, to the barest minimum, heterogeneity of outcomes from studies on PFPS.

Acknowledgments

The authors wish to acknowledge the authors of studies included in this review and authors who provided requested original data. We also acknowledge the staff at the Outpatient clinic, University of Potsdam.

Author Contributions

Adebisi Bisi-Balogun was tasked with preparation and finalisation of manuscript; statistical data analysis and interpretation of the results. Both authors conducted the electronic search process; quality ratings of the methodological process of included studies; data abstraction and revision of manuscript.

Conflicts of Interest

The author declares no conflicts of interest.

References

1. Boling, M.; Padua, D.; Marshall, S.; Guskiewicz, K.; Pyne, S.; Beutler, A. Gender differences in the incidence and prevalence of patellofemoral pain syndrome. *Scand. J. Med. Sci. Sports* **2010**, *20*, c723–c730.
2. Blond, L.; Hansen, L. Patellofemoral pain syndrome in athletes: A 5.7-year retrospective follow-up study of 250 athletes. *Acta Orthop. Belg.* **1998**, *644*, 393–400.
3. Callaghan, M.J.; Selfe, J. Has the incidence or prevalence of patellofemoral pain in the general population in the United Kingdom been properly evaluated? *Phys. Ther. Sport* **2007**, *81*, 37–43.
4. Wood, L.; Muller, S.; Peat, G. The epidemiology of patellofemoral disorders in adulthood: A review of routine general practice morbidity. *Prim. Health Care Res. Dev.* **2011**, *122*, 157–164.
5. Witvrouw, E.; Callaghan, M.J.; Stefanik, J.J.; Noehren, B.; Bazett-Jones, D.M.; Willson, J.D.; Earl-Boehm, J.E.; Davis, I.S.; Powers, C.M.; McConnell, J.; *et al.* Patellofemoral pain: Consensus statement from the 3rd International Patellofemoral Pain Research Retreat held in Vancouver, 2013. *Br. J. Sports Med.* **2014**, *48*, 411–414.
6. Thomee, R.; Augustsson, J.; Karlsson, J. Patellofemoral pain syndrome: A review of current issues. *Sports Med.* **1999**, *284*, 245–262.
7. Lankhorst, N.E.; Bierma-Zeinstra, S.; van Middelkoop, M. Factors associated with patellofemoral pain syndrome: A systematic review. *Br. J. Sports Med.* **2013**, *47*, 193–206.
8. Rothermich, M.; Glaviano, N.; Li, J.; Hart, J. Patellofemoral Pain Epidemiology, Pathophysiology, and Treatment Options. *Clin. Sports Med.* **2015**, *34*, 313–327.
9. Mascal, C.L.; Landel, R.; Powers, C. Management of patellofemoral pain targeting hip, pelvis, and trunk muscle function: 2 case reports. *J. Orthop. Sports Phys. Ther.* **2003**, *33*, 647–660.
10. Powers, C.M.; Ward, S.R.; Fredericson, M.; Guillet, M.; Shellock, F.G. Patellofemoral kinematics during weight-bearing and non-weight-bearing knee extension in persons with lateral subluxation of the patella: A preliminary study. *J. Orthop. Sports Phys. Ther.* **2003**, *33*, 677–685.
11. Ferber, R.; Davis, I.M.; Williams, D.S., III. Gender differences in lower extremity mechanics during running. *Clin. Biomech.* **2003**, *18*, 350–357.
12. Bolgla, L.A.; Malone, T.R.; Umberger, B.R.; Uhl, T.L. Hip strength and hip and knee kinematics during stair descent in females with and without patellofemoral pain syndrome. *J. Orthop. Sports Phys. Ther.* **2008**, *381*, 12–18.
13. Cichanowski, H.R.; Schmitt, J.S.; Johnson, R.J.; Niemuth, P.E. Hip strength in collegiate female athletes with patellofemoral pain. *Med. Sci. Sports Exerc.* **2007**, *398*, 1227–1232.
14. Lee, S.; Souza, R.; Powers, C. The influence of hip abductor muscle performance on dynamic postural stability in females with patellofemoral pain. *Gait Posture* **2012**, *36*, 425–429.
15. Gribble, P.A.; Hertel, J. Effect of hip and ankle muscle fatigue on unipedal postural control. *J. Electromyogr. Kinesiol.* **2004**, *146*, 641–646.
16. Chang, S.H.; Mercer, V.S.; Giuliani, C.A.; Sloane, P.D. Relationship between hip abductor rate of force development and mediolateral stability in older adults. *Arch. Phys. Med. Rehabil.* **2005**, *869*, 1843–1850.

17. Winter, D.A.; Prince, F.; Frank, J.S.; Powell, C.; Zabjek, K.F. Unified theory regarding A/P and M/L balance in quiet stance. *J. Neurophysiol.* **1996**, *756*, 2334–2343.
18. Watson, C.J.; Propps, M.; Ratner, J.; Zeigler, D.L.; Horton, P.; Smith, S.S. Reliability and responsiveness of the lower extremity functional scale and the anterior knee pain scale in patients withanterior knee pain. *J. Orthop. Sports Phys. Ther.* **2005**, *35*, 136–146.
19. Maher, C.; Sherrington, C.; Herbert, R.D.; Moseley, A.M.; Elkins, M. Reliability of the PEDro Scale for Rating Quality of Randomized Controlled Trials. *Phys. Ther.* **2003**, *838*, 713–721.
20. Higgins, J.P.T.; Green, S. *Cochrane Handbook for Systematic Reviews of Interventions (V5.0.2)*; The Cochrane Collaboration: London, UK, 2009.
21. Hedges, L.V.; Vevea, J.L. Fixed and random effects models in meta-analysis. *Psychol. Methods* **1998**, *3*, 486–504.
22. Van Tulder, M.; Furlan, A.; Bombardier, C.; Bouter, L.; Editorial Board of the Cochrane Collaboration Back Review Group. Updated method guidelines for systematic reviews in the Cochrane collaboration back review group. *Spine* **2003**, *28*, 1290–1299.
23. Nakagawa, T.; Batista Muniz, T.; Marche, R.; Menezes Reiff, R.; Serra, F. The effect of additional strengthening of hip abductor and lateral rotator muscles in patellofemoral pain syndrome: A randomized controlled pilot study. *Clin. Rehabil.* **2008**, *22*, 1051–1060.
24. Razeghi, M.; Etemadi, Y.; Taghizadeh, Sh.; Ghaem, H. Could Hip and Knee Muscle Strengthening Alter the Pain Intensity in Patellofemoral Pain Syndrome? *Iran. Red Crescent Med. J. IRCMJ* **2010**, *122*, 104–110.
25. Fukuda, T.; Rossetto, F.; Magalhães, E.; Fernandes Bryk, F.; Lucareli, P.R.; Carvalho, N. Short-Term Effects of Hip Abductors and Lateral Rotators Strengthening in Females with Patellofemoral Pain Syndrome: A Randomized Controlled Clinical Trial. *J. Orthop. Sports Phys. Ther.* **2010**, *40*, 736–740.
26. Fukuda, T.; Pagotti Melo, W.; Zaffalon, B.; Rossetto, F.; Magalhães, E.; Fernandes Bryk, F.; Martin, R. Hip Posterolateral Musculature Strengthening in Sedentary Women with Patellofemoral Pain Syndrome: A Randomized Controlled Clinical Trial with 1-Year Follow-up. *J. Orthop. Sports Phys. Ther.* **2012**, *42*, 823–830.
27. Khayambashi, K.; Fallah, A.; Movahed, A.; Bagwell, J.; Power, C. Posterolateral Hip Muscle Strengthening Versus Quadriceps Strengthening for Patellofemoral Pain: A Comparative Control Trial. *Arch. Phys. Med. Rehabil.* **2014**, *95*, 900–907.
28. Dolak, D.; Silkman, C.; Mckeon, M.J.; Hosey, R.; Lattermann, C.; Uhl, T. Hip Strengthening Prior to Functional Exercises Reduces Pain Sooner than Quadriceps Strengthening in Females with Patellofemoral Pain Syndrome: A Randomized Clinical Trial. *J. Orthop. Sports Phys. Ther.* **2011**, *418*, 23–32.
29. Regelski, C.; Ford, B.; Hoch, M. Hip Strengthening Compared with Quadriceps Strengthening in Conservative Treatment of Patients with Patellofemoral Pain: A Critically Appraised Topic. *Int. J. Athl. Ther. Train.* **2015**, *20*, 4–12.

8

Individual Responses for Muscle Activation, Repetitions, and Volume during Three Sets to Failure of High- (80% 1RM) *versus* Low-Load (30% 1RM) Forearm Flexion Resistance Exercise

Nathaniel D. M. Jenkins [1,*], Terry J. Housh [1], Samuel L. Buckner [2], Haley C. Bergstrom [3], Kristen C. Cochrane [1], Cory M. Smith [1], Ethan C. Hill [1], Richard J. Schmidt [1] and Joel T. Cramer [1,*]

[1] Department of Nutrition and Health Sciences, 211 Ruth Leverton Hall, University of Nebraska-Lincoln, Lincoln, NE 68583, USA; E-Mails: thoush1@unl.edu (T.J.H.); kcochrane@unl.edu (K.C.C.); csmith@unl.edu (C.M.S.); ethan.hill@unl.edu (E.C.H.); rschmidt1@unl.edu (R.J.S.)

[2] Department of Health, Exercise Science, and Recreation Management, University of Mississippi, Oxford, MS 38677, USA; E-Mail: bucknersamuel@gmail.com

[3] Department of Kinesiology and Health Promotion, University of Kentucky, Lexington, KY 40506-0219, USA; E-Mail: hbergstrom@uky.edu

* Authors to whom correspondence should be addressed; E-Mails: Nathaniel.jenkins@unl.edu (N.D.M.J.); jcramer@unl.edu (J.T.C.)

Academic Editor: Lee E. Brown

Abstract: This study compared electromyographic (EMG) amplitude, the number of repetitions completed, and exercise volume during three sets to failure of high- (80% 1RM) *versus* low-load (30% 1RM) forearm flexion resistance exercise on a subject-by-subject basis. Fifteen men were familiarized, completed forearm flexion 1RM testing. Forty-eight to 72 h later, the subjects completed three sets to failure of dumbbell forearm flexion resistance exercise with 80% (n = 8) or 30% (n = 7) 1RM. EMG amplitude was calculated for every repetition, and the number of repetitions performed and exercise volume were recorded. During sets 1, 2, and 3, one of eight subjects in the 80% 1RM group demonstrated a significant linear relationship for EMG amplitude *versus* repetition. For the 30% 1RM group, seven, five, and four of seven subjects demonstrated significant linear relationships during sets 1, 2, and 3, respectively. The mean EMG amplitude responses show that the fatigue-induced increases in EMG amplitude for the 30% 1RM group and no change in EMG amplitude for the 80% 1RM group resulted in similar levels of muscle activation in both groups. The numbers of repetitions completed were comparatively greater, while exercise volumes were similar in the 30% *versus* 80% 1RM group. Our results, in conjunction with those of previous studies in the leg extensors, suggest that there may be muscle specific differences in the responses to high- *versus* low-load exercise.

Keywords: electromyography; skeletal muscle; muscle fatigue; resistance training intensity; biceps brachii

1. Introduction

The current American College of Sports Medicine [1] and National Strength and Conditioning Association [2] guidelines recommend the utilization of resistance exercise loads corresponding to 60%–80% and 67%–85% of one repetition maximum (1RM), respectively, to maximize muscle hypertrophy. However, recent studies have challenged these recommendations [3–5]. For example, Burd *et al.* [3] demonstrated that acute resistance exercise performed to failure at 30% 1RM resulted in similar magnitudes of muscle protein synthesis and anabolic signaling as resistance exercise at 90% 1RM. In a follow-up study, Mitchell *et al.* [4] demonstrated that 10 weeks of leg extension resistance training to failure at 80% 1RM *versus* 30% 1RM resulted in comparable muscle hypertrophy. Similarly, Ogasawara *et al.* [5] showed that six weeks of bench press resistance training at 80% 1RM caused muscle hypertrophy equivalent to that observed after training at 30% 1RM. Therefore, the disparity between current resistance training recommendations and recent experimental results [3–5] has sparked a debate [6,7] regarding the most effective loads to prescribe to enhance muscle size with resistance training.

It has been suggested [8] that the recommendation of high-load resistance training (*i.e.*, ≥60% 1RM) to maximize muscle strength and hypertrophy is based on Henneman's size principle [9], which states that the recruitment of high-threshold motor units is dependent on the intensity of the stimulus [9]. Theoretically, therefore, motor unit recruitment is greater during resistance exercise at 80% 1RM than at 30% 1RM. While this may hold true for a single repetition in unfatigued muscle, the performance of submaximal contractions to volitional exhaustion may evoke the recruitment of additional motor units [10]. Accordingly, Burd *et al.* hypothesized that the similar acute increases in muscle protein synthesis and similar chronic muscle hypertrophy following low-load resistance training may be due to achieving "a similar degree of muscle fiber activation to that of high-intensity resistance exercise regimes." [11] (pp. 552–553). Burd *et al.* also suggested that the volume of exercise is "related to the degree of (muscle) fiber activation." [3] (pp. 7–8). However, while studies have examined muscle activation [12–15] and exercise volume [12] during high- *versus* low-load leg extension resistance exercise, we are unaware of previous studies that have compared muscle activation or exercise volume during high- *versus* low-load forearm flexion (*i.e.*, biceps curl) resistance exercise. Therefore, the purpose of this study was to compare electromyographic (EMG) amplitude, the number of repetitions completed, and exercise volume during three sets to failure of high- (80% 1RM) *versus* low-load (30% 1RM) forearm flexion resistance exercise on a subject-by-subject basis.

2. Materials and Methods

2.1. Subjects

Fifteen men (mean ± SD; age = 21.7 ± 2.4 years; height = 181.6 ± 7.5 cm; weight = 84.7 ± 23.5 kg) completed this study. Prior to any data collection, all subjects signed an informed consent form and completed a health history questionnaire. To be eligible, each participant must have been between the ages of 19 and 29, free from any current or ongoing musculoskeletal injuries or neuromuscular disorders involving the shoulders, elbows, or wrists, and could not have completed any regular or formal resistance training for at least six months prior to the start of the study. This study was approved by the university's Institutional Review Board for the protection of human subjects (IRB Approval #: 20140314046FB).

2.2. Experimental Design

A between-subjects design was utilized for this study, which consisted of three visits to the laboratory. During visits 1 and 2, subjects were familiarized with the exercises and procedures and forearm flexion (*i.e.*, biceps curl) 1RM was determined. The subjects were then randomized to either a high-load (80% 1RM; n = 8) or a low-load (30% 1RM; n = 7) resistance exercise group before returning to the laboratory 48 to 72 h later. During visit 3, subjects completed three sets to failure of bilateral dumbbell forearm flexion (e.g., biceps curl) resistance exercise with their assigned load. Each laboratory visit occurred at the same time of day (±2 h).

2.3. One Repetition Maximum

1RM testing was carried out according to the guidelines established by the National Strength and Conditioning Association [2]. Specifically, the subjects performed a light warm-up set with 5–10 repetitions at 50% of estimated 1RM, followed by 2–3 heavier warm-up sets of 2–5 repetitions with loads increasing by 10%–20% at each set. Subjects then began completing trials of 1 repetition with increasing loads (10%–20%) until they were no longer able to complete a single repetition. The highest load (kg) successfully lifted through the entire range of motion with the right arm with proper technique was denoted as the 1RM, which was determined in ≤4 trials for all subjects. Two to four min of rest were allowed between successive warm-up sets and 1RM trials. EMG and electrogoniometer signals were recorded from the right arm during the 1RM attempts.

2.4. Resistance Exercise

Subjects completed 3 sets of dumbbell forearm flexion resistance exercise to failure with loads corresponding (to the nearest 1.1 kg) to either 80% or 30% of 1RM. The subjects stood with their backs against a wall and their elbows supported by a brace (Bicep Bomber, Body Solid, Inc., Forest Park, IL, USA) to eliminate swinging of the torso or arms. Subjects were instructed to perform all repetitions through a complete range of motion. A metronome (Pro Metronome, EUMLab, Berlin, Germany) was set to 1 Hz, and participants were instructed to perform the concentric and eccentric phases corresponding with each tick of the metronome so that the concentric and eccentric phases were approximately 1 s. Verbal instruction and encouragement were provided during each set. Failure was defined as the inability to complete another concentric muscle action through the full range of motion. Two minutes of rest was provided between all sets for both groups. EMG and electrogoniometer signals were recorded from the right arm during all sets. In addition, the number of repetitions completed during each set was recorded and exercise volume was calculated as the product of the load (kg) and the number of repetitions completed during each set, summed across sets.

2.5. Electromyography

Pre-gelled bipolar surface electrodes (Ag/AgCl, AccuSensor, Lynn Medical, Wixom, MI, USA) were placed on the biceps brachii (BB) muscle of the right arm with an inter-electrode distance of 30 mm. The center of the bipolar electrode pair was placed at 33% of the distance between the fossa cubit and the medial acromion process [16]. A single pre-gelled surface electrode (Ag/AgCl, AccuSensor, Lynn Medical, Wixom, MI, USA) was placed on the lateral epicondyle of the humerus to serve as the reference electrode. To reduce inter-electrode impedance and increase the signal-to-noise ratio [17], local areas of the skin were shaved, abraded, and cleaned with isopropyl alcohol prior to the placement of the electrodes. Interelectrode impedance was kept below 2000 Ω [17].

2.6. Signal Processing

The EMG and goniometer signals were sampled at 2 kHz (MP150WSW, Biopac Systems, Inc., Santa Barbara, CA, USA), recorded on a personal computer, and processed off-line with custom software (Labview 12.0, National Instruments, Austin, TX, USA). The EMG signals were amplified (gain 1000) using a differential amplifier (EMG 100, Biopac Systems, Inc., Santa Barbara, CA, USA, bandwidth 1–5000 Hz) with a common mode rejection ratio of 110 dB min and an impedance of 2M Ω, digitally filtered (zero-phase shift 4th-order Butterworth filter) with a band-pass of 10–499 Hz, and rectified. The electrogoniometer signals were low-pass filtered (zero-phase shift 4th-order Butterworth filter) with a 15 Hz cutoff. The EMG amplitude was calculated as the time-averaged, integrated amplitude value ($\mu V \cdot s^{-1}$). EMG amplitude was quantified during the same 70° concentric portion of each repetition during each set, and then normalized to 1RM (expressed % 1RM). In addition, we compared EMG amplitude during the final common repetitions of sets 1, 2, and 3 for the 80% and 30% 1RM groups. The number of repetitions analyzed at the end of each set was established by the minimum number of repetitions achieved by any one subject within each group during sets 1, 2, and 3 (Table 1).

2.7. Statistics

Simple linear regression analyses were used to determine whether the slope coefficients for the individual EMG amplitude *versus* repetition relationships during sets 1, 2, and 3 were significantly different from zero. A type-I error rate of 5% was considered statistically significant for the linear regression analyses. Where applicable, 95% confidence intervals were calculated using the studentized t-distribution.

Table 1. The number of repetitions completed during sets 1, 2, and 3 and the volume (reps × load) completed across all sets, for each subject, as well as the mean (±95% confidence interval) volume completed for each group.

Group	Subject	Repetitions Completed			Individual Volume	Mean Volume
		Set 1	Set 2	Set 3	All sets	
80% 1RM	1	11	9	6	339.7	350.8 ± 72.8
	5	12	8	6	294.8	
	6	7	7	6	344.7	
	9	10	7	4	190.5	
	10	10	6	2	367.4	
	13	12	11	8	492.2	
	14	15	10	8	411.6	
	18	12	8	3	365.1	
30% 1RM	2	58	24	26	269.4	382.8 ± 101.4
	3	37	24	14	323.2	
	4	39	20	20	308.2	
	7	47	16	15	398.0	
	11	54	14	14	390.5	
	12	37	20	20	384.2	
	15	51	28	20	606.2	

3. Results

Table 1 displays the number of repetitions completed for each subject during each set, the total volume completed by each subject, and the mean (±95% confidence interval) volume completed by the 80% and 30% 1RM groups. The individual EMG amplitude *versus* repetition relationships for each subject during sets 1, 2, and 3 are depicted in Figure 1.

The results from the individual simple linear regression analyses for the EMG amplitude *versus* repetition relationships during sets 1, 2, 3 are depicted in Table 2. During sets 1, 2, and 3, one of eight subjects in the 80% 1RM group demonstrated a significant linear relationship. However, for the 30% 1RM group, seven of seven, five of seven, and four of seven subjects demonstrated significant linear relationships.

Figure 2 displays the EMG amplitude during the final common repetitions of sets 1, 2, and 3 for the 80% and 30% 1RM groups.

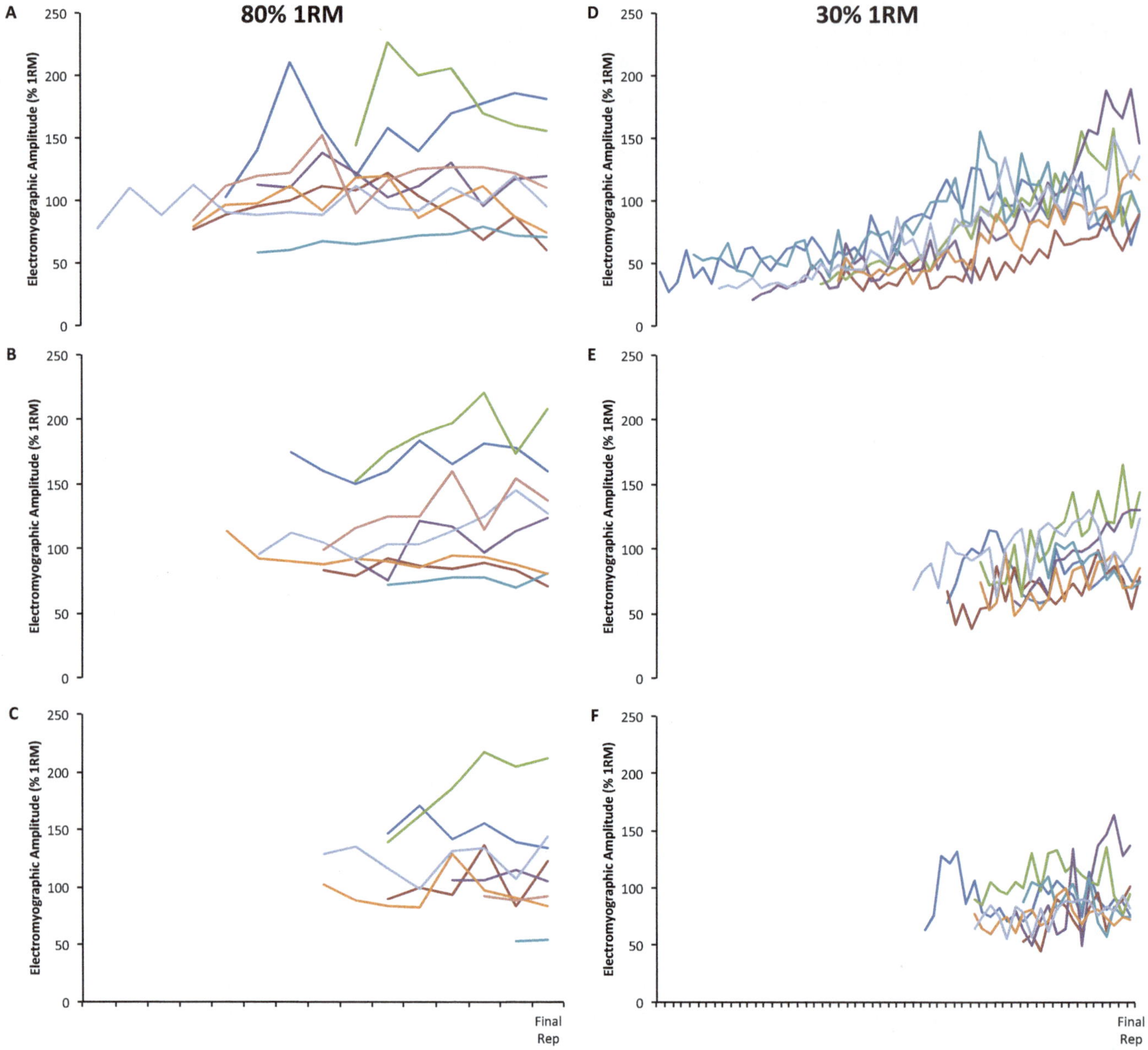

Figure 1. Individual electromyographic amplitude responses to resistance exercise at 80% one repetition maximum (1RM) during **(A)** set 1; **(B)** set 2; and **(C)** set 3 and at 30% 1RM during **(D)** set 1; **(E)** set 2; and **(F)** set 3.

Table 2. The individual simple linear regression analyses for the electromyographic (EMG) amplitude *versus* repetition relationships during sets 1, 2, and 3.

Group	Subject	Set 1				Set 2				Set 3			
		r	r^2	SEE	*p*-value	r	r^2	SEE	*p*-value	r	r^2	SEE	*p*-value
80% 1RM	1	0.50	0.25	28.36	0.11	0.24	0.06	12.11	0.54	0.58	0.34	12.13	0.23
	5	0.31	0.10	18.10	0.32	0.34	0.12	6.60	0.41	0.41	0.17	21.36	0.42
	6	0.32	0.10	31.90	0.48	0.66	0.44	19.08	0.11	0.90	0.82	14.95	0.01 *
	9	0.10	0.01	13.04	0.79	0.66	0.43	15.29	0.11	0.16	0.03	5.31	0.84
	10	0.84	0.71	3.56	<0.01 *	0.40	0.16	4.58	0.44	1.00	-	-	-
	13	0.08	0.01	15.80	0.80	0.59	0.35	6.95	0.05	0.07	<0.01	16.81	0.88
	14	0.33	0.11	11.80	0.23	0.77	0.59	11.09	<0.01 *	0.11	0.01	16.86	0.79
	18	0.28	0.08	17.90	0.37	0.66	0.43	16.71	0.08	0.06	<0.01	3.18	0.96
30% 1RM	2	0.76	0.58	16.70	<0.01 *	0.18	0.03	16.18	0.39	0.13	0.02	18.76	0.52
	3	0.85	0.73	9.12	<0.01 *	0.52	0.27	12.89	<0.01 *	0.66	0.44	13.35	0.01 *
	4	0.88	0.77	16.84	<0.01 *	0.80	0.64	16.91	<0.01 *	0.12	0.02	17.09	0.60
	7	0.90	0.80	21.50	<0.01 *	0.98	0.95	5.85	<0.01 *	0.77	0.59	26.43	<0.01 *
	11	0.76	0.58	19.26	<0.01 *	0.53	0.28	12.49	0.05	0.61	0.37	13.42	0.02 *
	12	0.92	0.84	10.26	<0.01 *	0.48	0.23	14.22	0.03 *	0.22	0.05	9.90	0.35
	15	0.93	0.86	12.91	<0.01 *	0.51	0.26	16.01	<0.01 *	0.50	0.25	9.72	0.03 *

r = correlation coefficient; r^2 = coefficient of determination; SEE = standard error of the estimate; * Indicates a significant relationship.

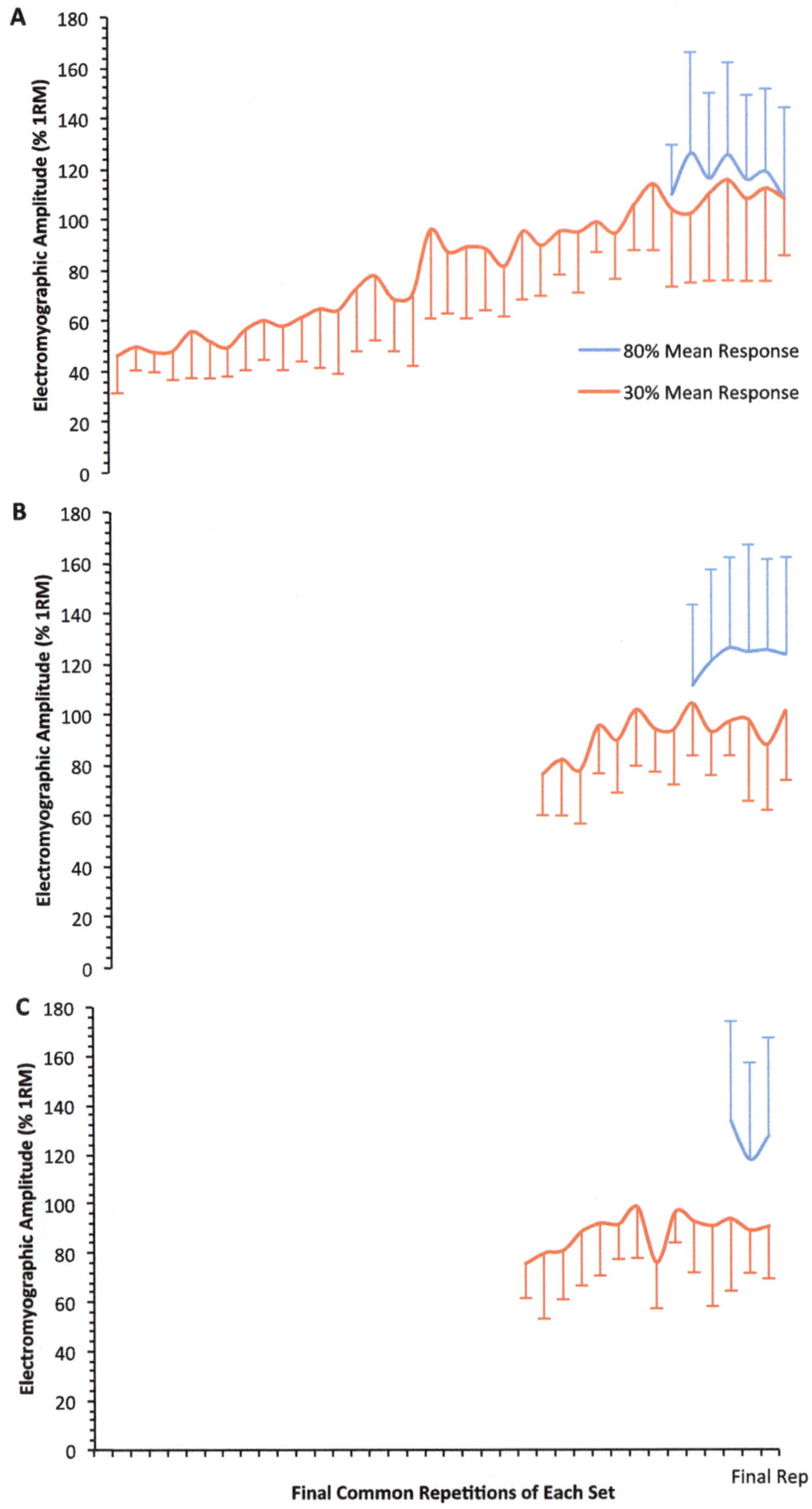

Figure 2. A comparison of the mean (±95% confidence interval) electromyographic amplitude responses during the final common repetitions for the 80% *versus* 30% 1RM groups during (**A**) set 1; (**B**) set 2; and (**C**) set 3. The number of repetitions analyzed for each set was based on the minimum number of repetitions achieved by any one subject in each group during sets 1, 2, and 3. For set 3, subject 10 was not included because he only completed two repetitions (see Table 1 for the repetitions completed by each subject during sets 1, 2, and 3).

4. Discussion

Mitchell *et al.* hypothesized that, "as lighter loads are repeated, the point of failure/fatigue ultimately necessitates near maximal motor unit recruitment to sustain muscle tension. Thus, relatively lighter loads lifted to the point of failure would result in a similar amount of muscle fiber activation compared with heavier loads lifted to failure" [4] (p. 75). Interestingly, our results supported this hypothesis [4]. The individual EMG amplitude *versus* repetition responses in our study indicated that muscle activation increased linearly for all subjects in the 30% 1RM group during set 1. Subsequently, however, EMG amplitude increased for five of seven and four of seven subjects during sets 2 and 3, respectively. In contrast, only one of eight subjects demonstrated an increase in EMG amplitude during the 80% 1RM group during sets 1, 2, and 3, which suggested that muscle activation started and remained at or near the same level across all repetitions and sets at 80% 1RM. Furthermore, the mean EMG amplitude responses (Figure 2) show that the fatigue-induced increases in EMG amplitude for the 30% 1RM group and no change in EMG amplitude for the 80% 1RM group resulted in similar levels of muscle activation in both groups. These results are in contrast to our recent study [12] and others [13,15,18] showing that muscle activation was higher during high- *versus* low-load leg extension resistance exercise to failure. The primary difference between the present study and those previous studies [12,13,15,18] is the muscle group studied. Factors such as location (*i.e.*, upper- *versus* lower-body), blood flow [19], architecture (*i.e.*, pennate *versus* fusiform), or fiber type composition [20,21] of the muscle may influence the activation responses to high- *versus* low-load resistance exercise. Therefore, the muscle activation achieved during high- compared to low-load resistance exercise to failure may be muscle specific.

The information provided by the amplitude of the surface EMG signal is considered a global measure of muscle activation [22]. Because traditional surface EMG is unable to isolate individual motor units, EMG amplitude is related to net motor unit activity, which is a function of both motor unit recruitment and motor unit firing rate [17,22]. Furthermore, EMG amplitude is influenced by peripheral (*i.e.*, fiber membranes properties, action potential shapes, *etc.*) factors [17,22]. Therefore, it is not possible to distinguish between alterations in motor unit recruitment and firing rate in the present study with EMG amplitude alone. However, the amplitude and frequency content of the surface mechanomyogram (MMG) are thought to reflect motor unit recruitment and global motor unit firing rate, respectively [23,24]. Therefore, future studies should examine the surface MMG signal in conjunction with surface EMG during high- *versus* low-load resistance exercise to failure to provide more specific information regarding changes in motor unit recruitment *versus* motor unit firing rate.

In the present study, the numbers of repetitions completed by the subjects in the 30% 1RM group were comparatively greater than the numbers completed by those in the 80% 1RM group (Table 1). This supports data presented by Jenkins *et al.* [12] who reported that the mean ± standard deviation for the numbers of repetitions completed during leg extension resistance training at 80% and 30% 1RM during sets 1, 2, and 3 were 8.9 ± 2.7 and 45.6 ± 14.3, 6.7 ± 1.9 and 26.8 ± 8.3, and 6.2 ± 1.7 and 22.2 ± 8.6 repetitions, respectively. Unexpectedly, however, the exercise volumes for the 80% and 30% 1RM groups were similar in the present study (Table 1). Previously, Jenkins *et al.* [12] showed that exercise volume during three sets of 30% 1RM leg extension resistance exercise was 58% greater than during three sets at 80% 1RM. Therefore, the volume of exercise performed during high- *versus* low-load training may be also be dependent on the muscle group studied, such that the exercise volume may be similar for high- and low-load exercise for the forearm flexors, but greater during low-load exercise for the leg extensors.

5. Conclusions

Overall, the results of the present study indicated that forearm flexion resistance exercise to failure at 30% 1RM caused fatigue-induced increases in EMG amplitude, whereas during 80% 1RM, EMG amplitude remained relatively constant (Figure 1). This load-dependent interaction for EMG amplitude led to similar levels of muscle activation during the final common repetitions at 80% and 30% 1RM (Figure 2). In addition, the numbers of repetitions achieved were comparatively greater for the 30% 1RM than the 80% 1RM group during sets 1, 2, and 3, while total exercise volume was similar between groups (Table 1). Thus, our results conflict with several previous studies [12,13,15,18] showing that muscle activation is greater, but exercise volume is lower [12], during 80% *versus* 30% 1RM resistance exercise in the leg-extensors. Future studies are needed with simultaneous examinations of EMG and MMG amplitude to better understand the interactions between motor unit recruitment and motor unit firing rate during these loading schemes. Based on the results of the present study, in conjunction with those of previous studies [12,13,15,18], the muscle activation responses and exercise volume completed during low-load training may be dependent on the location, blood flow, architecture, or fiber type composition of the muscle group studied.

Acknowledgments

The authors would like to thank Noelle M. Yeo and Jessie M. Miller for their help with data collection. This study was supported in part by the University of Nebraska Agricultural Research Division with funds provided through the Hatch Act (Agency: United States Department of Agriculture, National Institute of Food and Agriculture; Accession No: 1000080; Project No: NEB-36-078).

Author Contributions

Nathaniel D. M. Jenkins was the primary manuscript writer, and carried out data acquisition, data analysis, and data interpretation. Samuel L. Buckner, Haley C. Bergstrom, Kristen C. Cochrane, Cory M. Smith and Ethan C. Hill were significant contributors to data acquisition, read and approved the final manuscript, and were manuscript reviewers/revisers. Terry J. Housh and Richard J. Schmidt were significant manuscript reviewers/revisers. Joel T. Cramer was the primary manuscript reviewer/reviser, a substantial contributor to concept and design, and contributed to data analysis and interpretation.

Conflicts of Interest

The authors declare no conflict of interest.

References

1. Garber, C.E.; Blissmer, B.; Deschenes, M.R.; Franklin, B.A.; Lamonte, M.J.; Lee, I.M.; Nieman, D.C.; Swain, D.P. American college of sports medicine position stand. Quantity and quality of exercise for developing and maintaining cardiorespiratory, musculoskeletal, and neuromotor fitness in apparently healthy adults: Guidance for prescribing exercise. *Med. Sci. Sports Exerc.* **2011**, *43*, 1334–1359.
2. National Strength and Conditioning Association. *Essentials of Strength Training and Conditioning*, 3rd ed.; Human Kinetics: Champaign, IL, USA, 2008.
3. Burd, N.A.; West, D.W.; Staples, A.W.; Atherton, P.J.; Baker, J.M.; Moore, D.R.; Holwerda, A.M.; Parise, G.; Rennie, M.J.; Baker, S.K.; *et al.* Low-load high volume resistance exercise stimulates muscle protein synthesis more than high-load low volume resistance exercise in young men. *PLoS ONE* **2010**, *5*, doi:10.1371/journal.pone.0012033.
4. Mitchell, C.J.; Churchward-Venne, T.A.; West, D.W.; Burd, N.A.; Breen, L.; Baker, S.K.; Phillips, S.M. Resistance exercise load does not determine training-mediated hypertrophic gains in young men. *J. Appl. Physiol.* **2012**, *113*, 71–77.
5. Ogasawara, R.; Loenneke, J.P.; Thiebaud, R.S.; Abe, T. Low-load bench press training to fatigue results in muscle hypertrophy similar to high-load bench press training. *Int. J. Clin. Med.* **2013**, *4*, 114–121.
6. Burd, N.A.; Moore, D.R.; Mitchell, C.J.; Phillips, S.M. Big claims for big weights but with little evidence. *Eur. J. Appl. Physiol.* **2013**, *113*, 267–268.
7. Schuenke, M.D.; Herman, J.; Staron, R.S. Preponderance of evidence proves "big" weights optimize hypertrophic and strength adaptations. *Eur. J. Appl. Physiol.* **2013**, *113*, 269–271.
8. Carpinelli, R.N. The size principle and a critical analysis of the unsubstantiated heavier-is-better recommendation for resistance training. *J. Exerc. Sci. Fit.* **2008**, *6*, 67–86.
9. Henneman, E.; Somjen, G.; Carpenter, D.O. Functional significance of cell size in spinal motoneurons. *J. Neurophysiol.* **1965**, *28*, 560–580.
10. Conwit, R.A.; Stashuk, D.; Suzuki, H.; Lynch, N.; Schrager, M.; Metter, E.J. Fatigue effects on motor unit activity during submaximal contractions. *Arch. Phys. Med. Rehabil.* **2000**, *81*, 1211–1216.
11. Burd, N.A.; Mitchell, C.J.; Churchward-Venne, T.A.; Phillips, S.M. Bigger weights may not beget bigger muscles: Evidence from acute muscle protein synthetic responses after resistance exercise. *Appl. Physiol. Nutr. Metab.* **2012**, *37*, 551–554.
12. Jenkins, N.D.; Housh, T.J.; Bergstrom, H.C.; Cochrane, K.C.; Hill, E.C.; Smith, C.M.; Johnson, G.O.; Schmidt, R.J.; Cramer, J.T. Muscle activation during three sets to failure at 80% *vs.* 30% 1rm resistance exercise. *Eur. J. Appl. Physiol.* **2015**, in press.
13. Akima, H.; Saito, A. Activation of quadriceps femoris including vastus intermedius during fatiguing dynamic knee extensions. *Eur. J. Appl. Physiol.* **2013**, *113*, 2829–2840.
14. Schoenfeld, B.J. Potential mechanisms for a role of metabolic stress in hypertrophic adaptations to resistance training. *Sports Med.* **2013**, *43*, 179–194.
15. Cook, S.B.; Murphy, B.G.; Labarbera, K.E. Neuromuscular function after a bout of low-load blood flow-restricted exercise. *Med. Sci. Sports Exerc.* **2013**, *45*, 67–74.

16. Hermens, H.J.; Freriks, B.; Merletti, R.; Stegeman, D.; Blok, J.; Rau, G.; Disselhorst-Klug, C.; Hagg, G. *Seniam 8: European Recommendations for Surface Electromyography*; Roessngh Research and Development: Enschede, The Netherlands, 1999.
17. Beck, T.W.; Housh, T.J. Use of electromyography in studying human movement. In *Routledge Handbook of Biomechanics and Human Movement*; Hong, Y., Bartlett, R., Eds.; Routledge: New York, NY, USA, 2008; pp. 214–230.
18. Schoenfeld, B.J.; Contreras, B.; Willardson, J.M.; Fontana, F.; Tiryaki-Sonmez, G. Muscle activation during low- *versus* high-load resistance training in well-trained men. *Eur. J. Appl. Physiol.* **2014**, *114*, 2491–2497.
19. Samanek, M.; Goetzova, J.; Fiserova, J.; Skovranek, J. Differences in muscle blood flow in upper and lower extremities of patients after correction of coarctation of the aorta. *Circulation* **1976**, *54*, 377–381.
20. Ali, A.; Sundaraj, K.; Badlishah Ahmad, R.; Ahamed, N.U.; Islam, A.; Sundaraj, S. Muscle fatigue in the three heads of the triceps brachii during a controlled forceful hand grip task with full elbow extension using surface electromyography. *J. Hum. Kinet.* **2015**, *46*, 69–76.
21. Harwood, B.; Dalton, B.H.; Power, G.A.; Rice, C.L. Motor unit properties from three synergistic muscles during ramp isometric elbow extensions. *Exp. Brain Res.* **2013**, *231*, 501–510.
22. Farina, D.; Merletti, R.; Enoka, R.M. The extraction of neural strategies from the surface emg. *J. Appl. Physiol.* **2004**, *96*, 1486–1495.
23. Beck, T.W.; Housh, T.J.; Cramer, J.T.; Weir, J.P.; Johnson, G.O.; Coburn, J.W.; Malek, M.H.; Mielke, M. Mechanomyographic amplitude and frequency responses during dynamic muscle actions: A comprehensive review. *Biomed. Eng. Online* **2005**, *4*, doi:10.1186/1475-925X-4-67.
24. Gordon, G.; Holbourn, A.H. The sounds from single motor units in a contracting muscle. *J. Physiol.* **1948**, *107*, 456–464.

9

It's Not Me, It's You: The Disconnect of Physical Education Teachers to Physical Activity in the Gym

Dean Culpepper [1,*] and Lorraine Killion [2]

[1] Department of Health and Physical Education, Eastern New Mexico University, Portales, NM 88130, USA
[2] Department of Health and Kinesiology, Texas A and M University-Kingsville, Kingsville, TX 78363, USA; E-Mail: Lorraine.Killion@tamuk.edu

* Author to whom correspondence should be addressed; E-Mail: dean.culpepper@enmu.edu

Academic Editor: Eling de Bruin

Abstract: American adults and an increasing number of children, are not meeting the recommended amounts of daily physical activity. Research has documented the effects of low activity on health and increasingly new research has shown that low activity levels now impact academic achievement. Physical education (PE) can play an important role if the children participating are obtaining enough physical activity while in class and the PE program has not been targeted with cutbacks. The purpose of this study was to identify the amount and intensity of activity in PE classes. The results indicate that on average students at all levels are not meeting the activity requirements. In addition, PE teachers' perceptions of physical activity in their own class does not match actual activity levels. PE teachers must do a better job of increasing activity levels in their classrooms. Mounting research indicates students perform better academically if they are physically active. PE is the only subject where teachers can organize activities that meet both activity and intensity requirements.

Keywords: physical education; physical fitness; perceptions of PE teachers

---

1. Introduction

The report from the Surgeon General recommends that people of all ages perform 30 min of moderate physical activity on most days of the week [1]. This is due to the conclusive research for health benefits that are achieved from moderate levels of physical activity. Yet, many Americans do not receive the benefits of regular moderate physical activity. Healthy People 2010 reported that 85% do not engage in moderate activity on 5 or more days per week for 30 min. and 40% do not participate in any leisure-time physical activity [1]. Thus, in order to impact lifetime physical activity behavior, childhood has been identified as a critical period for nurturing lifetime activity behavior [1–3].

Recent studies have been able to identify when children are most active during the day so that interventions can be targeted to have the most effect. These studies have found that lunchtime physical activity (PA) represented the most important source of daily PA (15%–16%) obtained during school hours for both boys and girls, whereas recess accounted for 8%–9% and PE class accounted for 8%–11% of total steps per day [4]. While *unstructured play* is necessary and needed for growth and development, it is the *structured time* in physical education where continuous moderate to vigorous physical activity (which is needed for improvements to cardiorespiratory fitness) can be designed and monitored. It is also a time where health-related fitness concepts can be taught and applied [5]. Health-related fitness is the component measured by the PACER test administered by the FITNESSGRAM® (Cooper Institute, Dallas, TX, USA). Although the administration of this test has been in existence for over 30 years, results have shown a decline in students who scored in the Healthy Fitness Zone. This is an area of concern when children are becoming less active and healthy.

The results revealed age-related declines in the percentage of youth who achieved the HFZ standard for cardiovascular fitness (elementary school: 70%; middle school: 46%; high school: 34%). The increase in obesity levels has yielded a response in a number of research studies conducted evaluating the impact of physical activity (PA) on academic achievement. Significant improvement in academic achievement was found when physical activity was increased [6]. Additional studies have reported that increased fitness levels are positively associated with academic achievement [7,8]. The findings in this research are crucial because results indicate a consistent positive relationship between overall fitness and academic achievement. That is, as overall fitness scores improved, mean achievement scores also improved [6]. This is one of the most important findings to impact physical education in recent years because it is the only subject matter in schools where movement is the central theme. Physical education teachers can increase academic test performance by simply increasing movement time in their classes.

It is because of these findings that administrators, teachers, parents, and the government are calling for the increase in the physical education requirement for students [1]. The role of physical education and what schools can do to help increase physical activity among children are paramount. One of the national health objectives [1] is to increase physical activity in children. Researchers have recommended daily physical education to increase the knowledge and application of health-related physical fitness concepts [9–11]. Furthermore, it has been recommended that school-age youth should participate daily in 60 min or more of moderate to vigorous physical activity that is developmentally appropriate, enjoyable, and involves a variety of activities during their physical education class [12]. Some researchers recommend certain models or programs (e.g., CATCH, SPARK) to help PE teachers increase activity time in their classes. This has been a good recommendation; however, measuring the amount of activity time can be difficult for the average PE teacher.

Monitoring student activity levels can be accomplished via individual pedometers. Using such a measurement tool has been recommended [13]. According to Scruggs, *et al.*, 2005, "for a practical physical activity measurement tool, pedometry has been found to be valid and objective" (p. 174) [14]. By taking student steps per minute of physical education class, researchers can identify whether classes are meeting the physical activity needs of the students or whether changes must be implemented. Additionally, pedometers are a valid measure of moderate to vigorous physical activity and provide information on intensity [15]. This is of major importance since recent published research notes that physically active and fit children tend to have better academic achievement [16]. Additional research has found students with low levels of fitness also exhibit low academic scores on achievement tests [17,18]. In particular, it has been reported that children with low levels of fitness exhibit low scores for reading and/or math [19,20].

There is a strong correlation between a student's fitness level and his/her academic success [21]. A study conducted by the Cooper Institute in 2009 found that cardiovascular health, as measured by a walking/running test, had a higher correlation to school success than did Body Mass Index (BMI). Researchers investigated children in the third and fifth grades and the different contributions of the FITNESSGRAM® subcomponents. The study examined the individual contributions of aerobic capacity, muscle strength, muscle flexibility, and body composition to performance in reading and mathematics on the Illinois Standardized Achievement Test among a sample of 259 children [16]. The findings of this study were similar to those reported by the California Department of Education indicating a relationship between fitness and achievement performance [22]. When the individual components of the FITNESSGRAM® were broken down, the researchers concluded that only aerobic capacity was related to test performance.

Physical education teachers, regardless of how many days per week they see each student, should design and structure their classes to meet minimum activity requirements no matter what curriculum model the teacher selects. So the question that needs to be addressed now is: *do our students currently meet the activity requirements in physical education classes today?* There seems to be a misguided assumption that simply walking into a PE class achieves the activity recommendations that experts are calling for [14,23]. If they do, then daily physical education can play a vital role in helping our students to be healthy and improve their academic test performance. If they don't, then more work is needed in training teachers to monitor the activity levels of their students. PE teachers who believe, no matter what curriculum is being taught, that the students they teach are active may not make the necessary changes needed to improve the student scores on tests such as the FITNESSGRAM®. Simply increasing lunchtime PA is not enough to improve scores on these types of tests.

Purpose

The purpose of the study was to identify the activity time spent in physical education classes and compare the findings to the teachers' perception of the physical activity levels in their classes. In addition, steps per minute were assessed to identify if the activity intensity during the class was at the recommended level.

2. Methods

2.1. Participants

Participants were students enrolled in urban, suburban, and rural school districts in California, Minnesota, and Texas. The total number of schools involved was: 19 elementary, eight middle, and nine high schools. A total of 1111 students (445 elementary, 302 middle school, 364 high school students) were selected to participate in the study.

All classes were taught by physical education specialists with a minimum of five years of teaching experience (range = 5–20 years, mean = 12.3 years). The mean age was thirty-one years (range = 27–48 years). There were twelve elementary teachers (females = 9), eight middle school teachers (females = 3), and eleven high school (females = 8). Content in classes ranged from the: (a) Fitness Model consisting of aerobic/fitness games; (b) Skill Theme Model consisted of activities that developed and promoted fundamental skills and concepts (e.g., throwing to partners, hitting off tees, and progression to modified games); and (c) Game/Sport Model, consisting of team activities (e.g., soccer, basketball, flag-football). The Skill Theme approach is a method where teachers design experiences that encourage students to actively and successfully participate in class. Skill themes are the physical movement skills necessary to successfully participate and enjoy various activities and sports students participate during the school year. These experiences take place within themes such as locomotor skills (e.g., running, jumping, and skipping) dance (e.g., tapping, stomping, and shaking), gymnastics (e.g., rolling, spinning, and tumbling) and sports (e.g., basketball, volleyball, and soccer). Teachers whose classes exhibited this approach were categorized accordingly.

2.2. Data Collection

Teachers were contacted before the school year to volunteer their classes for the study. At this time each teacher was asked whether in general students obtain enough physical activity in physical education classes in their state. They were then asked if the children in their own classes obtained enough physical activity.

At the beginning of each class, investigators provided instruction on the correct placement for the pedometer. Correct placement for the pedometer is: (a) held firmly to the body; (b) clipped onto the belt or waistband; (c) in line with the knee; (d) worn so that it remains upright and not tilted forward or backward, and (e) worn so that it is level and not tilted to either side [24]. Students were reminded not to open the pedometers until the end of the class period. Class time is the "on paper" time assigned to the class, while activity time is the time spent in lesson, not transitioning between classes and changing.

The physical education teachers conducted their lessons as planned and the investigators moved around the perimeter of the gym and repositioned the pedometers as needed. The investigators documented the model and activity in which the students were engaged to be later analyzed for congruency. At the end of the class period, the investigators collected the pedometers and recorded the total number of steps accrued by each student.

2.3. Intervening Variables

Since gender might have an impact on the number of steps taken, it was used as a variable to explain potential differences [1]. Class time and grade level might also cause an effect since most elementary schools have 30-min classes and secondary schools have either a 50- or 90-min class period. The class time and grade level data were recorded and included in the analyses.

3. Results

Frequency data is presented in Table 1 regarding teacher perceptions of children physical activity. Descriptive statistics are presented in Table 2 for grade level, gender, curriculum model, total steps for the students controlled by class time, and the corresponding partial *eta* score. Steps per minute (SPM) were determined by dividing the total number of steps by class time [14]. Table 3 provides data for class time and SPM for grade level. Data on SPM for grade level by model are also presented. Significance exists ($p < 0.001$) across grades and models except for the Skill Theme Model between middle and high school ($p = 0.422$).

Table 1. Frequency statistics for teacher perceptions of physical activity time.

Grade Level	Does PE Provide Enough PA		Does Your Class Provide Enough PA	
	Yes	No	Yes	No
Elementary School	15.8%	84.2%	89.5%	10.5%
Middle School	6.3%	93.7%	74.6%	25.4%
High School	11.2%	88.8%	72.1%	27.9%

Table 2. Descriptive statistics for data controlled by class time.

Groups	N	Steps *M/SD*	h_p^2
Elementary School	445	1535.74/626.87 *	0.061
Middle School	302	1995.35/857.01 *	-
High School	364	2454.04/715.55 *	-
Class time*Grade	-	-	0.315
Males	576	2302.88/837.89 *	0.135
Females	535	1820.750.01 *	-
Class time*Gender	-	-	0.446
Game/Sport	13	2416.27/969.84 *	-
Fitness	14	1967.03/682.51 *	-
Skill Themes	09	1480.42/438.66 *	-
Class time*Model	-	-	0.336

Note: * $p < 0.001$.

A hierarchical multiple regression analysis (Table 4) was conducted to determine the influence of gender, the curriculum model, and grade level on total number of steps. Input for class time was entered using the "enter" function in block one first (as a covariate) followed by the remaining variables as a "stepwise" comparison in block two. The combination of variables was significantly related to total number of steps, ($F(5, 1106) = 202.51, p < 0.001$). Table 3 presents the regression data for the covariate of class time with curriculum, grade level, and gender. The regression model with only Class Time accounts for approximately 41% of the variance explained while the total model accounts for an estimated 50%.

Table 3. Class time, and SPM for grade level and model.

Grade Level	Class Time Min	Steps/Min
	M/SD	*M/SD*
Elementary School	27.67/2.54 *	51.19/20.89 *
Fitness	-	53.93/20.16 *
Game/Sport	-	57.64/15.02 *
Skill Themes	-	34.83/5.82 *
Middle School	71.46/24.42 *	27.84/10.92 *
Fitness	-	23.08/2.36 *
Game/Sport	-	32.36/8.30 *
Skill Themes	-	39.95/7.60$_a$ *
High School	81.18/18.15 *	31.24/8.99 *
Fitness	-	26.87/2.36 *
Game/Sport	-	32.36/8.30 *
Skill Themes	-	39.95/7.60$_a$ *

Notes: $_a$ No significant difference between middle and high school for the Skill Theme model; * $p < 0.001$

Table 4. Summary of hierarchical regression analysis for variables predicting steps.

Variable	*B*	*SE B*	β
Step 1 (Enter)	-	-	-
Class Time	−31.35	6.63	−1.05
Activity Time	85.76	10.70	1.86
Step 2 (Stepwise)	-	-	-
Gender	−461.87	40.80	−0.28
Curr. Model	−189.51	28.52	0.17
Grade Level	523.49	25.43	0.52

Notes: Class and activity time were controlled for in the regression analysis. $R = 0.663$ for Step 1; $R = 0.730$ for Step 2.

4. Discussion

The data represent some good news and some bad news and indicate some rather worrisome trends in physical education. High school students in this sample were not active in their classes (steps/min = 31.24). Scruggs, Mungen, and Oh [23] recommended 81.97 steps/min (traditional schedule = 82–88 steps/min; block schedule = 84.04–90.05 steps/min) and the current sample was not on track to meet this requirement. This is a discouraging finding since the high school years are when a traditional decline in overall physical activity is seen [2,3]. High school physical education (PE) teachers must be aware that their classes did not meet the minimum steps per minute to be considered as moderate intensity for the class period [23]. High school PE classes must redesign their classes so that they increase the amount of activity.

The middle school students only achieved approximately 27 steps per minute (SPM), and the elementary students had 51 SPM which is below the recommendation that Scruggs, *et al.*, [23] have published. The biggest concern raised is with the elementary students as the recommended SPM is approximately 60 SPM for elementary students and this sample had a mean of 51 SPM. This finding was surprising to the researchers as none of the elementary curriculum models achieved the level needed. The Fitness and Game/Sport Model were close, but were still short on activity levels.

A concerning trend that was found is that physical education teachers know that students are not obtaining enough physical activity in physical education; but only in other classes. A disconnect does seem to be occurring in teachers who believe they are doing an acceptable job in their classes when, in fact, the data does not support this conclusion.

The benefits of exercise on the body both psychologically [25] and physiologically [26–28] are well documented. Physical activity in PE classes has had a long history on what role it should play, from a strictly fitness standpoint to a motor development sport technique ideology. While this debate will most likely continue, mounting research on the benefits of physical activity on academic performance cannot be ignored. It is evident that PE teachers must use their classroom time to increase the activity levels of their students.

This study illustrated what many have thought, but have failed to publish: some classes are good at getting students moving, but most do not get their students' activity levels high enough. The demands placed on PE teachers are great and the stresses are increasing as PE is routinely being reduced or cut from schools' curricula. Teachers need an easy and efficient way to document the amount of activity students obtain. Unlike FITNESSGRAM®, where teachers measure HFZ once a year, pedometers and SPM offer the most valuable *real-time* data to increase physical activity. It is easy and teachers can use spot testing on two or three students to check SPM during a class, whereas, FITNESSGRAM® usually takes a week or more to conduct and can be difficult to administer to 60–100 students in a gym setting.

Increased physical activity can and should be accumulated throughout the school day. While it may seem that longer breaks (longer recess or lunch time) are the key, research consistently shows that the intensity of that PA is not enough. PE offers the structure needed to plan longer bouts of increased activity in various curriculum models [29].

A limitation for the study is the use of pedometers. Although, pedometers are a simple and inexpensive means for determining activity levels, these body-worn motion sensors have been used by teachers and researchers to assess and motivate physical activity behaviors. For healthy adults, 10,000 steps/day is a reasonable estimate of daily activity; however, recent evidence suggests that a goal of 10,000 steps/day is probably too low for children, particularly if the goal is to target the war against obesity. Recommendations have been made for Americans to accumulate a minimum of 150 min per week of moderate level intensity of physical activity. Studies support the use of pedometry steps per minute values as an accurate indicator of MVPA. Pedometry demonstrates a viable large-scale surveillance instrument for measuring MVPA in physical education [15]. The misconception that pedometers don't measure intensity is not generalizable. However, as new technology becomes available, devices such as Fitbit, Jawbone UP2, Moov, and Garmin Vivofit demonstrate the demand for interpreting physical activity more efficiently for teachers. These physical activity trackers measure more than just steps taken (as seen in pedometers), they offer the ability to measure distance, heart rate, and much more than just steps taken. Perhaps PA trackers could better increase school and public awareness of the health impacts of physical activity and interventions.

Research demonstrates students who perceive a supportive environment exhibit greater levels of competence and have higher levels of self-determination. Students should be motivated positively in PE [30]. Although P.E. teachers believe they are motivating their students to be actively engaged in their physical education setting, actual steps per minute counts demonstrate they fall short of that goal. PE teachers must do a better job of increasing activity levels in their classrooms. PE teachers should make a concerted effort to not only motivate their students to be physically active in gym class, but use measures such as pedometers for assessing the activities they plan as well as the activity levels achieved.

PE teachers must do a better job of increasing activity levels in their gyms and classrooms. Current research is mounting that indicates students perform better academically if they are physically active. PE is the only subject where teachers can organize activities that meet the SPM requirement. While recess/play time is important, it cannot be adjusted to meet the demands of individual students. As physical educators, we now stand at a crucial crossroad with vital decisions to be angry. The role of the schools is to produce healthy productive citizens. As obesity levels rise and physical activity levels decline, we must do a better job at keeping children active in our gyms/classrooms. PE can encourage (force) those students who lack motivation to move to start moving!

5. Conclusion

Previous research has confirmed many adolescents between the ages of 12 and 21 years of age do not engage in vigorous activity regularly and that physical activity (PA) declines as children reach adolescence. This is a primary time for promoting an active lifestyle. Concerted efforts should be made by physical educators to promote PA and strive to provide activities that increase the number of steps taken during their PE classes. Pedometers are not only inexpensive and easy to use, but provide a method for PE teachers to assess activity levels while promoting healthy activity. Taking advantage of modern technology by the use of pedometers can assist teachers in the evaluation of the children's activity levels in the lessons they provide.

Author Contributions

Lorraine Killion contributed to the review of literature, discussion, conclusion, and editing of this manuscript. Dean Culpepper contributed to the results, data anaylsis, and editing of the manuscript.

Conflicts of Interest

The authors declare no conflict of interest.

References

1. United States Department of Health and Human Services. *Healthy People 2010: Understanding and Improving Health*; Government Printing Office: Washington, DC, USA, 2000; pp. 1–1272.

2. Centers for Disease Control and Prevention. *Guidelines for School and Community Programs to Promote Lifelong Physical Activity among Young People*; *MMWR* 46(RR-6); U.S. Department of Health & Human Services: Atlanta, GA, USA, 1997, pp. 1–36.
3. United States Department of Health and Human Services. *Physical Activity and Health: A Report of the Surgeon General*; Government Printing Office: Washington, DC, USA, 1996; pp. 1–265.
4. Kang, M.; Bassett, D.; Barreira, T.; Tudor-Locke, C.; Ainsworth, B.; Reis, J.; Strath, S.; Swartz, A. How many days are enough? A study of 365 days of pedometer monitoring. *Res. Q. Exerc. Sport* **2009**, *80*, 445–453.
5. Kelly, L.E.; Melograno, V.J. *Developing the Physical Education Curriculum. An Achievement-Based Approach*; Human Kinetics: Champaign, IL, USA, 2004.
6. Sallis, J.F.; Owen, N. *Physical Activity and Behavioral Medicine*; Sage Publications: Thousand Oaks, CA, USA, 1999.
7. Shephard, R.J. Curricular physical activity and academic performance. *Pediatr. Exerc. Sci.* **1997**, *9*, 113–126.
8. Sibley, B.A.; Etnier, J.L. The relationship between physical activity and cognition in children: A meta analysis. *Pediatr. Exerc. Sci.* **2003**, *15*, 243–256.
9. McKenzie, T.L.; Sallis, J.F.; Kolody, B.; Faucette, N. Long-term effects of a physical education curriculum and staff development program: SPARK. *Res. Q. Exerc. Sport* **1997**, *68*, 280–291.
10. Simons-Morton B.G.; Parcel, G.S.; Baranowski, T.; Forthofer, R.; O'Hara, N.M. Promoting physical activity and a healthful diet among children: Results of a school-based intervention study. *Am. J. Public Health* **1991**, *81*, 986–991.
11. Strong, W.B.; Malina, R.M.; Blimkie, C.R.; Daniels, S.R.; Dishman, R.K.; Gutin, B.; Hergenroeder, A.C.; Must, A.; Nixon, P.A.; Pivarnik, J.M.; *et al.* Evidence-based physical activity for school-age youth. *J. Pediatr.* **2005**, *146*, 732–737.
12. Eston, R.G.; Rowlands, A.V.; Ingledew, D.K. Validity of heart rate, pedometry, and accelerometry for predicting the energy cost of children's activities. *J. Appl. Physiol.* **1998**, *84*, 362–371.
13. Scruggs, P.W.; Beveridge, S.K.; Watson, D.L.; Clocksin, B.D. Quantifying physical activity in first- through fourth-grade physical education via pedometry. *Res. Q. Exerc. Sport* **2005**, *76*, 166–175.
14. Scruggs, P.W; Beveridge S.K.; Eisenman, P.A.; Watson, D.L.; Shultz, B.B.; Ransdell, L.B. Quantifying physical activity via pedometry in elementary physical education. *Med. Sci. Sports Exerc.* **2003**, 35, 1065–1071.
15. Castelli, D.M.; Hillman, C.H.; Buck, S.M.; Erwin, H.E. Physical fitness and academic achievement in third- and fifth-grade students. *J. Sport Exerc. Psychol.* **2007**, *29*, 239–252.
16. Wittberg, R.A.; Northrup, K.I.; Cottrel, L. Children's physical fitness and academic achievement. *Am. J. Health Educ.* **2009**, *40*, 30–36.
17. Coe, D.P.; Pivarnik, J.M.; Womack, C.J.; Reeves, M.J.; Malina, R.M. Effect of physical education and activity levels on academic achievement in children. *Med. Sci. Sports Exerc.* **2006**, *38*, 1515–1519.
18. London, R.A.; Castrechini, S. A longitudinal examination of the link between youth physical fitness and academic achievement. *J. Sch. Health* **2011**, *81*, 400–408.

19. Van Dusen, D.P.; Kelder, S.H.; Kohl, H.W.; Ranjit, N.; Perry, C.L. Associations of physical fitness and academic performance among schoolchildren. *J. Sch. Health* **2011**, *81*, 733–740.
20. The Cooper Institute. *Associations between Health-Related Fitness and Academic Achievement: A Report from the Texas Youth Fitness Project*. Dallas, Texas, USA 2014; pp. 1–49
21. Grissom, J.B. Physical fitness and academic achievement. *J. Exerc. Physiol. Online* **2005**, *8*, 11–25.
22. Scruggs, P.W.; Mungen, J.D.; Oh, Y. Physical Activity Measurement Device Agreement: Pedometer Steps/Minute and Physical Activity Time. *Meas. Phys. Educ. Exerc. Sci.* **2010**, *14*, 151–163.
23. New Lifestyles. Using Your New Lifestyles Digi-Walker Pedometer [Brochure]. Available online: http://www.new-lifestyles.com/using_your_pedometer.pdf (accessed on 13 September 2014).
24. Weir, K. *The Exercise Effect*; American Psychological Association: Washington, USA, 2011; pp. 49–52.
25. Pate, R.R.; Ross, J.G. Factors associated with health-related fitness. *J. Phys. Educ. Recreat. Dance* **1987**, *58*, 93–95.
26. Sallis, J.F.; Patterson, T.L.; Buono, M.J.; Nader, P.R. Relation of cardiovascularfitness and physical activity to cardiovascular disease risk factors in children and adults. *Am. J. Epidemiol.* **1988**, *127*, 933–941.
27. McKenzie, T.L.; Nader, P.R.; Strikmiller, P.; Yang, M.; Stone, E.; Perry, C. School physical education: Effect of the child and adolescent trial for cardiovascular Health. *Prev. Med.* **1996**, *25*, 423–431.
28. Calfas, K.J.; Taylor, W.C. Effects of physical activity on psychological variables in adolescents. *Pediatr. Exerc. Sci.* **1994**, *6*, 406–423.
29. Pate, R.R.; Davis, M.G.; Robins, T.N.; Stone, E.J.; McKenzie, T.L.; Young, J.C. Promoting physical activity in children and youth: A leadership role for schools. *Circ.: J. Am. Heart Assoc.* **2006**, *114*, 1214–1224.
30. Standage, M.; Duda, J.; Ntoumanis, N. Students' motivational processes and their relationship to teacher ratings in school physical education. *Res. Q. Exerc. Sport* **2006**, *77*, 100–110.

10

Upper Extremity Muscle Activation during Bodyblade Exercises Following Six Weeks of Intervention Focusing on the Lumbopelvic-Hip Complex

Gretchen D. Oliver [1,†,*], Audrey J. Stone [2,†], Wendi H. Weimar [3,†], Lawrence Lemak [4,†], Jessica K. Washington [3,†] and Christopher P. Dougherty [5,†]

[1] School of Kinesiology, Auburn University, Auburn, AL 36849, USA; E-Mail: goliver@auburn.edu
[2] Heart and Vascular Institute Penn State College of Medicine, Hershey, PA 17033, USA; E-Mail: astone1@hmc.psu.edu
[3] School of Kinesiology, Auburn University, Auburn, AL 36849, USA; E-Mail: weimawh@auburn.edu (W.H.W.); jkw0011@auburn.edu (J.K.W.)
[4] Lemak Sports Medicine and Orthopedics, Birmingham, AL 35213, USA; E-Mail: llemak@thelemakgroup.com
[5] Agility Center, Orthopedics, Bentonville, AR 72712, USA; E-Mail: cptd12@gmail.com

† These authors contributed equally to this work.

* Author to whom correspondence should be addressed; E-Mail: goliver@auburn.edu;

Academic Editor: Eling de Bruin

Abstract: The current study examined the effects of a six-week lumbopelvic-hip complex (LPHC) strengthening program on muscle activation when performing the shoulder dump exercise. The shoulder dump is a total body exercise that includes overhead arm movements. A pre-post test with a control group was implemented. Twenty-seven graduate students (23.5 ± 1.34 yr; 174.4 ± 11.0 cm; 76.6 ± 16.9 kg) participated. Participants were randomly assigned to a control or intervention group where the intervention group performed LPHC exercises. Two-way analysis of variance (ANOVA) revealed a significant increase in muscle activation of the serratus anterior from pre- and post-LPHC intervention, ($t = 6.5, p < 0.001$). As presented by these data, incorporation of LPHC exercises may assist in facilitating greater activation in some of the scapula-stabilizing musculature that has traditionally been rehabilitated in prone or side-lying positions. It is, therefore, suggested that LPHC exercises be incorporated in a regular shoulder rehabilitation program.

Keywords: core; electromyography; functional shoulder rehabilitation; kinetic chain

---

1. Introduction

Often, shoulder rehabilitations focus on symptom resolution while restoration of total body function tends to be overlooked [1–4]. Kibler, *et al.* [4,5] emphasize the importance of a shoulder rehabilitation that addresses dysfunction at the proximal end of the kinetic chain in an attempt to facilitate efficient movement at the distal end. The kinetic chain has been described to have several functions, three of which are: (1) providing a proximal stable base for distal arm mobility [6], (2) maximizing force development from the lower extremity in an upward direction, through the lumbopelvic-hip complex (LPHC), and eventually to the hand [7–9], and (3) producing torques to decrease deceleration forces [10–12]. Thus, reiterating the commonly-accepted notion that optimal shoulder function relies on the kinetic chain [13–15].

The LPHC is the central link connecting the upper extremity to the lower extremity and is often referred to as the core. Additionally, it is the musculature of the LPHC that is active through the feed-forward mechanism for all extremity movements, indicating that LPHC musculature activation occurs in anticipation of limb movements [16,17]. It is the LPHC, therefore, that assists the body, functioning as a kinetic chain and facilitating efficient movement to meet the demands of the desired task [16,17].

The kinetic chain approach to dynamic upper extremity movement patterns focuses on glenohumeral motion, first through scapular control and then through hip stability [1]. It is the pelvis, essentially, providing a platform for the scapula which, in turn, provides a stable platform for the shoulder. Thus, it is accepted that scapula control is coordinated through a stable base of support from the trunk and pelvis [1,18], essentially allowing the musculature of the lumbopelvic-hip complex to initiate shoulder movement.

It has previously been established that implementing the Bodyblade (Mad Dogg Athletics, Venice, CA, USA) into a total body shoulder exercise allows for effective activation of not only the scapular stabilizing muscles, but also LPHC muscles [18,19]. As shoulder rehabilitation has shifted to more of a total body approach, exercises known to activate the musculature of the LPHC could be performed simultaneously with shoulder exercises [20]. If the LPHC is activated in an attempt to stabilize the pelvis, then the musculature that stabilizes the scapula will be more efficient due to the stable base of support of the pelvis. Therefore, it was the purpose of this study to determine if upper extremity muscle activation changes following a six-week intervention program focusing on LPHC exercises. It was hypothesized that those who were engaged in the intervention program would have greater upper extremity muscle activation during the shoulder dump than those in the control group.

2. Methods

2.1. Study Design

A pretest-posttest controlled laboratory study with repeated measures on time was used. The dependent variable was the percent of maximum voluntary isometric contraction (%MVIC) during the shoulder dump for each muscle (multifidus, latissimus dorsi, lower trapezius, middle trapezius, infraspinatus, serratus anterior) and the independent variables were time (pretest, posttest) and group (intervention and control).

2.2. Participants

Twenty-seven healthy collegiate graduate students (24 ± 1 yr; 174 ± 11 cm; 77 ± 17 kg), regardless of sex, consented to participate. "Healthy" was defined as having no history of any type of injury in the last six months, as well as currently participating in physical activity for at least 30 min, four times a week. In addition, participants were excluded if they were either currently performing a LPHC-strengthening program or if they reported a previous history of shoulder pain. The University Institutional Review Board approved testing protocols used in the current study and, prior to participation, the approved procedures, risks, and benefits were explained to all participants. All participants consented and the rights of the participants were protected according to the guidelines of the University's Institutional Review Board.

2.3. Procedure

Participants were randomly assigned to either the control or intervention group. All subjects participated in two EMG testing sessions that were separated by six weeks. During the six weeks between testing, the intervention group performed LPHC exercises. The LPHC exercises were based on a previous study validating the activation of the LPHC musculature [21]. All participants reported for pre- and post-testing prior to engaging in any vigorous activity for that day. Location of the dominant side multifidus, latissimus dorsi, lower trapezius, middle trapezius, infraspinatus, and serratus anterior were identified through palpation of the muscle belly. Prior to testing, the identified locations for surface electrode placement were shaved, abraded, and cleaned using standard medical alcohol swabs. Subsequent to surface preparation, adhesive 3M Red-Dot bipolar, 6 cm Ag/AgCl diameter disk-shaped, surface electrodes (3M, St. Paul, MN, USA) were attached over the muscle bellies and positioned parallel to muscle fibers using previously-published standardized methods [22–24]. The selected inter-electrode distance was 25 mm [25].

Electromyographic data were collected via a Noraxon Myopac 1400L 8-channel amplifier (Noraxon USA, Inc., Scottsdale, AZ, USA). The signal was full-wave rectified and root mean squared at 100 ms. Surface EMG data were sampled at a rate of 1000 Hz. The surface EMG data were notch filtered at frequencies of 59.5 and 60.5 Hz [26]. An additional electrode was placed on the contralateral anterior superior iliac spine (ASIS) to serve as a reference lead for the examined muscles. Following the application of surface electrodes, manual muscles testing (MMT) techniques by Kendal, *et al.* [27] were used to determine steady state contraction. A certified athletic trainer (AT), trained in performing MMTs, conducted all MMTs to ensure reliability throughout testing. Three MMTs lasting five seconds were performed for each muscle, with the first and last second of each test removed to obtain steady state results. The MMT provided baseline maximum voluntary isometric contraction (MVIC) data to which all surface EMG were compared. The aforementioned surface EMG methodologies were performed again during the post testing.

Manual Muscle Testing

The multifidus was tested with the participant prone, arms crossed over chest and attempting to perform back extension and rotation to the opposite side while the AT resisted. The latissimus dorsi was tested with the participant prone with arm adducted, extended, and medially rotated. The AT applied resistance against the forearm, in the direction of abduction and slight flexion of the arm. To test the lower trapezius, the participant was prone with arm diagonally overhead (extended and abducted approximately 30°, in the scapular plane), in line with the lower fibers of the trapezius. The AT applied pressure against the forearm, in a downward direction. To test the middle trapezius, the participant was prone, shoulder abducted to 90°, externally rotated so that thumb was pointed upward, and arm fully extended while the AT applied pressure against the forearm in a downward direction. For the infraspinatus, the participant was prone with arm resting on the table and elbow flexed to 90°. Participant attempted to laterally rotate the shoulder, with elbow held at 90° while the AT applied pressure in the direction of medial rotation

The serratus anterior was tested with the participant lying supine, shoulder forward flexed to 90°. The AT resisted force against the participant's fist as the participant attempted to protract.

Following MMTs, investigators instructed participants on the proper technique of the shoulder dump rehabilitation exercise, which was previously examined by McMullen and Uhl [1]. Participants were instructed to stand in a staggered stance with their left foot forward, left hip flexed, trunk flexed and rotated to the left, and right elbow at knee level. Participants were then instructed to shift weight to the right foot while extending and rotating the trunk to the right (Figure 1). All participants performed the shoulder dump exercise with a Bodyblade (Mad Dog Athletics, Venice, CA, USA) C × T (0.57 kg, 101.6 cm). The C × T model was chosen because it was applicable for beginners and was easier to control [18]. Before the participants began the EMG testing, they were given an average of three minutes to warm-up and become familiar with the Bodyblade (Mad Dogg Athletics, Venice, CA, USA) as well as the shoulder dump exercise. Participants were instructed on proper posture through verbal cues and visual aids provided by an AT. After participants were familiar with the exercise technique, they were instructed to perform three repetitions of the shoulder dump (Figure 1). The repetitions were on a time count provided by one of the investigators. The exercise's repetition count was 5 s to reach the middle of the shoulder dump and then 5 s to reach the end of the exercise, for a total time of 10 s.

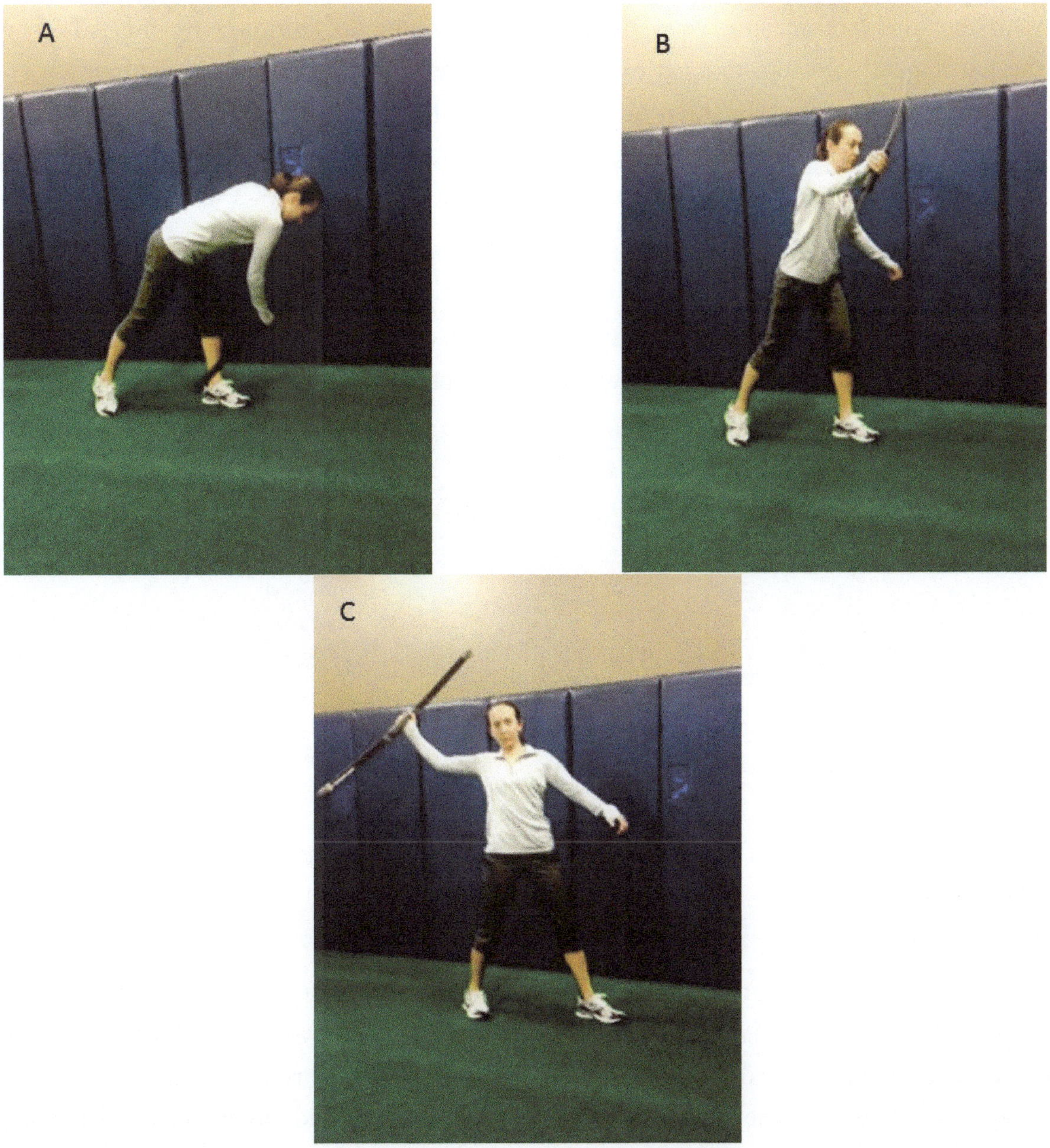

Figure 1. Shoulder Dump: (**A**) Start position of shoulder dump; (**B**) Middle of shoulder dump; (**C**) End position of shoulder dump.

2.4. Intervention Program

The intervention program consisted of a total of eight exercises (Figures 2–9), which were randomly alternated throughout the six weeks so that five exercises were performed every day of the intervention. The selection of eight consisted of isometric body weight exercises focusing on the LPHC. The participant had to choose five of the eight exercises and perform them two days a week for six weeks [28,29]. Eight exercises were given with only five being required in an attempt to allow for variation of exercise selection. Each exercise was performed for a duration of 30 s. After completion of the exercise, 15 s of rest was given before the next exercise was performed. An AT familiar with the intervention exercises supervised all intervention sessions. Participants enrolled in the intervention reported to perform the intervention program under supervision at the same time and place twice a week. All participants were compliant with the intervention and were monitored throughout the duration by the AT. The AT monitored the participant's posture in each exercise. If the participant could not maintain the correct posture, they were instructed to reposition and continue. All participants were able to complete the exercises with minimal instructional monitoring by the AT. The control group was instructed to continue their normal physical activity of at least 30 min of physical activity, four days a week.

Intervention Exercises

Side Plank: The participant supported their body on side with weight on their forearm and lateral aspect of foot. Body remained in a straight line, pelvis was held in neutral. Position was held for 30 s (Figure 2).

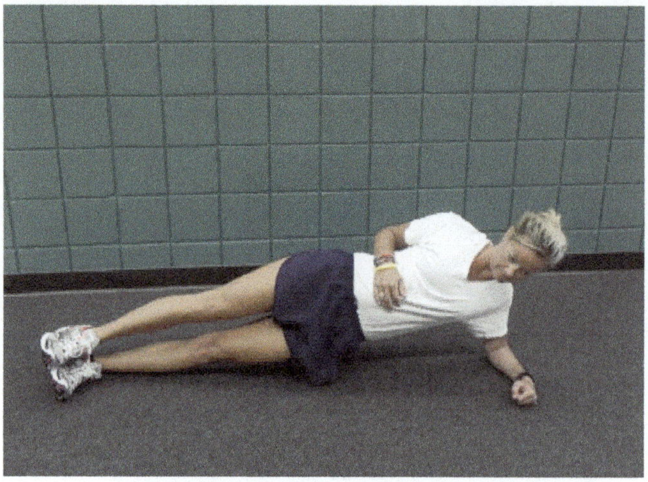

Figure 2. Side plank.

Front Plank: The participant supported their body on bilateral forearms and balls of feet. The body remained in a straight line and pelvis was held in neutral. This position was held for 30 s (Figure 3).
Flying Squirrel: Participant was prone with knees flexed, hips internally rotated and extended (legs off the floor), pelvis held in neutral. The shoulders were externally rotated and elbows flexed. This position was held for 30 s (Figure 4).
Bird Dog: The participant was on all fours and then extended contralateral arm and leg and maintained their pelvis in neutral. This position was held for 30 s (Figure 5).

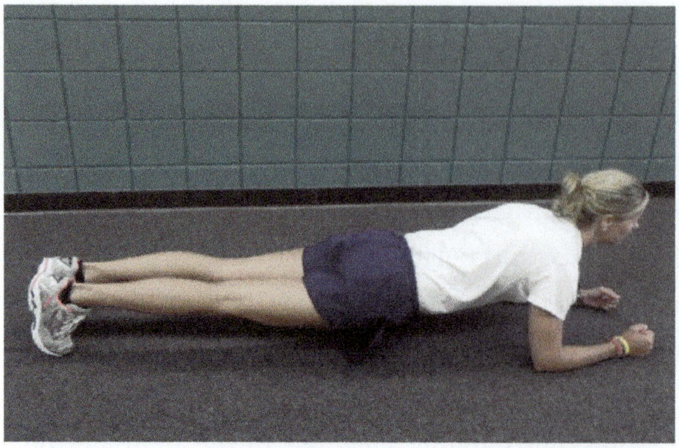

Figure 3. Front plank.

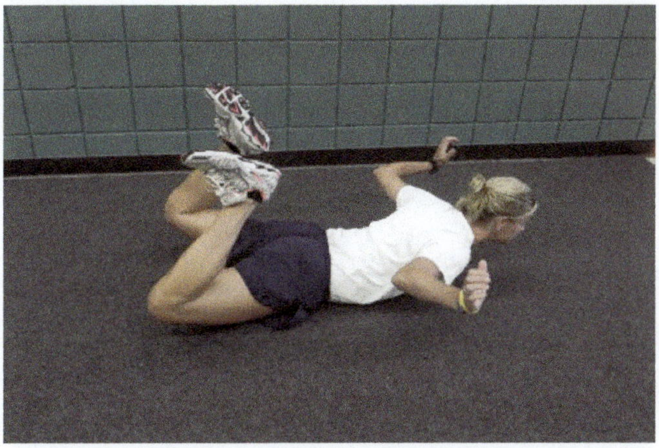

Figure 4. Flying squirrel.

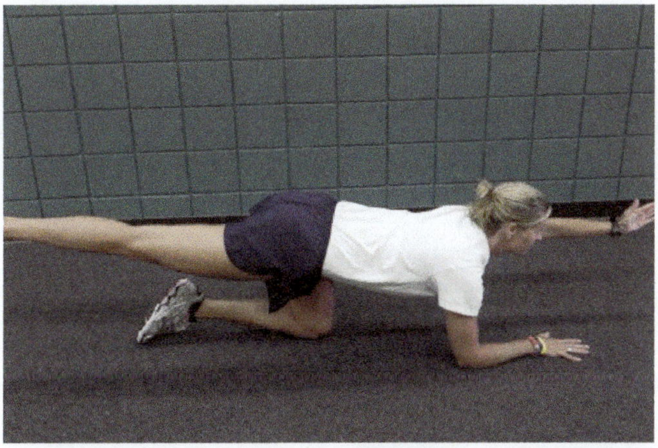

Figure 5. Bird dog.

Advanced Front Plank: Participant was in front plank position and extended contralateral arm and leg. The pelvis was held in neutral and the position was held for 30 s (Figure 6).

Single Leg Pelvic Tilt: The participant was supine. Participant's contralateral hip was in maximal flexion and held by participant with their hands. Ipsilateral foot was on ground. Ipsilateral foot pushed into floor to raise LPHC off floor. The participant's body remain in straight line and this position was held for 30 s (Figure 7).

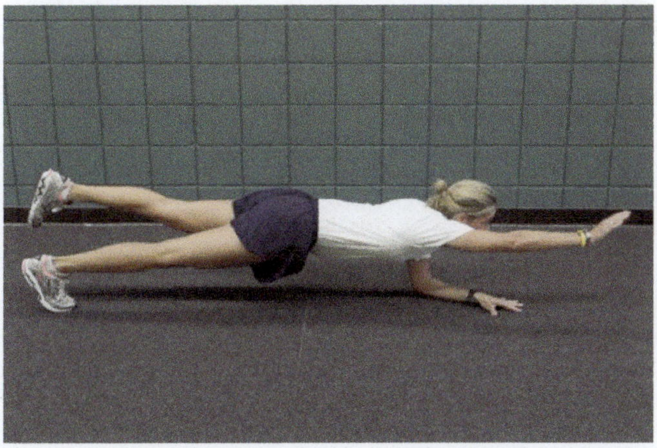

Figure 6. Advanced front plank.

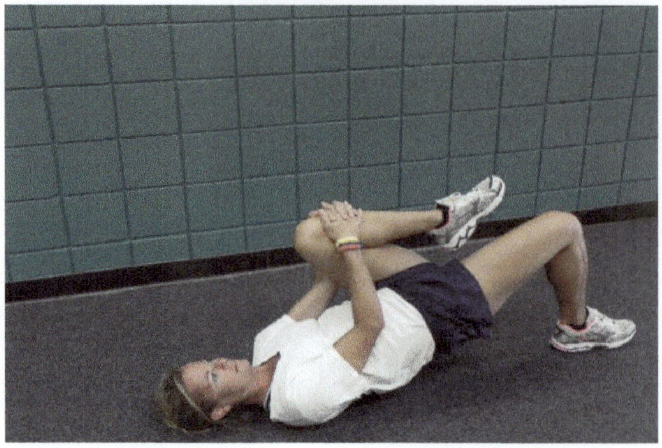

Figure 7. Single leg pelvic tilt.

Advanced Bird Dog: The participant positioned to perform the Bird Dog and then dropped into hip flexion while remaining in hip extension on the contralateral side. Position was held for 30 s (Figure 8).

Push-Up Hold: Participant was prone with weight supported on bilateral balls of feet and palms of hands. The participant's pelvis was in neutral and body was in a straight line, this position was held for 30 s (Figure 9).

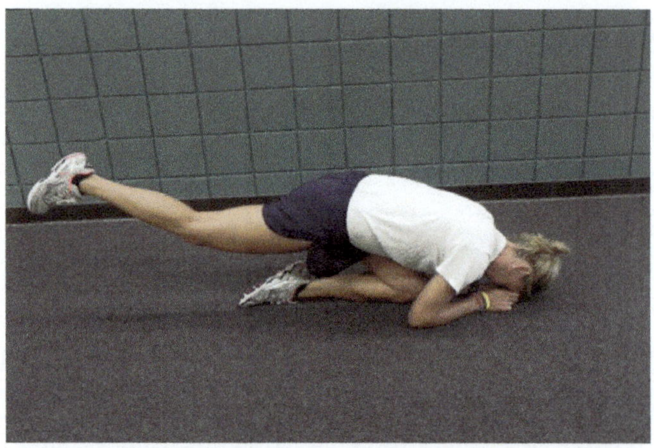

Figure 8. Advanced bird dog.

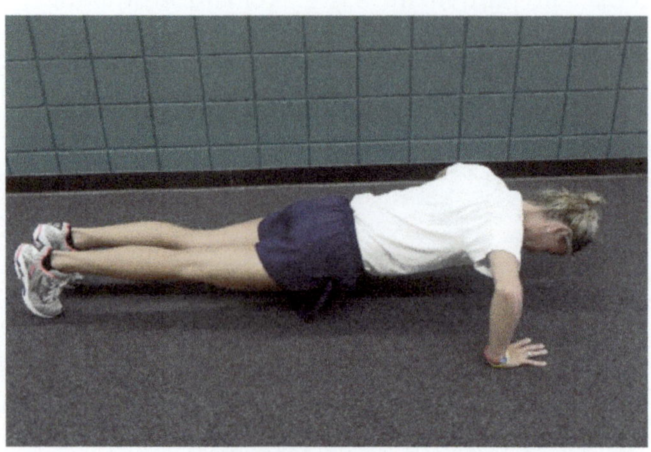

Figure 9. Push up hold.

2.5. Statistical Analysis

While performing the shoulder dump, mean activation from each muscle were normalized and expressed as a percent contribution of their %MVIC. Statistical analyses were performed using GraphPad Prism 6.0 software (GraphPad Software, Inc., La Jolla, CA, USA). Descriptive statistics were expressed by means and standard error of means (SEM). For each muscle group, a mixed model analysis of variance [ANOVA] was performed. An overall α-level was set *a priori* at $p \leq 0.05$. *Post hoc* analyses using Holm-Sidak for multiple comparisons were conducted when appropriate.

3. Results

Pre- and post-test %MVICs for each muscle group were analyzed between groups. There were no significant interactions between time (pre-test vs post-test) and group (intervention *vs*. control) for the lower trapezius, infraspinatus, multifidus, or latissimus dorsi muscles, $p > 0.05$ (Figure 10A–E). The statistical powers of the comparisons of %MVIC within each group are shown in Table 1. There was a significant main effect for time for the multifidus muscle (pre: 34.5 ± 5%MVIC; post: 23.6 ± 3%MVIC; $p = 0.025$) and the latissimus dorsi muscle (pre: 25.9 ± 4%MVIC; post: 12.9 ± 4%MVIC; $p = 0.026$). There was a significant interaction for the serratus anterior muscle, and *post hoc* analysis showed that, within the intervention group, the post-test (95.6 ± 13%MVIC) was significantly higher than the pre-test (28.3 ± 8%MVIC) (Figure 10F, $p < 0.05$).

Table 1. Statistical power of comparisons of %MVIC from pre- to post-test for each muscle within the control group and the intervention group.

	Control		Intervention	
Muscle	Power	*N*	Power	*N*
Lower trapezius	0.45	14	0.28	15
Middle trapezius	0.77	14	0.09	15
Infraspinatus	0.14	14	0.05	15
Mutifidus	0.84	14	0.21	15
Latissimus dorsi	0.98	14	0.33	15
Serratus Anterior	0.15	14	0.98	15

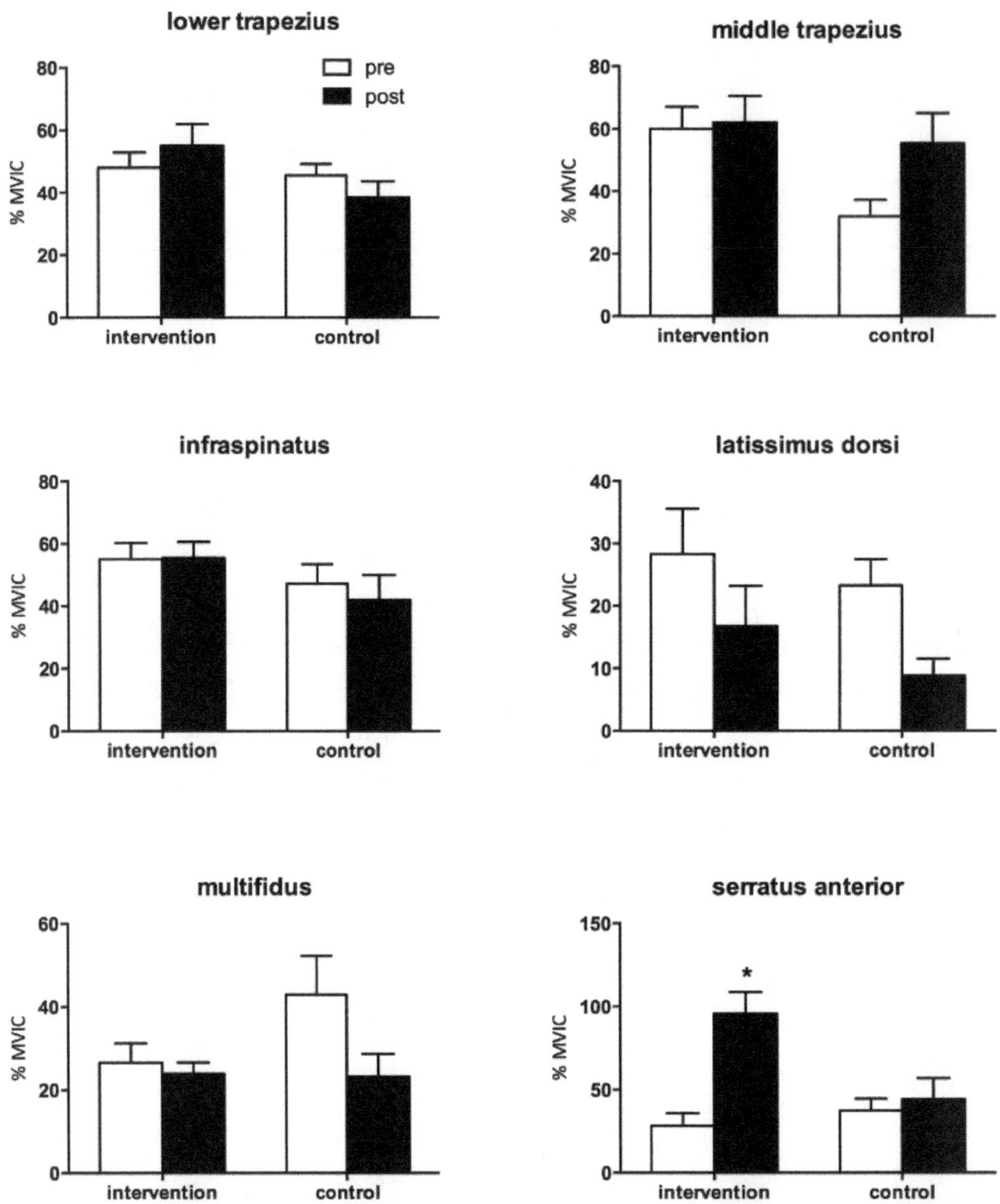

Figure 10. Percent MVIC of selected muscles presented as pre/post comparisons.

4. Discussion

The current study examined muscle activation of the upper extremity while performing the shoulder dump, pre- and post-intervention, as it was the aim of this study to present a LPHC intervention program to assist with achieving a total kinetic chain approach to shoulder rehabilitation. As the body functions as a kinetic chain, it works in a proximal to distal nature. Thus for efficient shoulder function, it is recommended that the proximal link, the LPHC in this case, demonstrate stability so that the distal link, the shoulder, has efficient mobility [4,5]. With the LPHC being the central link connecting the upper extremity to the lower extremity, it was hypothesized that a six-week intervention program focusing on the LPHC would result in greater upper extremity muscle activation during the shoulder dump than those in a control group. Though the only statistically significant change in muscle activation pre- and post-test was the serratus anterior, there is great clinical relevance from these results.

The current study revealed that, when performing the shoulder dump, there was moderately strong activation (35–50%MVIC) [30,31] of the lower trapezius, infraspinatus, and serratus anterior. This activation was consistent across the groups as well as pre- and post-testing. From a clinical standpoint, moderately strong activation has been an acceptable level for muscle strengthening [31], thus reiterating that the shoulder dump is an appropriate exercise to target the aforementioned scapular stabilizing musculature. These results are also in agreement with previously published work examining the shoulder dump exercise [18]. Additionally, it was noted that the two muscles, multifidus and latissimus dorsi, that both function in partial capacity to stabilize the pelvis, exhibited moderate to minimal (respectively) activation throughout the groups, as well as pre- and post-testing. This finding allows for clinicians to emphasis the shoulder dump, even though it is a total body activity, as more of a shoulder exercise. As for why there were decreases in activation of both the multifidus and latissimus dorsi, post-testing, is unknown. It is an intriguing find, especially with the intervention focusing on the LPHC. Thus, further investigation is needed to explain these findings.

The current study has demonstrated increased activation of scapular-stabilizing musculature, specifically the serratus anterior, in a standing posture while performing a total body functional movement pattern. Cools, *et al.* [32] advocates shoulder exercises where the patient is side-lying or prone as an attempt to gain the greatest lower trapezius and serratus anterior activation during the early phases of rehabilitation. However, the problem that arises is the need to have the rehabilitation mimic activities of daily living or sports-specific movement patterns. To perform the shoulder dump exercise, one has to incorporate diagonal patterns that mimic sport-specific movements. Therefore, the implementation of diagonal patterns while standing, as an attempt to engage the trunk and lower extremity, is desired in shoulder rehabilitation [1,4,18].

It should be noted that the current study only examined healthy subjects and further investigation into the injured population is needed. It is unknown if there is a need to correct a LPHC problem or do we just need to make the LPHC stronger. It is known that tissue injury, as well as anatomical deficits in the lower extremity, LPHC, or scapular stabilizers can lead to overuse shoulder injury [2,14]. Therefore, much more attention should be placed on the function of the LPHC and its relation with not only performance but also injury prevention. Our study was able to show increased activity in scapular stabilizing muscles, specifically serratus anterior, while incorporating the LPHC in a shoulder rehab exercise.

It also should be noted that the exercise, shoulder dump, was analyzed as a complete movement and not broken down into phases. Thus with further investigation, it would be advantageous to examine the shoulder dump into phases for further insight. Additionally, the shoulder dump was the only full-body dynamic exercise examined and introduced. Moreover, other exercises could also give insight into the LPHC intervention that was introduced in this study.

In conclusion, this study was able to demonstrate that the shoulder dump exercise performed after a six-week intervention resulted in significantly greater activation of the serratus anterior. As a periscapular muscle, the serratus anterior functions as one of the scapula stabilizers during overhead movements [32–37]. The shoulder dump is a total body exercise that includes overhead arm movements. As presented by these data, incorporation of LPHC exercises may assist in facilitating greater activation in some of the scapula-stabilizing musculature that has traditionally been rehabilitated in prone or side-lying positions.

The authors thus suggest incorporation of LPHC exercises into a regular shoulder pre-rehabilitation program in an attempt to facilitate great upper extremity muscle activation.

Author Contributions

Gretchen Oliver and Christopher Dougherty conceived and designed the experiments, Gretchen Oliver and Audrey Stone performed the experiments. Gretchen Oliver analyzed the data. Audrey Stone, Wendi Weimar, Jessica Washington, Lawrence Lemak contributed analysis tools and further analysis. Gretchen Oliver wrote the paper.

Conflicts of Interest

The authors declare no conflict of interest.

References

1. McMullen, J.; Uhl T.L. A kinetic chain approach for shoulder rehabilitation. *J Athl. Train.* **2000**, *35*, 329–337.
2. Kibler, W.B.; Press, J.; Sciascia, A. The role of core stability in athletic function. *Sports Med.* **2006**, *36*, 189–198.
3. Kibler, W.B.; Sciascia, A.D.; Uhl, T.L.; Tambay, N.; Cunningham, T. Electromyographic analysis of specific exercises for scapular control in early phases of shoulder rehabilitation. *Am. J. Sports Med.* **2008**, *36*, 1789–1798.
4. Kibler, W.B.; McMullen, J.; Uhl, T. Shoulder rehabilitation strategies, guidance and practice. *Oper. Tech. Sports Med.* **2012**, *20*, 103–112.
5. Kibler, W.B. The role of the scapula in athletic shoulder function. *Am. J. Sports Med.* **1998**, *26*, 325–337.
6. Kibler, W.B.; Kuhn, J.E.; Wilk, K.; Sciascia, A.; Moore, S.; Laudner, K.; Ellenbecker, T.; Thigpen, C.; Uhl, T. The disabled throwing shoulder: Spectrum of pathology-10year update. *Arthroscopy* **2013**, *29*, 141–161.
7. Elliott, B.C.; Marshall, R.; Noffal, G. Contributions of upper limb segment rotation during the power serve in tennis. *J. Appl. Biomech.* **1995**, *11*, 443–447.
8. Linter, D.; Noonan, T.J.; Kibler, W.B. Injury patterns and biomechanics of the athlete's shoulder. *Clin. Sports Med.* **2008**, *27*, 527–552.
9. Toyoshima, S.; Miyashita, M. Force-velocity relation in throwing. *Res. Quart.* **1973**, *44*, 86–95.
10. Putnam, C.A. Sequential motions of body segments in striking and throwing skills: Description and explanations. *J. Biomech.* **1993**, *26*, 125–135.
11. Fleisig, G.S.; Andrews, J.R.; Dillman, C.J.; Escamilla, R.F. Kinetics of baseball pitching with implications about injury mechanisms. *Am. J. Sports Med.* **1995**, *23*, 233–239.
12. Fleisig, G.S.; Barrentine, S.W.; Escamilla, R.F.; Andrews, J.R. Biomechanics of overhead throwing implications for injury. *Sports Med.* **1996**, *21*, 421–437.
13. Cordo, P.J.; Nashner, L.M. Properties of postural adjustments associated with rapid arm movements. *J. Neurophysiol.* **1982**, *47*, 287–308.

14. Sciascia, A.; Thigpen, C.; Namdair, S.; Baldwin, K. Kinetic chain abnormalities in the athletic shoulder. *Sports Med. Arthrosc. Rev.* **2012**, *20*, 16–21.
15. Sewick, A.; Kelly, J.D.; Rubin, B. Physical examination of the overhead athlete's shoulder. *Sports Med. Arthrosc. Rev.* **2012**, *20*, 11–15.
16. Hodges, P.W.; Richardson, C.A. Relationship between limb movement speed and associated contraction of the trunk. *Ergonomics* **1997**, *40*, 1220–1230.
17. Hodges, P.W.; Richardson, C.A. Feedforward contraction of transversus abdominis is not influenced by the direction of arm movement. *Exp. Brain Res.* **1997**, *114*, 362–370.
18. Oliver, G.D.; Sola, M.; Dougherty, C.P.; Huddleston, S. Quantitative examination of upper and lower extremity muscle activation during common shoulder rehabilitation exercises using the Bodyblade. *J. Strength Cond. Res.* **2013**, *27*, 2509–2517.
19. Moreside, J.M.; Vera-Garacia, F.J.; McGill, S.M. Trunk muscle activation patterns, lumbar compressive force, and spine stability when using the Bodyblade. *Phys. Ther.* **2007**, *87*, 153–521.
20. Brumitt, J.; Dale, R.B. Integrating shoulder and core exercises when rehabilitating athletes performing overhead activities. *N. Am. J. Sports Phys. Ther.* **2009**, *4*, 132–138.
21. Oliver, G.D.; Stone, A.J.; Plummer, H. Electromyographic examination of selected muscle activation during isometric exercises. *Clin. J. Sports Med.* **2010**, *20*, 452–457.
22. Basmajian, J.V.; Deluca, C.J. Apparatus, detection, and recording techniques. In *Muscles Alive, Their Functions Revealed by Electromyography*, 5th ed.; Butler, J.P., Ed.; Williams and Wilkins: Baltimore, MD, USA, 1985; pp. 19–64.
23. Cram, J.R.; Kasman, G.S.; Holtz, J. (Eds.) Electrode placement. In *Introduction to Surface Electromyography*; Aspen Publishers: Gaithersburg, MD, USA, 1998; pp. 237–383.
24. Zipp, P. Recommendations for the standardization of lead positions in surface electromyography. *Eur. J. Appl. Physiol.* **1982**, *50*, 41–54.
25. Hintermeister, R.A.; Lange, G.A.; Schultheis, J.M.; Bey, M.J.; Hawkins, R.J. Electromyographic activity and applied load during shoulder rehabilitation exercises using elastic resistance. *Am. J. Sports Med.* **1982**, *26*, 210–220.
26. Oliver, G.D.; Plummer, H.A. Ground reaction forces, kinematics, and muscle activation during the windmill softball pitch. *J. Sport Sci.* **2011**, *29*, 1071–1077.
27. Kendall, F.P.; McCreary, E.K.; Provance, P.G. *Muscles: Testing and Function*, 4th ed.; Williams and Wilkins: Baltimore, MD, USA, 1993.
28. Oliver, G.D.; Adams-Blair, H.R.; Dougherty, C.P. Implementation of a core stability program for elementary school children. *Athl. Train. Sports Health Care* **2010**, *2*, 261–266.
29. Roling, K.; Oliver, G.D.; Dittmore, S.; Moiseichik, M. The effects of a lumpopelvic-hip strengthening intervention program on functional testing in collegiate female tennis players. *Clin. Kinesiol.* **2012**, *66*, 13–18.
30. Campbell, B.M.; Stodden, D.F.; Nixon, M.K. Lower extremity muscle activation during baseball pitching. *J. Strength Cond. Res.* **2010**, *24*, 964–971.
31. Tucker, S.; Armstrong, C.W.; Swartz, E.E.; Campbell, B.; Rankin, J.M. An electromyographic analysis of the cuff link rehabilitation device. *J Sport Rehabil.* **2005**, 14, 124–136.

32. Cools, A.M.; Lanszweert, F.; Notebaert, D.; Roets, A.; Soetens, B.; Cagnie, B.; Witvrouw, E.E. Rehabilitation of scapular muscle balance. Which exercise to prescribe. *Am. J. Sports Med.* **2007**, *35*, 1744–1751.
33. Cools, A.M.; Witurouw, E.E.; Declercq, G.; Danneels, L.A.; Cambier, D.C. Scapular muscle recruitment patterns: Trapezius muscle latency with and without impingement symptoms. *Am. J. Sports Med.* **2003**, *31*, 542–549.
34. Cools, A.M.; Witurouw, E.E.; Declercq, G.; Vanderstraeten, G.G.; Cambier, D.C. Evaluation of isokinetic force production and associated muscle activity in the scapular rotators during a protraction-retraction movement in overhead athletes with impingement syndrome. *Br. J. Sports Med.* **2004**, *38*, 64–68.
35. Cools, A.M.; Witurouw, E.E.; Mahieu, N.N.; Danneels, L.A. Isokinetic scapular muscle performance in overhead athletes with and without impingement symptoms. *J. Athl. Train.* **2005**, *40*, 104–110.
36. Ludewig, P.; Cook, T. Alterations in shoulder kinematics and associated muscle activity in people with symptoms of shoulder impingement. *Phys. Ther.* **2000**, *80*, 276–291.
37. Wadsworth, D.J.S.; Bullock-Saxton, J.E. Recruitment patterns of the scapular rotator muscles in freestyle swimmers with subacromial impingement. *Int. J. Sports Med.* **1997**, *18*, 618–624.

11

Effect of Level and Downhill Running on Breathing Efficiency

Matthew D. Cook, Stephen D. Myers, John S. M. Kelly and Mark E. T. Willems *

Department of Sport & Exercise Sciences, University of Chichester, West Sussex PO19 6PE, UK;
E-Mails: m.cook@chi.ac.uk (M.D.C.); s.myers@chi.ac.uk (S.D.M.); j.kelly@chi.ac.uk (J.S.M.K.)

* Author to whom correspondence should be addressed; E-Mail: m.willems@chi.ac.uk;

Academic Editor: Arno Schmidt-Trucksäss

Abstract: Ventilatory equivalents for oxygen and carbon dioxide are physiological measures of breathing efficiency, and are known to be affected by the intensity and mode of exercise. We examined the effect of level running (gradient 0%) and muscle-damaging downhill running (−12%), matched for oxygen uptake, on the ventilatory equivalents for oxygen ($\dot{V}E/\dot{V}O_2$) and carbon dioxide ($\dot{V}E/\dot{V}CO_2$). Nine men (27 ± 9 years, 179 ± 7 cm, 75 ± 12 kg, $\dot{V}O_{2max}$: 52.0 ± 7.7 mL·kg^{-1}·min^{-1}) completed two 40-min running bouts (5 × 8-min with 2-min inter-bout rest), one level and one downhill. Running intensity was matched at 60% of maximal metabolic equivalent. Maximal isometric force of *m.quadriceps femoris* was measured before and after the running bouts. Data was analyzed with 2-way ANOVA or paired samples *t*-tests. Running speed (downhill: 13.5 ± 3.2, level: 9.6 ± 2.2 km·h^{-1}) and isometric force deficits (downhill: 17.2 ± 7.6%, level: 2.0 ± 6.9%) were higher for downhill running. Running bouts for level and downhill gradients had $\dot{V}O_2$, heart rates and respiratory exchange ratio values that were not different indicating matched intensity and metabolic demands. During downhill running, the $\dot{V}E/\dot{V}O_2$, (downhill: 29.7 ± 3.3, level: 27.2 ± 1.6) and $\dot{V}E/\dot{V}CO_2$ (downhill: 33.3 ± 2.7, level: 30.4 ± 1.9) were 7.1% and 8.3% higher ($p < 0.05$) than level running. In conclusion, breathing efficiency appears lower during downhill running (*i.e.*, muscle-damaging exercise) compared to level running at a similar moderate intensity.

Keywords: eccentric exercise; muscle damage; ventilatory equivalent; metabolic equivalent; moderate intensity; treadmill running

1. Introduction

During dynamic whole-body exercise, the main function of the respiratory system is to supply oxygen (O_2) to the blood and eliminate the carbon dioxide (CO_2) produced in the working skeletal muscles. Over a broad range of exercise intensities, a change in exercise intensity is associated with a change in breathing responses, e.g., a change in minute ventilation, *i.e.*, the volume of exhaled air per minute, allowing increased oxygen consumption and carbon dioxide elimination. Measures of breathing efficiency are the ventilatory equivalents for oxygen (O_2) and carbon dioxide (CO_2) which are the ratios of minute ventilation to O_2 consumption ($\dot{V}E/\dot{V}O_2$), and minute ventilation to CO_2 output ($\dot{V}E/\dot{V}CO_2$), respectively [1].

Breathing efficiency and exercise intensity are related [2]. Breathing efficiency decreases from low-intensity exercise reaching a plateau value at moderate to high intensities [2]. Breathing efficiency is also related to the exercise modality. For example, higher $\dot{V}E/\dot{V}O_2$ were reported for arm exercise compared to leg exercise [3]. Additionally, running had a higher $\dot{V}E/\dot{V}O_2$ ratio than simulated swimming [4], the $\dot{V}E/\dot{V}CO_2$ during treadmill running was higher than cycle ergometry at submaximal intensity [5], but higher for cycle ergometry than uphill treadmill running at maximum intensity [6].

Running is a common exercise modality, with the gradient determining whether the exercise consists mainly of concentric or eccentric contractions. Running exercise at a negative gradient (*i.e.*, downhill running) is an activity that requires primarily eccentric contractions of skeletal muscles (*i.e.*, lengthening muscle actions). When running at similar speeds, the eccentric contractions of skeletal muscles will require a lower oxygen demand than level running with concentric contractions [7]. In addition, the physiological responses by the cardiovascular and respiratory systems during eccentric exercise are lower compared to concentric exercise. This lower response may be partly due to recruitment of motor units being less for eccentric compared to concentric contractions at any given force [8]. Eccentric contractions are also known to have higher force production, and the combination of high force and low fibre recruitment makes contractile proteins more susceptible to muscle damage because of increased mechanical stress applied per cross-bridge. When individuals are not accustomed to the eccentric exercise, muscle damage occurs. Muscle damage is observed by acute force loss during maximal voluntary contractions (MVC), and measurement of maximal voluntary force is considered the best method to establish muscle damage [9].

Because the exercise modality is related to breathing efficiency and downhill running known to be muscle-damaging exercise, it is possible that the ventilatory equivalents during level running and downhill running are different. Previous studies, using countermovement jumps [10] or squat exercise [11] to induce muscle damage, demonstrated increased ventilatory equivalents for O_2 48 h later. These observations clearly demonstrate that the presence of muscle damage influences breathing efficiency. The exact mechanisms for the decrease in breathing efficiency are unknown, yet are postulated to relate to the process of muscle damage. It is not known whether there is an acute effect of muscle-damaging exercise with primarily eccentric contractions on breathing efficiency.

Therefore, the aim of the present study was to examine the effects of muscle-damaging downhill treadmill running and non-damaging level treadmill running, matched for intensity on the ventilatory equivalents for O_2 and CO_2. It was hypothesized that the ventilator equivalents for O_2 and CO_2 would be higher for downhill treadmill running compared to level running at similar intensity.

2. Subjects and Methods

2.1. Participants

Nine healthy men (age 27 ± 9 years, height 179 ± 7 cm, body mass 75.3 ± 12.0 kg, $\dot{V}O_{2max}$ 52.0 ± 7.7 mL·kg^{-1}·min^{-1}) volunteered for the study and provided written informed consent. Participants were physically active, had within the last two months no activities with unaccustomed eccentric contractions of knee extensor muscles, and were free from musculoskeletal injury. The study was approved by the University of Chichester Research Ethics Committee with all procedures performed in accordance with the 1964 World Medical Association Declaration of Helsinki.

2.2. Study Design

Participants attended the laboratory for five visits, all completed at a similar time of the morning (<2 h difference). In brief, in the first visit, participants were familiarized for the performance of an isometric voluntary maximal contraction (iMVC) of the *m.quadriceps femoris* of both legs. In the same session, participants also completed an incremental submaximal treadmill (0% gradient) test for determination of level running speed and metabolic equivalent (MET) and a maximal oxygen uptake test ($\dot{V}O_{2max}$). In the second visit, participants arrived at the laboratory following a 12 h fast and sat resting for 10 min before a 10-min collection of expired gas for determination of the oxygen cost during quiet sitting (*i.e.*, resting metabolic equivalent, 1-MET, 3.1 ± 0.8 mL·kg^{-1}·min^{-1}, resting heart rate 57 ± 8 beats·min^{-1}). In the third visit, participants completed an incremental submaximal treadmill tests (−12% gradient) for determination of the relationship between downhill running speed and MET. In the fourth and fifth visit, performed at least 2 weeks later with at least 1 week between the 4th and 5th visit, participants performed 40 min level (0% gradient) and downhill (−12% gradient) running at 60% maximal MET, respectively. The same treadmill was used for all testing.

2.3. Maximal Voluntary Contraction

Force with isometric maximal voluntary contractions of the *m.quadriceps femoris* was assessed on a custom built chair (University of Chichester, Chichester, UK) with 90° hip and knee flexion. Participants were instructed to maintain upper body position during contractions of the *m.quadriceps femoris* which was facilitated with Velcro straps secured around the chest and waist. A cuff was positioned around the ankle of the participants (proximal to the fibular notch and medial malleolus) and attached via a steel chain to a s-beam load cell (RS 250 kg, Tedea-Huntleigh, Cardiff, UK). Participants received standard instructions in preparation of a maximal voluntary isometric contraction including strong verbal encouragement during the task [12]. Force was recorded on a computer with a sampling frequency of 1000 Hz using Chart 4 V4.1.2 (ADInstruments, Oxford, UK) and displayed at 1.5 m in front of the participants. Prior to performing the iMVC, participants performed three 5-second sub-maximal contractions (~200 N) to become accustomed to the experimental set up. Participants performed three voluntary maximal isometric contractions with the maximal isometric force quantified as the highest mean over a time period of 0.5 s. The highest force values were taken for analysis. Participants rested for 2 min between each maximal contraction. The measurement of iMVC was practiced in Visit 1 and performed immediately before and following the running bouts in Visits 4 and 5. Coefficient of variation of repeated maximal isometric force measurements was 4.6%.

2.4. Maximal Oxygen Consumption

Maximal oxygen uptake was established using an incremental exercise test on a motorized treadmill (HP Cosmos Pulsar, Bodycare Direct, Southam, UK). Expired gas samples were collected using Douglas Bags (Cranlea Human Performance Ltd., Birmingham, UK). Starting speed was 9 $km \cdot h^{-1}$ with a gradient of 1% [13]; the gradient was increased by $1\% \cdot min^{-1}$ during for the first five min after which speed was increased by 0.1 $km \cdot h^{-1}$ every five seconds until the participant reached volitional exhaustion. Expired gas was collected in separate bags for the last 3-min of the test. The last collection bag was only analyzed when collection time and expired volume was greater than 30 s and 65 L, respectively. Expired and inspired fractions of oxygen and carbon dioxide were measured using a gas analyzer (Series 1400 gas analyzer, Servomex, Crowborough, UK), calibrated using three- and two-point calibration for oxygen and carbon dioxide, respectively (Linde Gas UK Ltd., West Bromwich, UK) and volumes measured with a calibrated Harvard dry gas meter (Harvard Apparatus Ltd., Edenbridge, UK). Volumes were standardized to STPD conditions and Haldane transformation used for calculation of gas volumes. Participants $\dot{V}O_{2max}$ was converted in MET (*i.e.*, maximal MET, 16.7 ± 5.8) to allow intensity matching of running for experimental Visits 4 and 5.

2.5. Level and Downhill Running

The level (0% gradient) and downhill (−12% gradient) running bouts in Visits 4 and 5 were performed following an overnight fast. For all participants, in Visits 1 and 3, the MET value for level and downhill running at speeds of 8, 9, 10 and 11 $km \cdot h^{-1}$ (each speed for 5 min) were measured. Subsequently, the relationship between running speed and MET was calculated with linear regression to allow matched-intensity exercise for level and downhill running. Exercise intensity for the 40 min level and downhill running (*i.e.*, 5 stages of 8-min with 2-min rest between stages) was set at 60% maximal MET with heart rate recording. In the last minute of each 8-min stage, expired gas was collected using the Douglas Bag technique and similar techniques for analysis and calculations were used as for the expired air samples collected during the maximum oxygen uptake test. The heart rate at end of each expired air collection was recorded (FS1, Polar, Kempele, Finland).

2.6. Statistical Analysis

All statistical analyses were completed using SPSS 20.0 (SPSS, Chicago, IL, USA). Sample size was based on mean ± SD for ventilatory equivalent for oxygen at 60% P_{max} [10] (alpha error level is 0.05 and statistical power is 0.8) to detect a 4% difference in the downhill running group. Data normality assumptions were assessed using Kolmogorov-Smirnov test. A two-way ANOVA (time and condition) was used to examine the difference in force of the iMVC, with differences located with pre-planned Bonferroni corrected paired samples *t*-tests. For the five expired air collections during each level and downhill running bout, oxygen consumption, respiratory exchange ratio, and ventilatory equivalents for oxygen and carbon dioxide were calculated, averaged and analyzed with a paired sample *t*-test.

Heart rate measured during the expired air collections were averaged and analyzed with a paired sample t-test. All data are reported as mean ± SD and significance was set at alpha level of $p < 0.05$.

3. Results

3.1. Isometric Force of Knee Extensors

The force during iMVC at baseline for both conditions were not different (downhill: 571 ± 97, level: 568 ± 99 N, $p > 0.05$). The maximal isometric force was not different immediately following level running (Post: 554 ± 94 N, $p > 0.05$), but was reduced following downhill running (Post: 467 ± 200 N, $p < 0.05$). The decrease in force for the iMVC was 17.2 ± 7.6% after downhill running.

3.2. Level and Downhill Running Comparison

The running speed was higher for downhill running (downhill: 13.5 ± 3.2, level: 9.6 ± 2.2 km·h^{-1}, $p < 0.05$). Downhill and level running bouts had $\dot{V}O_2$ (2.20 ± 0.33 *vs.* 2.28 ± 0.51 L·min^{-1}, $p > 0.05$), $\dot{V}CO_2$ (2.0 ± 0.3 *vs.* 2.0 ± 0.5 L·min^{-1}, $p > 0.05$), respiratory exchange ratio (RER) (0.89 ± 0.05 *vs.* 0.89 ± 0.03, $p > 0.05$) and heart rates (147 ± 19 *vs.* 143 ± 16 beats·min^{-1}, $p > 0.05$) that were not different indicating matched intensity and metabolic demands.

Figure 1a,b show the ventilatory equivalents for O_2 and CO_2 for downhill and level running, respectively. Ventilatory equivalents for O_2 (downhill: 29.7 ± 3.3, level: 27.2 ± 1.6, $p < 0.05$) and CO_2 (downhill: 33.2 ± 2.7, level: 30.4 ± 1.9, $p < 0.05$) were 7.1% and 8.3% higher for downhill running, respectively.

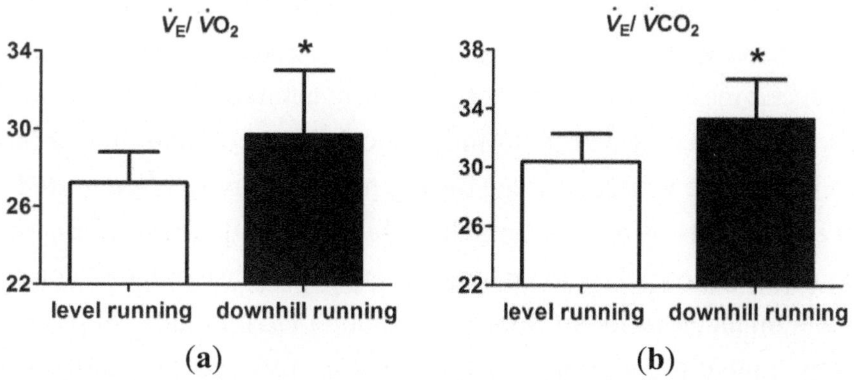

Figure 1. (**a**) Ventilatory equivalent for oxygen during intensity matched level and downhill running at 60% of maximal MET. Values are mean ± SD. * indicates the ventilatory equivalent is significantly elevated in the downhill compared to the level running condition ($p < 0.05$); (**b**) Ventilatory equivalent for carbon dioxide during intensity matched level and downhill running at 60% of maximal MET. Values are mean ± SD. * indicates the ventilatory equivalent is significantly elevated in the downhill compared to the level running condition ($p < 0.05$).

4. Discussion

The major finding of the present study was that whole-body moderate intensity exercise (*i.e.*, 60% of maximal MET) with primarily eccentric contractions of *m.quadriceps femoris* (*i.e.*, downhill running) was performed with lower breathing efficiency than matched-intensity exercise with primarily concentric contractions (*i.e.*, level running). Similarity in physiological ($\dot{V}O_2$, $\dot{V}CO_2$, and heart rate) and metabolic responses (*i.e.*, RER) confirmed that the level and downhill running bouts were performed with matched intensity and metabolic demands. The successful matching of exercise intensities resulted in a higher downhill running speed as the oxygen demand during downhill running is normally less than that for level running at the same speed [14]. Downhill running resulted in substantial isometric force deficits of the *m.quadriceps femoris* (17 ± 7.6%), which is comparable to other studies using downhill running [15–17]. For both running bouts, the ability of participants to produce maximal isometric force was measured immediately post-exercise suggesting that fatigue may have caused some of the force deficits. However, because the bout of level running did not affect the ability to produce maximal isometric force, this supports the suggestion that the force deficits following the downhill running bout were primarily the result of muscle damage.

Reduced breathing efficiency during moderate-intensity muscle-damaging downhill running exercise may be related to different mechanical and neural events compared to non-damaging level running. Interestingly, analysis of the ventilatory equivalents over time during the running bouts indicated a time effect for the ventilatory equivalent for CO_2 for both level and downhill running (unpublished observations). In general, cardiovascular and ventilatory adaptations during exercise may result from responding to mechanical distortion or metabolic by-products from exercising skeletal muscle through thinly myelinated (group III) and unmyelinated (group IV) muscle afferents [18]. Because the exercise intensity was matched for level and downhill running bouts, greater mechanical distortion from the higher downhill running speed may have occurred, as eccentric contractions are also known to produce higher forces. Group III afferents are sensitive to mechanical distortion and have a large response to muscle stretch [19]. In addition, the ventilation rate during muscle activity is suggested to be related to activity of group III and IV afferents by distension of blood vessels [20]. This observation can be linked with potential disruption of the microcirculation during eccentric exercise induced muscle damage [21], and this could have resulted in an elevation of minute ventilation [22]. Finally, impairment of group III and IV muscle afferents by lumbar intrathecal fentanyl injections reduced the ventilatory equivalent for CO_2 during steady state cycling [23], thus damage-inducing downhill running exercise may occur with elevated discharge of group III and IV afferents, in turn elevating the ventilatory equivalents for O_2 and CO_2. Therefore, it is possible in the present study that the type III and IV afferents had increased discharge during downhill running affecting the ventilatory response. This neurophysiological response is further supported by the observation that contraction type during fatiguing tasks can affect group III and IV afferent fibres after the activity, with eccentric contractions affecting afferent activity more than concentric contractions [24]. Additional support of increased afferent discharge may come from the perception of muscle discomfort experienced during the downhill running. All participants reported increased muscle discomfort during the downhill running, while no such reports were given during the level running. The muscle discomfort may provide a stimulus for the ventilatory response via mechanical stimulation of nociceptive muscle afferents [25,26] with a large number of group IV afferents also being nociceptors [27].

It needs to be acknowledged that no measurements of breathing frequency and tidal volume were taken. It cannot be excluded that higher breathing frequency values during downhill running may have resulted in reduced tidal volume, increased dead space volume and inefficient alveolar ventilation. Such respiratory events could explain the higher ventilatory equivalents for downhill running.

5. Conclusions

This is the first study to examine the breathing efficiency during intensity-matched whole-body dynamic exercise with primarily eccentric and concentric contractions at moderate intensity (*i.e.*, 60% of maximal MET). Future work should examine the breathing efficiency at low and high exercise intensities of matched-intensity non muscle-damaging and muscle-damaging running protocols. It would also be of interest to examine the breathing efficiency of level and downhill running at similar speeds. In addition, it would be of interest to examine the discharge patterns of group III and IV afferents for matched-intensity whole-body dynamic exercise. It is concluded that breathing is less efficient during muscle damage-inducing downhill treadmill running at moderate intensity than intensity matched level treadmill running. These findings may have implications when using downhill treadmill exercise in clinical populations with respiratory diseases where breathing efficiency is already compromised.

Author Contributions

All authors were involved in study design, data collection, data interpretation, and manuscript writing. Willems and Cook were involved in data analysis.

Conflicts of Interest

The authors declare no conflict of interest.

References

1. Cooper, C.B.; Storer, T.W. *Exercise and Testing and Interpretation: A Practical Guide*; Cambridge University Press: Cambridge, UK, 2001.
2. Ofir, D.; Laveneziana, P.; Webb, K.A.; Lam, Y.M.; O'Donnell, D.E. Sex differences in the perceived intensity of breathlessness during exercise with advancing age. *J. Appl. Physiol.* **2007**, *104*, 1583–1593.
3. Rasmussen, B.; Klausen, K.; Clausen, J.P.; Trap-Jensen, J. Pulmonary ventilation, blood gases, and blood pH after training of the arms or the legs. *J. Appl. Physiol.* **1975**, *38*, 250–256.
4. Armstrong, N.; Davies, B. An ergometric analysis of age group swimmers. *Br. J. Sports Med.* **1981**, *15*, 20–26.
5. Laursen, P.B.; Rhodes, E.C.; Langill, R.H.; Taunton, J.E.; McKenzie, D.C. Exercise-induced arterial hypoxemia is not different during cycling and running in triathletes. *Scand. J. Med. Sci. Sports* **2005**, *15*, 113–117.

6. Gavin, T.P.; Stager, J.M. The effect of exercise modality on exercise-induced hypoxemia. *Respir. Physiol.* **1999**, *115*, 317–323.
7. Minetti, A.E.; Moia, C.; Roi, G.S.; Susta, D.; Ferretti, G. Energy cost of walking and running at extreme uphill and downhill slopes. *J. Appl. Physiol.* **2002**, *93*, 1039–1046.
8. Bigland-Ritchie, B.; Woods, J.J. Integrated electromyogram and oxygen uptake during positive and negative work. *J. Physiol.* **1976**, *260*, 267–277.
9. Warren, G.L.; Lowe, D.A.; Armstrong, R.B. Measurement tools used in the study of eccentric contraction-induced injury. *Sports Med.* **1999**, *27*, 43–59.
10. Twist, C.; Eston, R.G. The effect of exercise-induced muscle damage on perceived exertion and cycling endurance performance. *Eur. J. Appl. Physiol.* **2009**, *105*, 559–567.
11. Davies, R.C.; Eston, R.G.; Poole, D.C.; Rowlands, A.V.; DiMenna, F.; Wilkerson, D.P.; Twist, C.; Jones, A.M. Effect of eccentric exercise-induced muscle damage on the dynamics of muscle oxygenation and pulmonary oxygen uptake. *J. Appl. Physiol.* **2008**, *105*, 1413–1421.
12. Gandevia, S.C. Spinal and supraspinal factors in human muscle fatigue. *Physiol. Rev.* **2001**, *81*, 1725–1789.
13. Jones, A.M.; Doust, J.H. A 1% treadmill grade most accurately reflects the energetic cost of outdoor running. *J. Sport Sci.* **1996**, *14*, 321–327.
14. Robergs, R.A.; Wagner, D.R.; Skemp, K.M. Oxygen consumption and energy expenditure of level versus downhill running. *J. Sports Med. Phys. Fitness* **1997**, *37*, 168–174.
15. Eston, R.G.; Lemmey, A.B.; McHugh, P.; Byrne, C.; Walsh, S.E. Effect of stride length on symptoms of exercise-induced muscle damage during a repeated bout of downhill running. *Scand. J. Med. Sci. Sports* **2000**, *10*, 199–204.
16. Chen, T.C.; Nosaka, K.; Tu, J.H. Changes in running economy following downhill running. *J. Sports Sci.* **2007**, *25*, 55–63.
17. Green, M.S.; Doyle, J.A.; Ingalls, C.P.; Benardot, D.; Rupp, J.C.; Corona, B.T. Adaptation of insulin-resistance indicators to a repeated bout of eccentric exercise in human skeletal muscle. *Int. J. Sport Nutr. Exerc. Metab.* **2010**, *20*, 181–190.
18. Kaufman, M.P.; Hayes, S.G.; Adreani, C.M.; Pickar, J.G. Discharge properties of group III and IV muscle afferents. *Adv. Exp. Med. Biol.* **2002**, *508*, 25–32.
19. Kaufman, M.P.; Longhurst, J.C.; Rybicki, K.J.; Wallach, J.H.; Mitchell, J.H. Effects of static muscular contraction on impulse activity of groups III and IV afferents in cats. *J. Appl. Physiol. Respir. Environ. Exerc. Physiol.* **1983**, *55*, 105–112.
20. Haouzi, P. Tracking pulmonary gas exchange by breathing control during exercise: Role of muscle blood flow muscle blood flow. *J. Physiol.* **2014**, *592*, 453–461.
21. Kano, Y.; Padilla, D.J.; Behnke, B.J.; Hageman, K.S.; Musch, T.I.; Poole, D.C. Effects of eccentric exercise on microcirculation and microvascular oxygen pressures in rat spinotrapezius muscle. *J. Appl. Physiol.* **2005**, *99*, 1516–1522.
22. Haouzi, P.; Chenuel, B.; Huszczuk, A. Sensing vascular distension in skeletal muscle by slow conducting afferent fibers: Neurophysiological basis and implication for respiratory control. *J. Appl. Physiol.* **2004**, *96*, 407–418.

23. Amann, M.; Blain, G.M.; Proctor, L.T.; Sebranek, J.J.; Pegelow, D.F.; Dempsey, J.A. Group III and IV muscle afferents contribute to ventilatory and cardiovascular response to rhythmic exercise in humans. *J. Appl. Physiol.* **2010**, *109*, 966–976.
24. Martin, V.; Dousset, E.; Laurin, J.; Gondin, J.; Gautier, M.; Decherchi, P. Group III and IV muscle afferent discharge patterns after repeated lengthening and shortening actions. *Muscle Nerve* **2009**, *40*, 827–837.
25. Duranti, R.; Pantaleo, T.; Bellini, F.; Bongianni, F.; Scano, G. Respiratory responses induced by the activation of somatic nociceptive afferents in humans. *J. Appl. Physiol.* **1991**, *71*, 2440–2448.
26. Gleeson, M.; Blannin, A.K.; Walsh, N.P.; Field, C.N.; Pritchard, J.C. Effect of exercise-induced muscle damage on the blood lactate response to incremental exercise in humans. *Eur. J. Appl. Physiol. Occup. Physiol.* **1998**, *77*, 292–295.
27. Mense, S. Nociception from skeletal muscle in relation to clinical muscle pain. *Pain* **1993**, *54*, 241–289.

12

Relationship between the Pedaling Biomechanics and Strain of Bicycle Frame during Submaximal Tests

Aneliya V. Manolova, Samuel Crequy †, Philippe Lestriez †, Pierre Debraux and William M. Bertucci *

Groupe de Recherche En Sciences Pour l'Ingénieur (GRESPI, EA4694), Université de Reims-Champagne-Ardenne (URCA), Moulin de la Housse 51687 Reims cedex 2, France; E-Mails: aneliya.manolova@sci-sport.com (A.V.M.); samuel.crequy@univ-reims.fr (S.C.); philippe.lestriez@univ-reims.fr (P.L.); pierre.debraux@sci-sport.com (P.D.)

† These authors contributed equally to this work.

* Author to whom correspondence should be addressed; E-Mail: william.bertucci@univ-reims.fr;

Academic Editor: Eling de Bruin

Abstract: The aim of this study was to analyse the effect of forces applied to pedals and cranks on the strain imposed to an instrumented bicycle motocross (BMX) frame. Using results from a finite element analysis to determine the localisation of highest stress, eight strain gauges were located on the down tube, the seat tube and the right chain stay. Before the pedaling tests, static loads were applied to the frame during bench tests. Two pedaling conditions have been analysed. In the first, the rider was in static standing position on the pedals and applied maximal muscular isometric force to the right pedal. The second pedaling condition corresponds to three pedaling sprint tests at submaximal intensities at 150, 300 and 550 W on a cycle-trainer. The results showed that smaller strain was observed in the pedaling condition than in the rider static standing position condition. The highest strains were located in the seat tube and the right chain stay near the bottom bracket area. The maximum stress observed through all conditions was 41 MPa on the right chain stay. This stress was 11 times lower than the yield stress of the frame material (460 MPa). This protocol could help to adapt the frame design to the riders as a function of their force and mechanical power output. These results could also help design BMX frames for specific populations (females) and rider morphology.

Keywords: biomechanics; cycling; BMX frame; pedal forces

1. Introduction

Bicycle Motocross (BMX) racing was introduced at the 2008 Olympics Games in Beijing, China. The BMX race takes place on a specific track of 300 to 400 m with jumps and berms. The start is stationary on top of an inclined ramp (starting hill). It is followed by a straight line of 40 m long before the first obstacle. During the race, it is difficult to overtake opponents and the position of the riders at the end of the straight line usually determines the final order [1–4]. Thus, an explosive start is required to succeed. As a result of this explosive start, the forces applied to the pedals and the mechanical power output during the first straight line can be high, with peak power output in excess of 2000 W for high-level male athletes [5,6].

2. Context

The transfer of the mechanical energy produced by the rider from the pedal to the rear wheel is achieved by the bicycle frame [7]. The frame is the main component of a bicycle; it provides a structural function by linking the various mechanical parts, and supports the rider. A highly efficient frame has to deliver the mechanical power output of the rider to the drive train while minimizing energy loss due to the strain [8].

Watt *et al.* [9] showed that a significant positive correlation exists between the power output and the strain observed in the bicycle frame. Under high-level BMX race conditions, the frame is expected to experience high levels of strain due to the elevated power output. To develop frames capable of efficiently transferring mechanical power, it is necessary to analyse frame response as a function of the force applied to the pedals during all pedaling conditions (standing position, isometric muscular contraction, *etc.*). The use of 3-axis dynamometric pedals allows measurement of the forces directly applied by the cyclist to the pedals and cranks (Figure 1). Providing information on the relationship between forces applied to the pedals and resultant tube strain could be useful to optimise the BMX frame design. In fact, since BMX racing became an Olympic sport, no study has focused on whether the current BMX frame design is optimised for racing at this level. In high-level competitions, races can be won or lost in 0.01 s. Additional research has ascertained that the margin between 1st and 2nd place in the 2012 BMX world cup series was 0.49 ± 0.36 s [10]. Clearly, any optimisation of the frame could be an important factor in future world championships or Olympics games. The major aim of this study was to discuss of the optimisation of bicycle frames from analysis of the relationship between local frame loads measured on an instrumented BMX and pedal forces applied by a rider measured by 3-axis dynamometric pedals in different conditions.

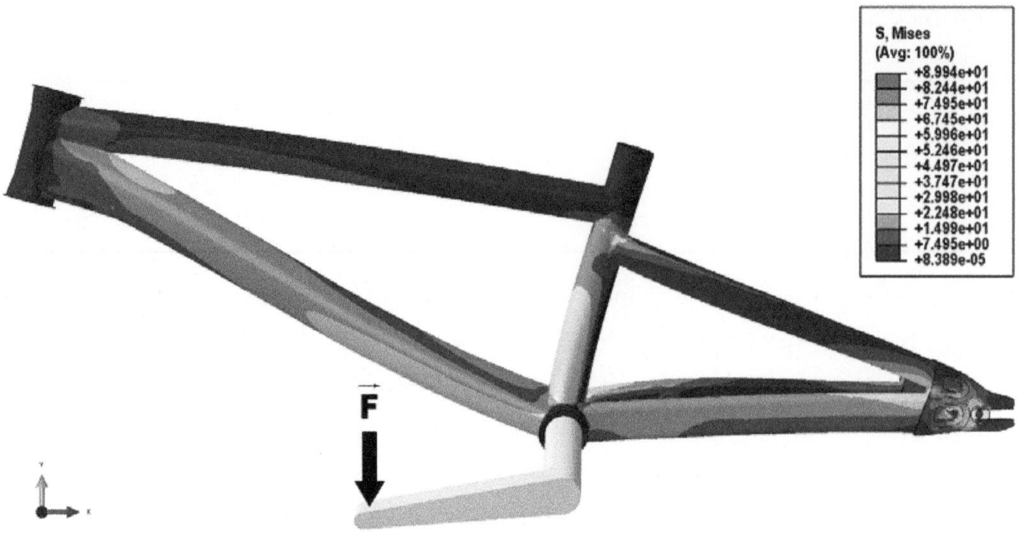

Figure 1. Stress (von Mises) analysis performed with finite element analysis to identify the location of higher strain in the frame.

3. Method

3.1. Participant and Procedures

One competitive male cyclist of national level (age = 24 years, body mass = 77.5 kg, body height = 1.75 m) volunteered as a participant for this study. The cyclist read and signed an informed consent form prior to his involvement in the study. This research was approved by our academic Human Subjects Review Committee and in accordance with the Declaration of Helsinki.

To study the influence of the applied forces on the frame strain, different tests were conducted: (1) A bar system was designed to simulate the forces applied to the pedals by the rider in static standing condition; (2) the BMX bicycle was placed on a cycle-trainer and the rider applied a maximal muscular isometric force on one pedal (during this exercise, the rider had his hands on the handlebars); and (3) the rider performed three submaximal pedaling exercises at the following different pedaling cadences 60, 100 and 200 revolutions per minute (revs·min^{-1}), corresponding to a mean power output at the crank of 150, 300 and 550 W, respectively.

3.2. Instrumentation of the Frame with Strain Gauges

To quantify the strain during the different conditions of this protocol, the BMX frame (aluminum alloy 7005) was fitted with eight uniaxial strain gauges (CEA-13-125UN-350, Vishay Measurements, France). The gauge had lengths of 3.18 mm and a nominal resistance of 350% ± 0.3% Ω. At 24 °C, the gauge factor and transverse sensitivity were 2.125% ± 0.5% and 0.5% ± 0.2%, respectively.

In order to place the strain gauges on the BMX frame, a finite element analysis was performed to locate the areas of highest strain. A numerical model of the frame was designed using Pro/ENGINEER® Wildfire™ 2.0, PTC, USA. All dimensions of the framework components (lengths and diameters of tubes) were measured using a caliper (±0.01 mm sensitivity). The welds were not taken into account. The 3D model of the BMX frame was imported into a finite element analysis software package

(ABAQUS™, SIMULIA, Dassault Systems, France). A mesh was created consisting of 184,091 nodes and 646,209 tetrahedral 3D elements to four nodes (C3D4-Abaqus). This mesh permitted the study of the exact locations of the strain gauges on the frame. The material used in this modeling is an aluminum alloy whose main characteristics (Young's modulus (E) of 72,000 MPa and a Poisson's ratio (v) of 0.33) were similar to the BMX frame alloy (Aluminum 7005).

The finite element analysis consisted of applying a force of 1200 N on a system with two lever arms fixed in the center of the bottom bracket to represent the crank (Figure 1). The lever arms lengths were 0.14 and 0.175 m. The frame was fixed at the head tube and the axis of the rear wheels with zero degrees of freedom. The areas with the highest strain are shown in Figure 1.

With respect to the finite element analysis results, the eight strain gauges used in this study were placed on the frame as shown in Figure 2. The gauges were fixed according to the recommendations of the manufacturer (CEA-13-125UN-350, Vishay Measurements, France). Three pairs of gauges were located on the top of the down tube, on the left lateral side of the seat tube, and on the medial side of the right chain stay. Gauges were paired, with one placed parallel to the axis of the tube to analyse the strain in tension/compression, and the other oriented at 45° to the axis of the tube to analyse the strain in torsion. The gauges were located to have at least 30 mm of clearance from the weld. This distance was chosen to avoid strain concentrations at the joints and a changing strain field under the strain gauges [11].

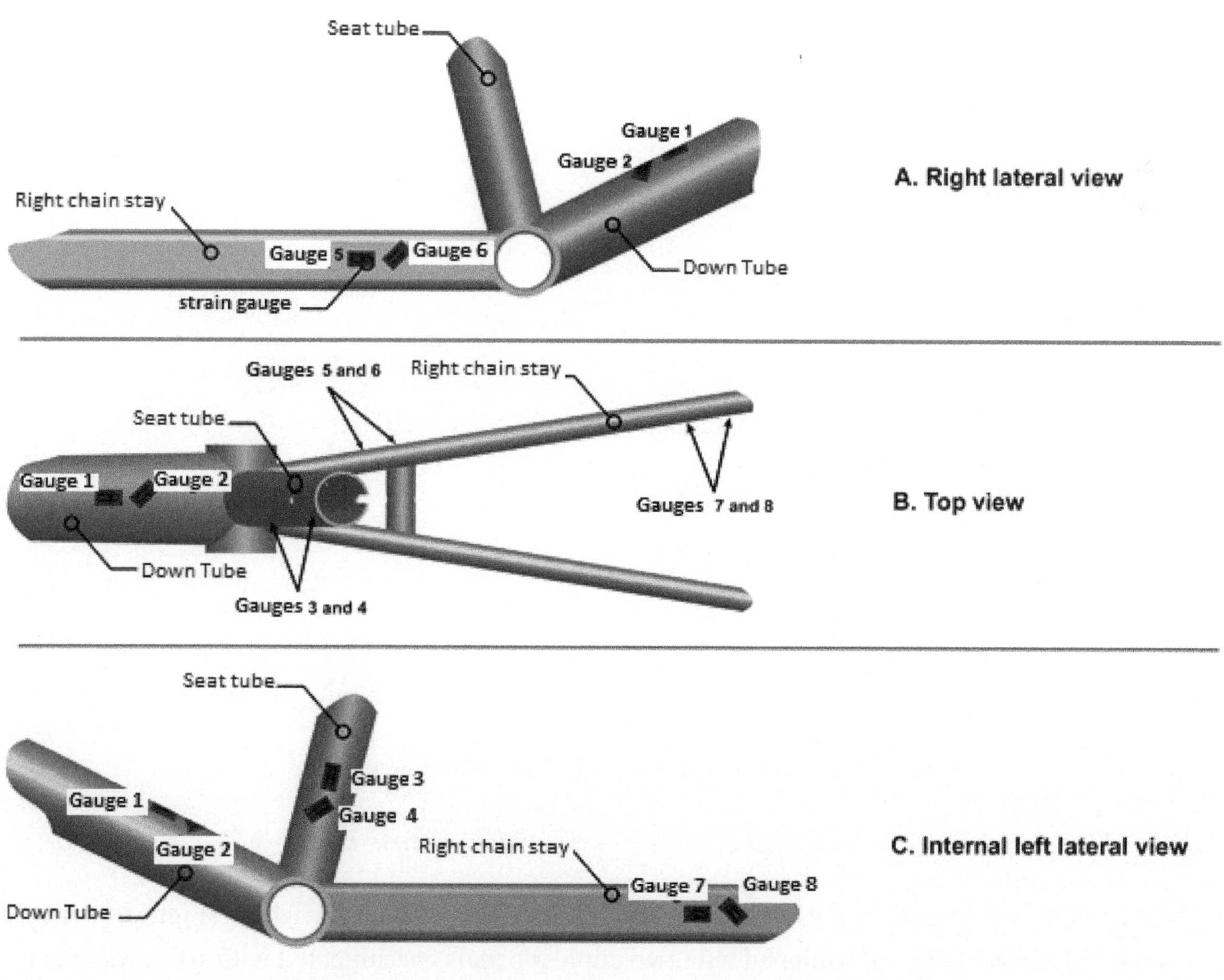

Figure 2. Strain gauge locations on the BMX frame.

3.3. Static Experiment

The bicycle frame instrumented with strain gauges was mounted on a test bench with boundary conditions (0 degree of freedom) at the front and rear of the frame. To simulate the perpendicular force applied at the pedal by the rider during pedaling, a system of two manufactured bars (Steel XC 38) was designed and screwed into the bottom bracket. This bar system (Figure 3) represents the two lever arms (*i.e.*, crank arm and pedal) applied during the pedaling. The bar that was screwed directly into the bottom bracket, and which is transversal to the frame, represents the distance perpendicular to the frame between the point of force application on the pedal and the center of the bottom bracket (0.14 m). The second bar, parallel to the frame and to the ground, represents the crank length (0.175 m). To simulate perpendicular forces applied on a right pedal by a rider under actual conditions from 40 to 880 N (Personal data), loads from 1 to 18 kg were applied on the bar system (on the right side of the frame) using a steel cable and the resultant strain was recorded. In this test configuration, a load of 18 kg in the bench test corresponds to a force of 880 N applied perpendicularly to the BMX pedal. In the present study, we have chosen to test extreme condition and we have used a maximal load up to 21 kg that corresponds at a perpendicularly pedal force of 1044 N and a crank torque of 179 N.m.

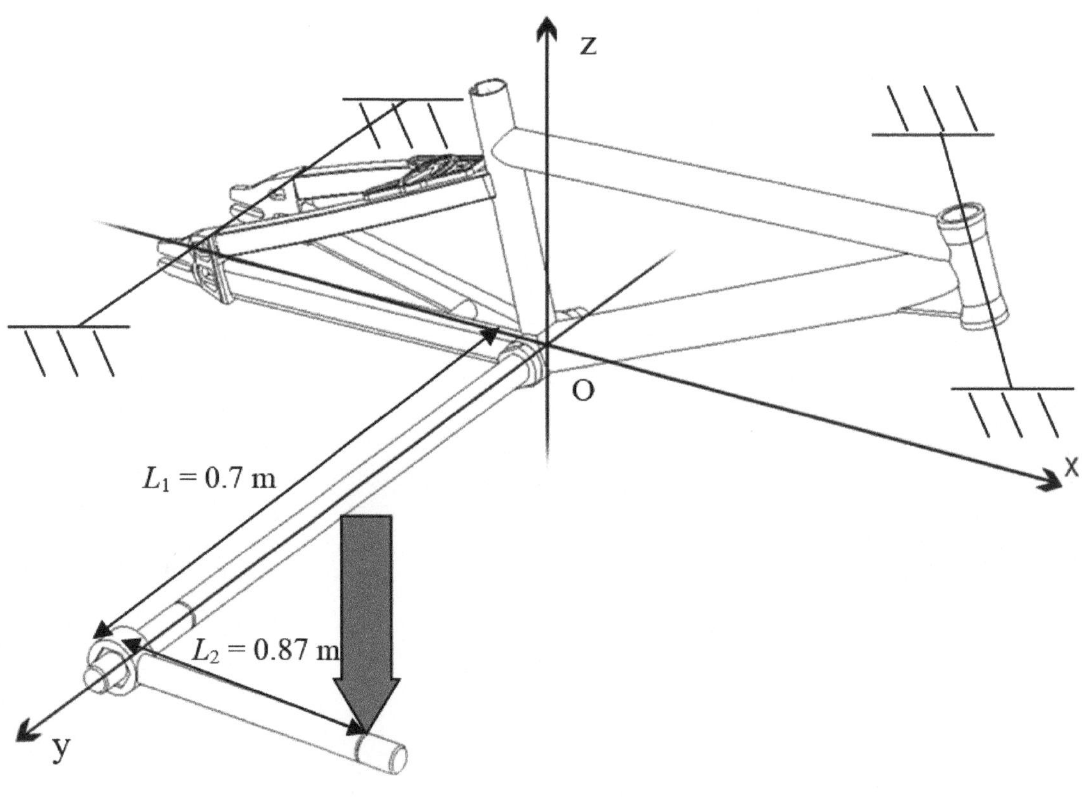

Figure 3. BMX frame during the static bench test.

3.4. Maximal Muscular Isometric Force Applied on a 3-Axis Dynamometric Pedal

The BMX bicycle was placed on a cycle-trainer through the axis of the rear wheel (Figure 4). The bicycle was leveled horizontally and equipped with two clipless pedals instrumented with six-component force sensors (Sensix, France). The sampling frequency of these sensors was 250 Hz. These pedals measured antero-posterior and vertical forces applied on the right pedal (F_{XP} and F_{ZP}, in N) and the right crank (F_{XC} and F_{ZC}, in N) as a function of time. During the trials, the strain as a function of time was recorded with the help of a computer and a dynamic data acquisition system (Model 5100A scanner, Vishay Instruments Division, France) whose sampling frequency was 10 Hz. The rider in standing position was instructed to apply a maximal muscular isometric force on the right pedal. During this exercise, the rider had his hands on the handlebars as in actual conditions. In order to compare the results with the experimental static condition, the cranks (0.175 m) were horizontal, with the right pedal forward. In standing pedaling, the maximal force is applied to the pedal when the angle of the crank is about 140 degrees forward [12]. However, to allow a maximal muscular isometric force to be applied, the rider had to place the crank in a horizontal position allowing a better configuration for the muscular length of the right leg. The rear wheel was locked. The rider was wearing shoes with an automatic attachment system (*i.e.*, clipless pedals). The inflation pressure for the front and rear tires were 200 and 250 kPa, respectively.

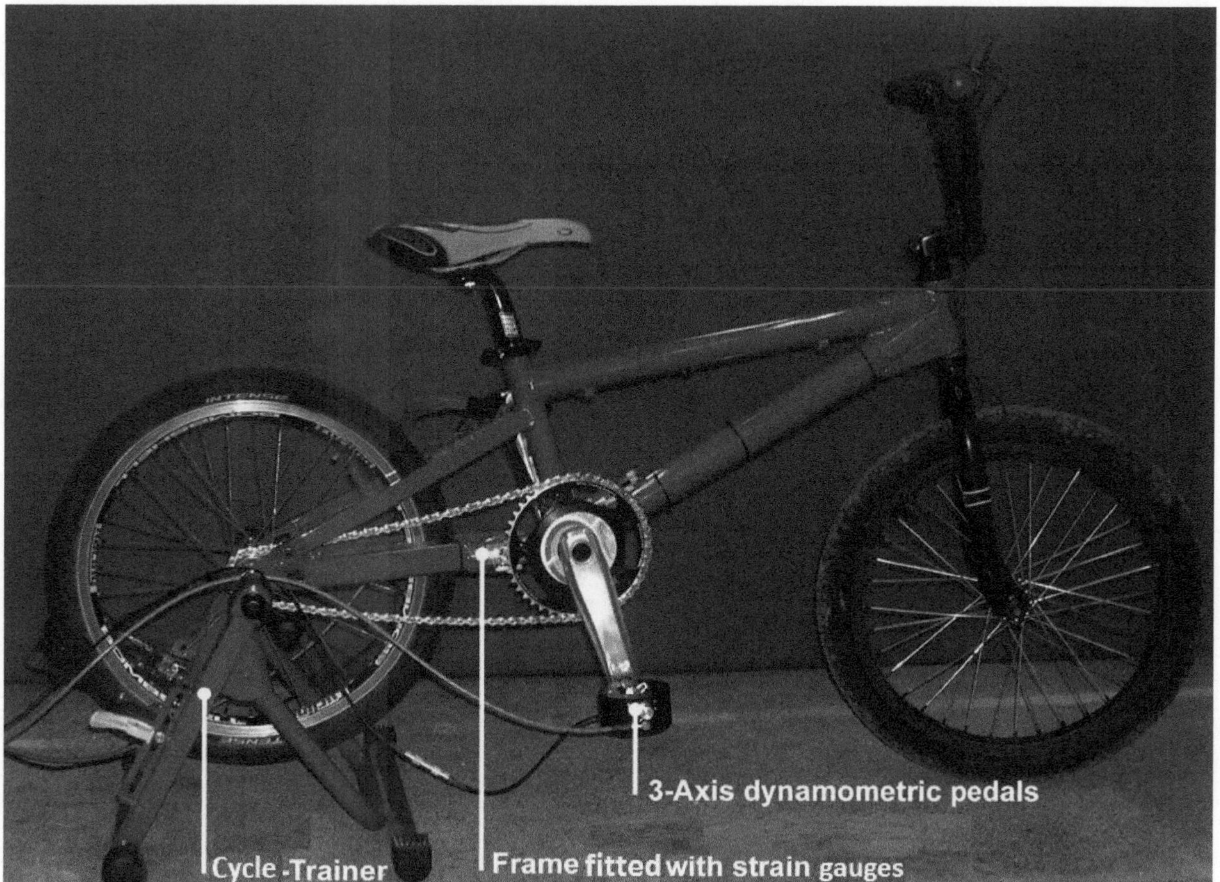

Figure 4. BMX bike on cycle-trainer with 3-axis dynamometric pedals and a frame with strain gauges.

3.5. Pedaling Tests on a Cycle-Trainer

On the cycle-trainer with the same equipment as described previously, the rider pedaled for 10 s in steady-state while in a standing position on the 3-axis dynamometric pedals. The rider was instructed to pedal at three different submaximal intensities: 150, 300 and 550 W at a mean pedaling cadence of 60,

100 and 200 revs·min^{-1}, respectively. Power outputs (W) and pedaling cadences were monitored using a BMX powermeter (SRM Training system, Schoberer Rad Messtechnik, Germany). In order to study the influence of the applied forces by the rider on the frame during pedaling, the vertical and antero-posterior forces were applied on the pedals (F_{ZP} and F_{XP}, respectively) and on the cranks (F_{ZC} and F_{XC}, respectively) and the frame strains were simultaneously measured as a function of time.

3.6. Statistical Analyses

A matrix of Pearson product-moment correlation coefficients (r) was used to determine the significance between the right peak F_{ZP}, F_{ZC}, F_{XP}, F_{XC}, the mechanical power output and the peak strain during the pedaling tests on the cycle-trainer. This correlation matrix was performed using the software Statistica 7.1 (StatSoft, France). The significance level was set at $p < 0.05$. Data are presented as mean values ± SD.

4. Results

For the static test, the strain increased with applied force (Figure 5). Strain gauges 2, 5, 7 and 8 measured strain in compression, and gauges 1, 3, and 6 measured strain in tension. The highest strains were recorded on the seat tube (gauge 3), the down tube (gauge 1) and the internal rear right chain stay (gauge 7), with maximal values of 468, 185 and 180 μm/m, respectively (Table 1).

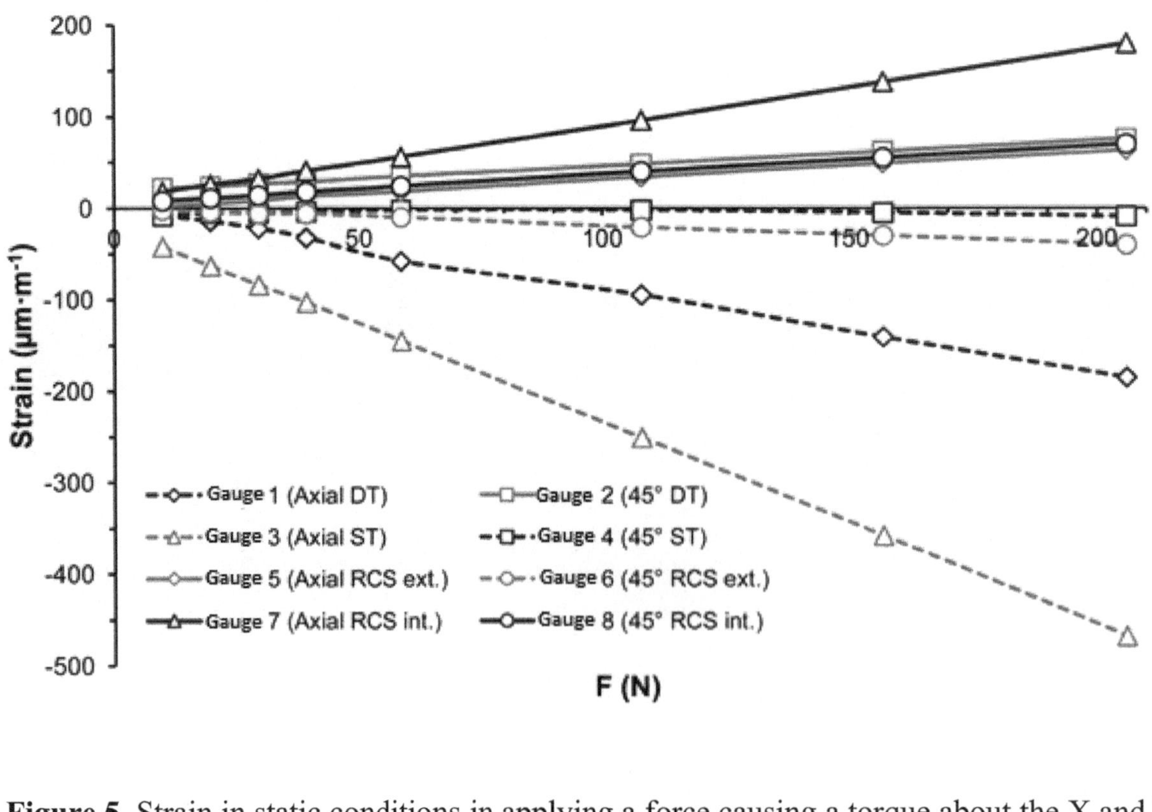

Figure 5. Strain in static conditions in applying a force causing a torque about the X and Y axes. DT: Down Tube; ST: Seat Tube; RCS: Right Chain Stay; ext.: external; int.: internal. Positive and negative values represent compression and tension, respectively.

Table 1. Maximum strain and stress measured with strain gauges placed on a bicycle motocross (BMX) frame for different conditions.

	Bar System		**Maximal isometric force**		**Pedaling tests**	
	Strain ($\mu m \cdot m^{-1}$)	Stress (MPa)	Strain ($\mu m \cdot m^{-1}$)	Stress (MPa)	Strain ($\mu m \cdot m^{-1}$)	Stress (MPa)
Gauge 1 (Axial DT)	185^T	13.3	52^T	3.7	6^C	0.4
Gauge 2 (45° DT)	76^C	5.5	328^C	23.6	69^T	5
Gauge 3 (Axial ST)	468^T	33.7	408^T	29.4	301^C	21.7
Gauge 4 (45° ST)	9^T	0.6	42^C	3	48^T	3.5
Gauge 5 (Axial RCS ext.)	63^C	4.5	573^T	41.3	58^C	4.2
Gauge 6 (45° RCS ext.)	40^T	2.9	316^T	22.7	62^C	4.5
Gauge 7 (Axial RCS int.)	180^C	13	221^T	15.9	155^T	11.2
Gauge 8 (45° RCS int.)	70^C	5	32^C	2.3	22^T	1.6

DT: Down Tube; ST: Seat Tube; RCS: Right Chain Stay; ext.: external; int.: internal; ^{T}: Tension; ^{C}: Compression.

For the maximal muscular isometric effort on the right pedal, F_{ZP} and F_{ZC} (vertical forces applied on the right pedal and right crank, respectively) reached maximal peak force of 1344 N and 1035 N (Figure 6A,B), respectively. At $t = 0.6$ s, the rider started to apply a muscular isometric force on the pedal until the maximal force was reached. The frame strains (Figure 6C) increased with F_{ZP} and F_{ZC}, except for gauge 7, located in the rear of the right chain stay. Three gauges measured strain in compression (gauges 2, 4 and 8), and five gauges measured strain in tension (gauges 1, 3, 5, 6 and 7). The largest strains were recorded on the right chain stay (gauges 5, 6 and 7), the seat tube (gauge 3) and the down tube (gauge 2). The maximal strain values recorded were 573, 408, 328, 316 and 221 $\mu m \cdot m^{-1}$ for gauges 5, 3, 2, 6 and 7, respectively (Table 1).

For the pedaling tests on the cycle-trainer, we observed that F_{ZP}, F_{ZC} and the peak strains were the highest during the 200 revs·min^{-1} pedaling cadence condition (Table 2). Figure 7 illustrates three cycles during each condition with the corresponding frame strain. For each pedaling condition, gauge 3 (seat tube) and gauge 7 (internal right chain stay) recorded the highest strains. The Figure 8 shows the linear regression of the mean strain of a BMX frame as function of the mean mechanical power output during pedaling on a cycle-trainer.

The matrix of Pearson product-moment correlation coefficients show that F_{ZP}, F_{XP}, F_{ZC}, F_{XC} and P during pedaling tests were significantly correlated with the frame strain for almost all gauges (Table 3). No correlation has been observed with the strain in gauge 1 (down tube), between F_{ZP} and the strain in gauge 5 (external right chain stay) and between power output and the strain in gauge 8 (internal right chain stay).

Table 2. Mean values (SD) of the forces applied to the right pedal and crank during pedaling tests on a cycle-trainer. All forces are in N, and strains in $\mu m \cdot m^{-1}$.

	Pedaling Conditions		
	60 rpm 150 W	100 rpm 300 W	200 rpm 500 W
F_{ZP}	449 ± 9	556 ± 22	1177 ± 45
F_{XP}	18 ± 8	18 ± 2	41 ± 9
F_{ZC}	388 ± 53	271 ± 156	970 ± 51
F_{XC}	210 ± 89	466 ± 74	667 ± 24
Gauge 1 (Axial DT)	5 ± 1	5 ± 1	6 ± 3
Gauge 2 (45° Axial DT)	30 ± 5	36 ± 5	69 ± 30
Gauge 3 (Axial ST)	73 ± 3	132 ± 6	301 ± 25
Gauge 4 (45° ST)	18 ± 2	36 ± 3	48 ± 5
Gauge 5 (Axial RCS ext.)	23 ± 1	41 ± 7	58 ± 25
Gauge 6 (45° RCS ext.)	17 ± 2	30 ± 7	62 ± 8
Gauge 7 (Axial RCS int.)	43 ± 2	69 ± 1	155 ± 27
Gauge 8 (45° RCS int.)	8 ± 1	13 ± 2	22 ± 4

F_{ZP}: Force perpendicular to pedal; F_{XP}: Force antero-posterior to pedal; F_{ZC}: Force perpendicular to crank; F_{XC}: Force antero-posterior to crank; DT: Down Tube; ST: Seat Tube; RCS: Right Chain Stay; ext.: external; int.: internal.

Table 3. Correlation coefficients during pedaling tests on a cycle-trainer.

	F_{ZP} (N)	F_{XP} (N)	F_{ZC} (N)	F_{XC} (N)	P (W)
Gauge 1 (Axial DT) ($\mu m \cdot m^{-1}$)	0.29	0.37	0.22	0.37	-0.09
Gauge 2 (45° Axial DT) ($\mu m \cdot m^{-1}$)	0.76*	0.79*	0.70*	0.69*	0.53*
Gauge 3 (Axial ST) ($\mu m \cdot m^{-1}$)	0.98*	0.83*	0.88*	0.89*	0.76*
Gauge 4 (45° ST) ($\mu m \cdot m^{-1}$)	0.84*	0.72*	0.68*	0.90*	0.42*
Gauge 5 (Axial RCS ext.) ($\mu m \cdot m^{-1}$)	0.70*	0.67*	0.58	0.74*	0.64*
Gauge 6 (45° RCS ext.) (μm/m)	0.96*	0.88*	0.86*	0.89*	0.48*
Gauge 7 (Axial RCS int.) ($\mu m \cdot m^{-1}$)	0.97*	0.75*	0.88*	0.86*	0.62*
Gauge 8 (45° RCS int.) ($\mu m \cdot m^{-1}$)	0.89*	0.90*	0.75*	0.87*	0.22

* $p < 0.05$, significant correlation; F_{ZP}: Force perpendicular to pedal; F_{XP}: Force antero-posterior to pedal; F_{ZC}: Force perpendicular to crank; F_{XC}: Force antero-posterior to crank; P: Mechanical power output; DT: Down Tube; ST: Seat Tube; RCS: Right Chain Stay; ext.: external; int.: internal.

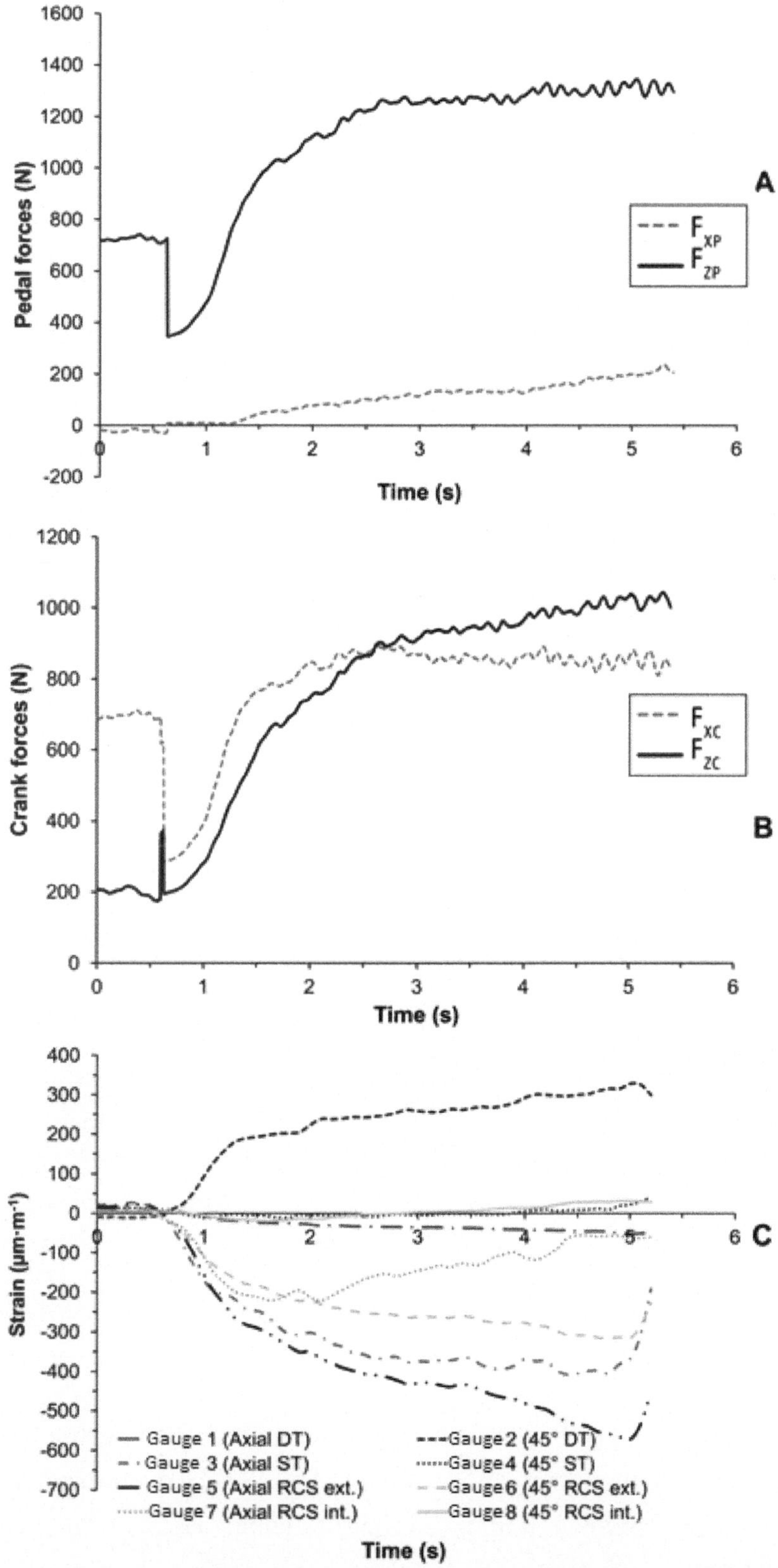

Figure 6. Antero-posterior and vertical forces on right pedal (F_{XP} and F_{ZP}) (**A**) and crank (F_{XC} and F_{ZC}) (**B**) and frame strain recorded (**C**) during maximal isometric effort on the right pedal with help of the handlebars. DT: Down Tube; ST: Seat Tube; RCS: Right Chain Stay; ext.: external; int.: internal.

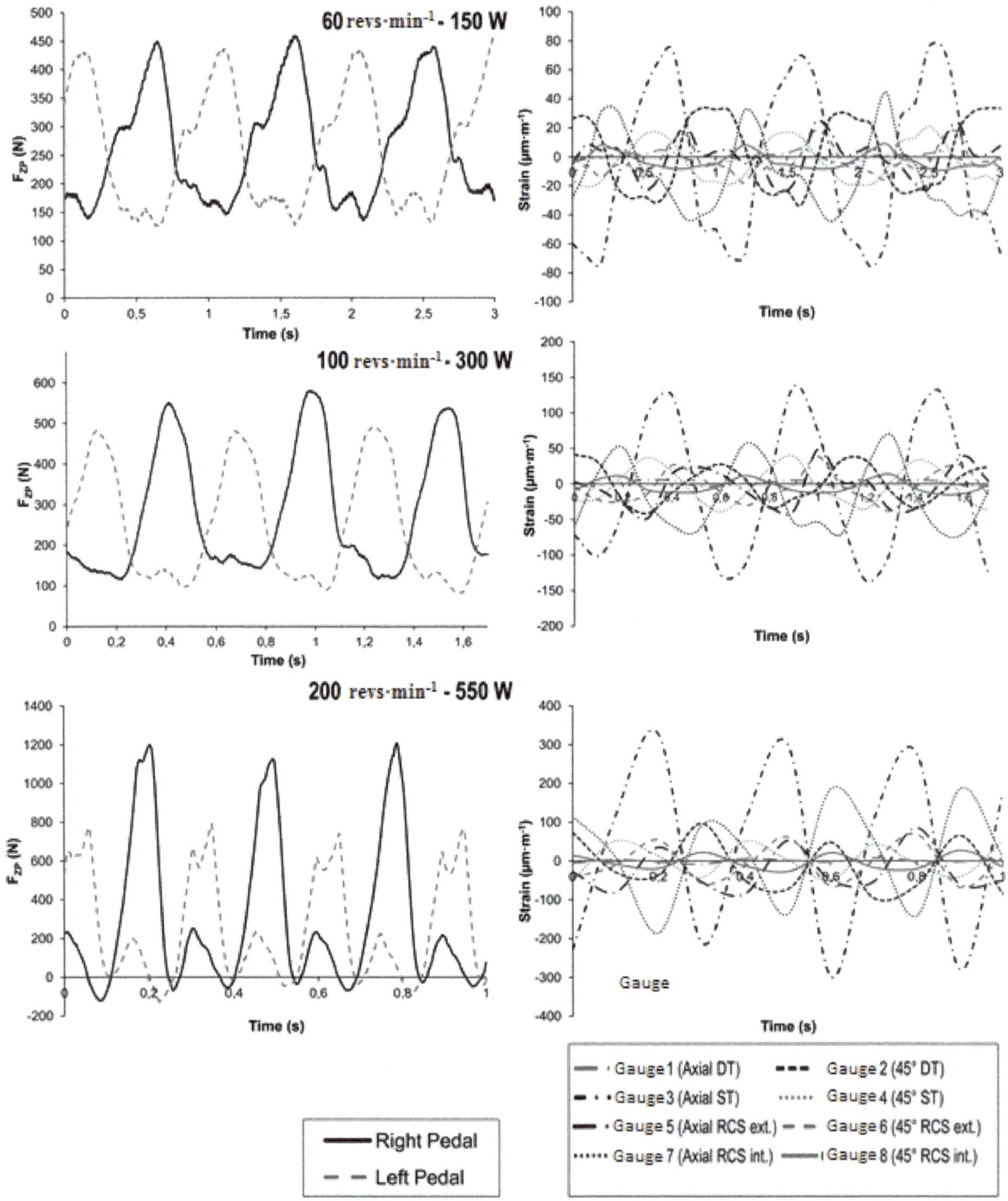

Figure 7. Perpendicular forces to right pedal and frame strain recorded during three bouts of steady-state pedaling at different intensity: 150, 300 and 550 W on a cycle-trainer. F_{ZP}: Force perpendicular to pedal; DT: Down Tube; ST: Seat Tube; RCS: Right Chain Stay; ext.: external; int.: internal.

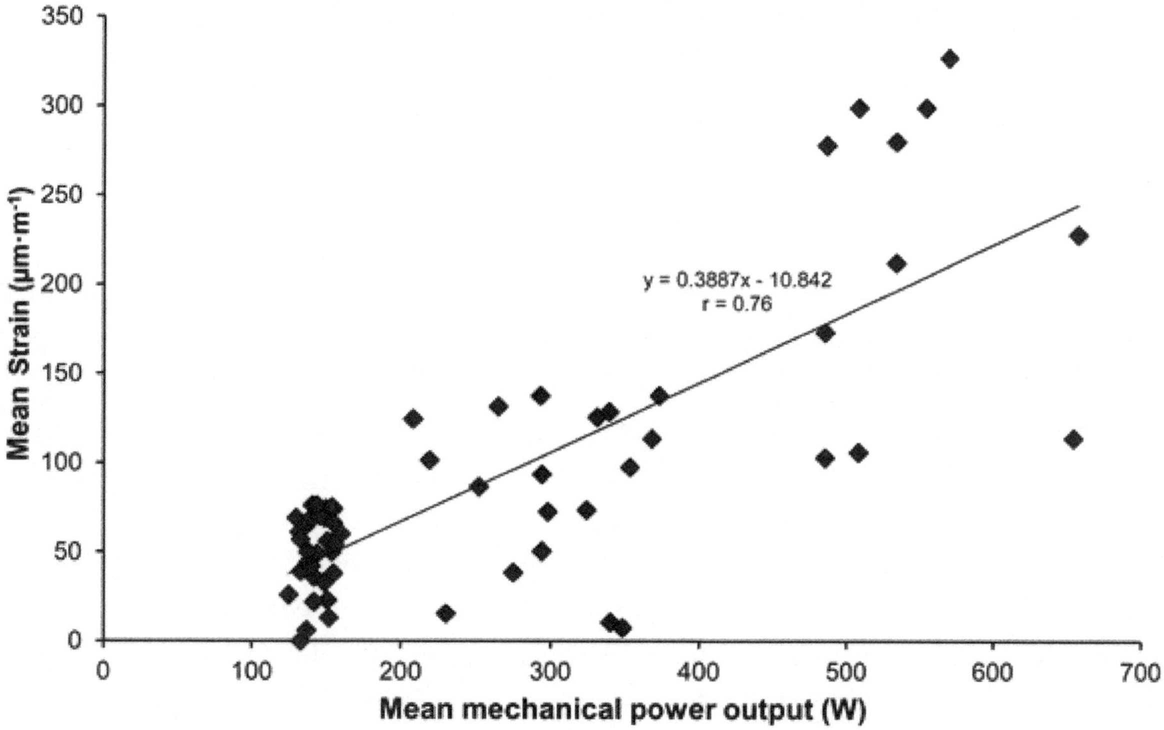

Figure 8. Linear regression of the mean strain of a BMX frame as function of the mean mechanical power output during pedaling on a cycle-trainer.

5. Discussion

The aim of this study was to investigate the effect of forces applied to 3-axis dynamometric pedals on the local strain response of an instrumented BMX frame under various conditions. These results have been analysed and compared to other studies e.g., [7–9,13]. The strain observed in the frame tubes increases with the forces perpendicular to the pedal and crank applied by the rider, for all conditions. The absolute maximum strain values were observed under the conditions of maximal muscular isometric effort (Table 1). These values were observed in the seat tube (gauge 3: 468 $\mu m \cdot m^{-1}$) and the right chain stay (gauge 5: 573 $\mu m \cdot m^{-1}$), with corresponding forces F_{ZP} of 880 and 1350 N, respectively. The maximum stress calculated according to the Von Mises criterion is equal to 41 MPa for the right chain stay (gauge 5), during the maximal isometric effort condition (Figure 6 and Table 1). The yield strength of the aluminum alloy used is 460 MPa so the measured stress is 11 times smaller than the yield strength so that the system remains elastic. At this stress, there is no possibility for the frame tubes to break, assuming critical flaws are not present. For a static load of 445 N, applied to a horizontal crank, Davis and Hull [7] observed the strain in the bottom bracket area with gauges on an aluminum road bicycle frame. They measured stresses from 30.4 to 39.7 MPa. These values are consistent with our results even though the applied force was two times greater in our study. This can be explain by difference in muscular characteristics of the cyclist that have participated at these two studies. In our study, the subject was a BMX rider with high force muscular capacity contrary to the Davis and Hull study [7]. This can also be explained by the difference in the materials of the studied frames. The road bicycle frame was aluminum 6061-T6, with a Young's modulus of 69 GPa and a yield strength of 250 MPa, whereas in our study the aluminum alloy was 7005 with a Young's modulus of 72 GPa and a yield strength of 460 MPa.

Moreover, the road bicycle frame tubes are thinner and lighter than those in a BMX frame. These reasons can explain the higher stress observed by Davis and Hull (1981) in the bottom bracket area.

Arola *et al.* [8] studied the static strain in a BMX bicycle frame composed of titanium alloy (Ti6Al4V) for most tubes and aluminum alloy (6061-T6) for the head tube and bottom bracket. Loads were applied vertically on the pedals but the position of the crank was not specified. The strain observed in the joint between the down tube and the head tube was approximately 110 $\mu m \cdot m^{-1}$ for 910 N. This value seems consistent with our result even though we did not study the head tube area. Moreover, the yield strength of the titanium alloy is 830 MPa with a Young's modulus of 105-120 GPa, so smaller strains are expected for comparable geometries.

During the pedaling tests (Tables 1 and 2, Figure 7), the maximum strain values were observed for the 200 $revs \cdot min^{-1}$ pedaling cadence test condition (550 W) in the seat tube (gauge 3: 301 ± 25 $\mu m \cdot m^{-1}$). We also observed a significant correlation (Table 3, Figure 8) between the power output at the crank and the frame strain. Watt *et al.* [9] found a similar correlation, but they did not mention the measured strain during their experiment. Despite a high value of perpendicular force on the pedal, from 1200 to 1350 N, most of the frame tubes show a relative low strain. The bench tests have exhibited more strain than the dynamic ones. During the pedaling test, the front wheel was not fixed and static contrary during the bench test where the front fork was rigidly connected. This difference could be explained, in part, by the difference between the two experimental conditions.

During a BMX race, jumps and landings from different heights occur and could cause high strain in the frame. The results of Arola *et al.* [8] mean that if an impact occurs at a speed of 10 $m.s^{-1}$, the BMX frame will be destroyed, even though the frontal impact on the front wheel is not a current event in a BMX race. In actual competition, the height jumps can be higher than 2 m. However, the technical skills of the riders enables the impact on landing to be reduced. Landings from high jumps are usually made on inclined planes, which further reduces the impact. A high impact would mean a failed landing, a loss of time, and, thus, a lost race. To verify this assumption, further study of the frame strain during a complete lap on a BMX track should be undertaken.

The different conditions highlighted the localisation of the highest strain in the tubes near the bottom bracket and the rear wheel axis. The use of 3-axis dynamometric pedals and strain gauges allow measurement of the input forces and knowledge of the corresponding stresses on the bicycle frame as function of the force applied to the pedal and crank. This information can be important for the process of frame design. Moreover, the results suggest that the vertical and antero-posterior forces on the pedal and crank show significant correlation with the frame strain during pedaling. The highest correlations were observed in the seat tube and the right chain stay with the force perpendicular to pedal. Although the force perpendicular to the crank is the motor force which contributes to crank rotation, it appears that the correlation is stronger between the frame and the force perpendicular to pedal. However, there is no way to distinguish the effect of a specific force on the frame strain although the pedaling condition was executed on a cycle-trainer, which does not allow a lateral tilt of the frame. The lateral tilt is encountered during standing pedaling in BMX and it could change the force pattern. This hypothesis is confirmed by the fact that the sprint performances in standing position were lower in laboratory conditions with no lateral tilt [14]. Indeed, some riders could produce high forces on pedals but with a low index of efficiency [12]. These inefficient pedaling forces could contribute to the largest strain, and the loss of energy to the frame could be a significant source of reduced performance. Studies should be conducted under actual conditions to determine the correlation between frame strain and the applied forces on the pedals and cranks and in order to see if frame tilt has an influence on frame strain. De Lorenzo and Hull have analysed the strain on the handlebar and on the hubs of both wheels on mountain bike in actual condition. However, it is difficult to compare their results with our study because they didn't instrument the frame and they didn't specifically explore the link between frame load and pedal forces.

For a perpendicular pedal force greater than 1300 N, the maximum stress observed during these tests was 11 times smaller than the yield strength of the aluminum alloy 7005. One of the major results of this study was that the safety coefficient of this bicycle frame is high. The mass of this frame is equal to approximately 2 kg. It would be interesting to lower the safety coefficient by decreasing the mass and/or by changing the material since, for a given material, decreasing the quantity of the material will result in an increase of the strain for a given geometry. Furthermore, the force applied by a female or a male athlete is different. The maximal mechanical power output for a male and a female high-level BMX athlete is approximately 2270 and 1500 W (personal data), respectively. Based on the pedaling tests, the relationship of the mean strain in the seat tube to the mean mechanical power output was determined (Figure 8). It is important to point out that this relationship is valid specifically for the frame studied in the present study; for other frames (e.g., geometry, composition), this relationship could be determined using the same methods. Under the conditions of the present study, for 2270 and 1500 W, the mean strain would be 968 and 631 $\mu m \cdot m^{-1}$, respectively. For the frame studied in this study, the corresponding stress would be equal to 70 and 45 MPa, respectively. In this case, the BMX frame could be lighter for a woman. In analysing the forces applied on pedals, this protocol could be useful in testing the frames and in finding a better compromise between safety coefficient, mass, strain, and performance for each rider as a function of his/her force and competition level. However, our results are based on laboratory tests and the location of the strain gauges was chosen according to a finite element analysis. Although numerical analyses are recognized to be effective, a 3D model of the frame could be more accurate in taking into account the weld, for example. Moreover, eight uniaxial strain gauges were used to study the bottom bracket area and the rear axis, more gauges could be placed on the frame to study the strain in all tubes and the use of three-gauge rosettes could amplify the accuracy of the results. More research on the frame strain should be done in actual conditions during an all-out sprint. The supplementary information obtained would allow a more complete understanding of the strain and could provide a better basis for the design of a race frame. The present study has several limits. Firstly, further studies should be performed with a greater sample size to confirm the present results. Secondly, even though it is difficult to perform high intensity exercise on a specific BMX cycle-trainer, further tests should be performed at higher intensities of exercise to better reflect the actual BMX condition. Thirdly, the results of this study should be considered specific to the BMX frame characteristics used in this study and should be used with caution for other BMX frames. Even if this study has several limits, the present study provides original findings illuminating the mechanical behavior of the BMX frame under different conditions of tests and pedaling and provides a methodology that could be used to test different cycle frames type (e.g., road, mountain bike). The results could give information for the riders or coaches for the choice of BMX frame or manufacturer.

In the future, the transfer of energy could be analysed by comparing the power output measured at the instrumented pedals and those transmitted to the ground. This data could be obtained using a force platform. Moreover, the 3-axis pedal system could facilitate the study of the frame strain as a function of the pedaling index of efficiency.

6. Conclusions

The principal results are that the maximum stress observed was about 11 times lower than the yield stress of the material and that the frame strain observed was greater under static loading than dynamic loading, *i.e.*, while pedaling. In actual competition, this ratio could be decreased by reducing the mass of the frame. Thus, the choice of the material for the frame would be relevant. The results obtained should be confirmed during an actual sprint on a BMX track. Such a measurement would be useful in finding the best compromise between safety coefficients, mass, energy transfer, and performance. The establishment of a protocol to optimise the design of frames is important because the behavior of the structure should be studied under conditions close to actual racing so the human factor and the rider-frame interaction can be taken into account. The testing protocol using 3-axis pedals and strain gauges could give information about the integrated performance of the whole system so that factors leading to inadequate design can be identified. The mechanical power output, and the antero-posterior and vertical forces on cranks and pedals were significantly correlated with the frame strain while pedaling on a cycle-trainer. For high-level riders, the 3-axis pedals could provide information about the pedaling pattern of the riders in order to adapt the design of the frame as a function of the level of force and mechanical power output.

Author Contributions

Aneliya Manolova and William Bertucci have conceived and designed the experiments, analysed the data and wrote the paper, Pierre Debraux, Samuel Crequy have performed the experiments, and Philippe Lestriez has contributed reagents/materials/analysis tools and analyzed the finite element analysis data.

Conflicts of Interest

The authors declare no conflict of interest.

References

1. Bertucci, W.; Hourde, C.; Manolova, A.; Vettoretti, F. Mechanical performance factors of the BMX acceleration phase in trained riders. *Sci. Sports* **2007**, *22*, 179–181.
2. Zabala, M.; Sanchez-Munoz, C.; Mateo, M. Effects of the administration of feedback on performance of the BMX cycling gate start. *J. Sports Sci. Med.* **2009**, *8*, 393–400.
3. Mateo, M.; Blasco-Lafarga, C.; Zabala, M. Pedaling Power and Speed Production *vs.* Technical Factors and Track Difficulty in Bicycle Motocross Cycling. *J Strength Cond Res*. **2011**, *25*, 3248–3256.
4. Rylands, L.; Roberts, S.J. Relationship between starting and finishing position in World Cup BMX racing. *Int. J. Perform. Anal. Sport* **2014**, *14*, 14–23.
5. Bertucci, W.M.; Hourde, C. Laboratory testing and field performance in BMX riders. *J. Sports Sci. Med.* 2011 *10*, 417–419.

6. Debraux, P.; Manolova, A.; Soudain-Pineau, M.; Hourde, C.; Bertucci, W. Maximal torque and power pedaling rate relationships for high level BMX riders in field tests. *J. Sci. Cycl.* **2013**, *2*, 51–57.
7. Davis, R.R.; Hull, M.L. Design of Aluminium bicycle frames. *J. Mech. Design.* **1981**, *103*, 901–907.
8. Arola, D.; Reinhall, P.G.; Jenkins, M.G.; Iverson, S.C. An experimental analysis of a hybrid bicycle frame. *Exp. Tech.* **1999**, *23*, 21–24.
9. Watt, J.B; Reiser, R.F., 2nd.; Peterson, M.L.; Walrath, D.E. Quantifying power output during cycling through measuring strain energy in a bicycle frame. *Biomed. Sci. Instrum.* **2002**, *38*, 417–421.
10. Rylands, L.; Roberts, S.J.; Hurst, H.T. Bentley, I. Effect of cadence selection on peak power and time of power production in elite BMX riders: A laboratory based study. *J. Sports Sci.* **2015**, in process.
11. Stone, C.; Hull, M.L. Rider/Bicycle interaction loads during standing treadmill cycling. *J. Appl. Biomech.* **1993**, *9*, 202–218.
12. Coyle, E.F.; Sidossis, L.S.; Horowitz, J.F.; Beltz, J.D. Cycling efficiency is related to the percentage of type I muscle fibers. *Med. Sci. Sports Exerc.* **1992**, *24*, 782–788.
13. De Lorenzo, D.S.; Hull, M.L. Quantification of structural loading during off-road cycling. *J Biomech. Eng.* **1999**, *121*, 399–405.
14. Bertucci, W.; Taiar, R.; Grappe, F. Differences between sprint tests under laboratory and actual cycling conditions. *J. Sports Med. Phys. Fit.* **2005**, *45*, 277–283.

13

Recommendations for Recruiting and Retaining Adolescent Girls in Chronic Exercise (Training) Research Studies

Rachel Massie, Brett Smith and Keith Tolfrey *

School of Sport, Exercise and Health Sciences, Loughborough University, Loughborough, Leicestershire LE11 3TU, UK; E-Mails: r.c.massie@lboro.ac.uk (R.M.); b.m.smith@lboro.ac.uk (B.S.)

* Author to whom correspondence should be addressed; E-Mail: k.tolfrey@lboro.ac.uk

Academic Editor: Eling de Bruin

Abstract: Extensive challenges are often encountered when recruiting participants to chronic exercise (training) studies. High participant burden during chronic exercise training programmes can result in low uptake to and/or poor compliance with the study. The aim of this qualitative study was to identify factors affecting adolescent girls' recruitment and adherence to chronic exercise training research studies. Twenty-six adolescent girls (aged 12 to 15 years) participated in one of five focus groups discussing recruitment and retention to exercise physiology research involving a chronic exercise training programme. A thematic analysis was used to analyse the data and eight final themes were inductively identified. Seven evidence-based practical recommendations are suggested to improve the recruitment and retention of participants for prospective, chronic exercise training studies. Successful recruitment requires: (i) the defining of exercise-related terms; (ii) appropriate choice of recruitment material; and (iii) an understanding of participant motivations. Retention strategies include: (iv) regular monitoring of participant motives; and (v) small groups which foster peer and researcher support. Finally, (vi) friendship and ability groups were favoured in addition to (vii) a variety of activities to promote adherence to an exercise training programme.

Keywords: adolescent; exercise; focus groups; health promotion; research participation

---

1. Introduction

Cardiorespiratory fitness (CRF) levels are important for both adults and young people when completing everyday activities to athletic performance. However, there appears to be a decline in CRF during adolescence in girls [1]. Low CRF levels have been shown to be associated with adiposity and cardiovascular disease risk factors [2]. Exercise training could be used to prevent this reduction in CRF and could, consequently, promote improved mental health, quality of life and academic performance [2]. Yet, recruiting adolescents to exercise research studies can be very challenging [3,4]. Adolescent girls can be particularly difficult to recruit, due, in part, to gender-specific challenges (e.g., body image concerns, social comparison [5] and conflicting activities [6]).

Recruitment and retention of human participants in research studies is vital to obtain the highest quality of evidence possible with external validity [7–9]. Recruitment is the process encompassing the presentation of the study to the target population, obtaining consent, screening for eligibility and allocation of participants to the study [7]. Successful recruitment in research means minimising systematic and random error by recruiting a large enough sample "that adequately represents the target population" being studied and of sufficient power [10]. Retention of the participants can also be a challenge, for chronic exercise studies requiring a sustained commitment particularly and depends, in part, on a strong researcher–participant relationship, comprised with a sense of worthiness and achievement for the participant [8,11]. Poor participant retention can have a detrimental impact on research findings and their validity. For example, dropout or missing data points may bias the sample; which, in addition to a smaller sample size, can reduce the power of the study. Many interacting factors, both individual and social, affect and complicate the process of recruitment and retention [9].

Comprehensive accounts of retention problems and strategies to overcome these in longitudinal behavioural interventions have been detailed previously [12,13]. However, the majority of the participants in these studies were adults, in which responses to various barriers might differ to those of adolescents. Exploring the attitudes of the target group and the incorporation of their views and preferences when developing complex interventions is of great importance [12,14–16]. Correlates of adolescents' physical activity have been studied previously and used to improve physical activity interventions [17,18]. These correlates do not though provide the specific details associated with recruitment and retention to a supervised chronic exercise training programme. Jago *et al.* [19] provided useful, practical ideas to enhance recruitment, such as highlighting the enjoyment factor and offering taster sessions to increase activity engagement with girls. Although these findings can be applied to physical activity interventions, they are specific to a dance intervention and may be limited in terms of their application to chronic exercise training programmes with a physiological research purpose because of the associated challenges to accurately measure outcome variables embedded within the study (e.g., cardiorespiratory fitness, body composition and blood pressure).

Exercise physiology research is often constrained by the strict standard controls that must be adhered to. As a result, chronic exercise training programmes often place great demands on the participants, which can lead to low uptake to and/or poor compliance with the study [3]. This means the success of the research might be hindered from the outset. Therefore, it is important to attempt to minimise participant burden [9]. One way to achieve this might be to adapt the way in which exercise training programmes are planned. While ensuring compliance with the research protocols, patient and public involvement (PPI) with the research design could benefit the external validity of the research through improved participant recruitment and retention to the study. Affording participants greater autonomy and ownership during the planning process might enhance recruitment and adherence to a study compared with the researcher-led training programmes employed traditionally [3,14]. With recent technological advancements in the measurement of behaviours such as free-living energy expenditure, it should be possible to still measure outcome variables with more novel and inventive exercise programmes. Direct discussion with intended participants might enhance the relevance of the training programme to the target group and help alleviate difficulties recruiting and retaining participants.

The aim of this qualitative study was to identify factors affecting adolescent girls' recruitment and adherence to a chronic exercise training programme. This aim is vital to inform the recruitment and retention process to prospective exercise training studies and provide practical solutions to problems researchers face regularly when undertaking chronic studies with a substantial exercise component.

2. Methods

2.1. Context

The present study is part of a series of studies designed to support the recruitment, retention and data collection of adolescent girls' participation in a chronic exercise training programme with physiological outcome variables (e.g., body composition, cardiorespiratory fitness and resting metabolic rate). The outcomes of this study were used to devise the supervised exercise training component.

2.2. Participants

A purposive sampling strategy was used to identify adolescent girls who wanted to be more physically active and enhance their cardiorespiratory fitness. All girls in years 8 to 10 from a local secondary school attended a presentation detailing the study and were invited to participate in the focus groups. All girls had the opportunity to take an information pack home including the project details, consent forms and an interview guide. Twenty-six girls aged 12 to 15 years volunteered to participate in the study. Six participants were involved with regular sport and exercise currently, 14 participants took part in some physical activity (1 or 2 times per week), while the remaining six participants self-selected themselves as inactive. After providing written assent and parental consent the participants attended one focus group. The University Ethical Advisory Committee approved the study prior to data collection.

2.3. Data Collection

Focus groups were utilised to collect data. This method was considered appropriate for young people because of the interactional component of focus groups and that this group of people could engage in a discussion in a relaxed atmosphere with peers, rather than talking simply to an adult in a one-to-one interview [20]. Each focus group consisted of four to six girls and was homogenous in group composition for school year group and self-reported physical activity. This ensured all participants had the opportunity to share their opinion and could feel comfortable doing so as recommended by Heary and Henessey [21]. A moderator facilitated the sessions, while a second researcher took field notes. The focus groups were digitally recorded using two Olympus dictaphone voice recorders and lasted, on average, one hour. Data saturation was achieved after conducting five focus groups.

At the beginning of each focus group, participants were provided with a verbal and written explanation of the study. Additionally issues regarding confidentiality and respect for others were discussed. A semi-structured design based on the following four sections was employed to moderate the focus groups. Opening background questions regarding current physical activity levels and previous experience with research were used to promote participation. Next, thoughts about the factors which motivated and prohibited adolescent girls to exercise were sought, followed by general opinions about exercise and engaging girls with exercise-based research. Finally, participants were given ownership of an exercise training programme and asked to note down ideas and create a mind map of their ideal programme, including preferred activities, location, timing and any other specific and relevant details. A number of practical elicitation techniques, such as photographs of different people exercising and scenario tasks, were delivered throughout the focus group to supplement verbal questions, promote discussion and increase enjoyment [22]. To elicit richer data, probing questions were also used throughout each focus group interview.

2.4. Data Analysis

All focus group recordings were transcribed verbatim. Transcription occurred immediately after each focus group and prior to the next focus group. An inductive thematic analysis was used to identify the main patterns within the data. This approach enables the development of future exercise physiology interventions to be informed by the data collected. The six-phase procedure used is described in detail by Braun and Clarke [23]. After familiarisation with the data through data collection, transcription and re-reading, initial codes to describe the data were generated. These codes were then grouped into broader categories, before being refined to collate eight coherently meaningful themes. Once checked against the data set, themes were defined and named.

3. Results

The thematic analysis led to the development of eight main themes and twelve subthemes. The first three main themes relate to recruitment and were termed dynamics of communication, presentation of content and motives to participate. The final five themes explain participation and retention in an exercise training programme. These were termed barriers, exercise training programme, benefits of participation, peer relationships and instructor qualities.

3.1. Dynamics of Communication

The girls suggested the initial communication of the study is an important factor when recruiting adolescent girls to a chronic exercise training programme. Communication from both the research team and peers can impact on the girls' decision making process regarding their participation and is captured in the following two subthemes.

3.1.1. Presenter

Participants identified the presenters' characteristics and personality to be important when delivering a recruitment presentation. Participants reported that recruitment would benefit from the researcher communicating the study details in a positive, enthusiastic, honest, clear and realistic manner. For example one girl stated, "tell them exactly what happened there because if you like make stuff up and say over exaggerate things then, it, they might be a bit confused when they actually get there; so if you tell them exactly what you do and what to expect then they should be more persuaded".

3.1.2. Peers

Participants suggested successful recruitment is, in part, dependent on the response of their friends and peers. Issues relating to dominance, age and interest were raised. The impact of peer dominance was captured in the following comment, "if you had like a positive dominant person [within a friendship group] then that would be good but if they were quite negative it wouldn't really help encourage people to take part." It was also suggested that separate presentations for each year group might be more effective than one large presentation which combined year groups. Finally, one group proposed asking girls who had an initial interest in the study to attend an assembly to learn more. They perceived separating these girls from others who are not interested to be advantageous in recruitment by minimising disruption. The girls suggested an initial letter providing an overview of the study or a brief explanation by the teacher would help the girls decide whether they wished to attend the presentation.

3.2. Presentation of Content

How the study is communicated through the content of the presentation was identified as another important element of the recruitment process. Individual interpretation of the content was reiterated through all focus groups and its impact on recruitment is captured in the following two subthemes.

3.2.1. Images

The choice of images used in the presentation is crucial when recruiting adolescent girls to an exercise training programme. Participants suggested images displaying exercise in a positive manner, for example happy facial expressions, and not what they perceive to be negative, such as sweat, would aid recruitment as explained in the following two quotes. One girl stated; "I think it would be better if you had a photo of her cheering and celebrating because that makes her look upset and sad and it might just think oh, if that's what it's going to make me feel like do I really want to put myself through that and do it?"

Another girl commented; "That one [photo of a sweaty tennis player] would really put you off because she's sweaty, she looks tired and if you're not a fan of getting sweaty, or getting tired, or running or anything that would really put you off and not want you to join in".

The ability of the girls to relate to the images and visualise themselves participating in the activity was also an influential factor in recruitment to an exercise study. Preference of celebrities *versus* ordinary people pictured exercising to promote recruitment with adolescent girls returned a mixed response.

3.2.2. Choice of Words and Phrases

The choice and interpretation of words used to explain the programme was also suggested to influence the success of recruitment drives with adolescent girls. The meaning and relevance of the words to an individual were identified as key aspects of language impacting successful recruitment. For example, the words exercise and sport, often used interchangeably, were open to a wide variation of interpretations. The opinions of three different girls were as follows, "I prefer the word sport to exercise, because exercise seems like you are working really hard but sport seems like there is a lot of different sports and activities"; "Sport is like basically the same as exercise"; "They see the word sport and they say no and just think of horrible hours of running".

Additionally, the phrasing of the exercise component of the study can affect decisions to participate. Both year groups suggested strong, persuasive phrases would aid recruitment. However, one participant highlighted the need for careful consideration of these phrases, stating, "Well it's different for everyone isn't it". While both year groups agreed that conveying the potential for social interactions was important, other key differences were raised. Many year 9's suggested phrases such as "you'll look fit" and "you'll lose weight" to be attractive. Whereas, a discussion between two year 8 participants suggested these words and phrases would put them off volunteering to participate in an exercise research study.

Participant (P) 1: If you said lots of stuff about losing weight, it would put me off because it's like you are trying to change me;

Participant (P) 2: Yeh, if someone just came up to me and said, "hey join my thing for weight loss scheme", I would be like I don't really want to do that to lose weight. If you'd come up and said "hey do you want to join this club—it's fun and it's active", I would do it because I don't really care about weight loss I just care about having fun and doing something worthwhile;

Participant (P) 1: Yeh, if they phrased it a different way. "I've just had loads of fun with my friends doing my sport". It phrases differently and attracts you.

3.3. Motives to Participate

The final recruitment theme captures the reasons why adolescent girls choose to participate. Fun and enjoyment were suggested as the main reasons why adolescent girls would engage in such an exercise programme. One girl stated, "If you enjoy it then you're going to do it". Nevertheless, it was clear that these thoughts were entwined with the enjoyment from the social element of group exercise as reported in the following three quotes, "because I enjoy sport when I'm doing it with someone I know"; "it's like in PE like, it's harder to do when you're on your own. But if you've got friends it kind of makes you want to do it, and makes it more fun, and encourages you as well"; "I put fun, that's probably because you meet new people". While social and enjoyment factors dominated the year 8 discussions; body image and aesthetics were another key incentive for some girls, year 9's predominantly. Improvements in self-confidence and health were identified as another motivational influence to recruit adolescent girls to exercise. The majority of girls indicated the opportunity for days off school to be in the laboratory, to meet athletes and their own autonomy within the exercise training programme were external drivers promoting recruitment.

3.4. Barriers

The participants identified a number of key barriers that increase the difficulty for girls to engage in a chronic exercise training programme. These are explained in the following two subthemes.

3.4.1. Logistical Barriers

Participants cited several difficulties associated with continued participation in an exercise training programme. Lack of time, arranging transport and activity cost were identified frequently as participation barriers. Numerous activities were identified which compete with young people's spare time. For example one girl said "with school work and home work and things like that you don't really have enough time to do it (exercise)". Another girl stated "they like want to do something else, like, I don't know, shopping or something". Time commitments of family members can also affect regular participation in a research exercise programme. For example, "If you've got single parents as well it's really hard, if you've got younger brothers and sisters who are like asleep and then you are going to have to wake them just for them to go and collect you." Some participants said that arranging transport to and from activities could be difficult as a result of their parents work commitments. One group suggested organised transport to the exercise training sessions could help overcome this challenge. Finally, cost was a well discussed topic with girls being deterred by expensive activities and additional expenses during the programme, such as buying specific sports clothing.

3.4.2. Comparative Barriers

The comparative barriers adolescent girls encounter include social comparisons and peer pressure. Peer pressure is discussed further under the theme 'participant characteristics and peer relationships'. For adolescent girls the process of social comparison can lead to barriers to participating in exercise. Concerns about feeling judged, embarrassed or self-conscious when exercising were suggested to result in lack of retention to the programme. Feelings of embarrassment were associated, in particular, with clothing and fitness levels. One girl commented, "It's embarrassing with some of the stuff you have to wear…like leggings that suck to you. And when you sweat, it makes you feel uncomfortable". When discussing reasons why adolescent girls might drop-out of an exercise programme one girl reported that they might be embarrassed or they might not be as fit as everyone else, "people are there and they are watching me and I don't like it. If you put them with more friends rather than feeling embarrassed with people they don't know. Especially in year groups where it's hard. Like we don't really want to go in front of them, but then year 9s (8th grade) are alright to come in front of us because they are obviously older and comparing us".

Participants suggested flexibility within the programme to overcome some of the logistical barriers and concurrent acknowledgment of the presence of comparative barriers could aid retention rates.

3.5. Exercise Training Programme

The exercise training programme was identified as a crucial factor when recruiting and retaining adolescent girls to an exercise-based research study. The following subthemes capture specific components of the exercise programme with the potential to affect retention.

3.5.1. Activity Characteristics

The variety of exercise activities were identified as a key component to promote participation in a chronic exercise training programme. Participants suggested that a range of different activities would afford girls greater autonomy and choice during the programme, maintain interest and prevent boredom. One girl reported that, "there should be a variety of sports, where, if they may not like this sport one day they might like the one the next day, so they can still carry on and enjoy it, but may not enjoy the others as much, because you can't please everyone at every time".

Novel activities, such as water sports and roller-skating, were reported favourably. Dance was also cited repeatedly, "things you can do as a group with music like Zumba and yoga and exercises". Using gym equipment, including weights and a variety of machines were discussed by some year 9s; while expensive gym memberships were reported as the main deterrent for the remaining girls. Numerous team sports were also reported in the discussions of an ideal exercise programme (*i.e.*, netball, football, hockey and rounders). The girls added, however, that an appropriate intensity and skill level of all activities, reflecting individual differences, is vital to maintain engagement. The girls acknowledged that when performing team activities, individual differences can separate the group, for example, "some people wouldn't say they were good at netball, so wouldn't bother and would just stand on the side-lines."

3.5.2. Group Composition

For many participants structuring the exercise training programme to promote a positive, flexible, fun and social atmosphere was important. The girls suggested group exercise sessions provide the enjoyment and social support necessary to improve girls' participation retention. One year 9 girl said, "That (group exercise class) would be quite good because you could go with your friends and still help each other and have fun and stuff." This view was supported by another girl who stated "if it was an individual activity—that would put me off more because I don't want to work alone without anyone to like support me."

The selection and composition of these groups were identified as crucial factors for achieving high participant retention rates. The first group composition discussed related to ability levels. With reference to a previous sports club experience, one girl stated, "They did groups ranging from like 10 year olds to like 14 year olds and you're all different standards so they were just going by the top and we were really struggling". A discussion between two year 9 students also supported the benefits of dividing exercise groups by ability.

P3: Some would be like trying to show off because they are so fast;
P4: Yeh, so only let the slow people come;
P3: Or have different ability groups.

Second, grouping according to age was reported positively by both year groups. One year 9 student stated, "I don't like the idea of being in year 8's clubs because I don't like them. I just get really angry with the year 8's if you decided to combine our groups"; whereas, as stated previously, year 8 students do not like exercising in front of year 9's because they can perceive social comparison pressures.

3.5.3. Session Details

The session context was reported to influence both participation and retention in a chronic exercise training programme. Participants stated the location, facilities, length and timing of the training sessions were key features of the exercise programme. The University was suggested as an attractive location with appropriate facilities. Other reasons why the girls favoured exercise at the University included "we are at school too often" and "if they did it in a local area or school they might not take it seriously because they think they can overpower adults".

The ideal number and duration of individual training sessions were variable; preferred session frequency ranged from 1 to 3 sessions a week, while preferred duration ranged between 30 min and 2 h. The girls indicated their preference was closely related to maintained enjoyment and interest. One girl suggested "Once or twice a week I would say because you don't want it to be too often because then you might get fed up with it." Likewise, another girl considering the duration of the programme stated, "About an hour…but if you made it too long, they might end up getting bored and then not wanting to come because it's too long". There was a mixed preference regarding indoor or outdoor activities; yet, all girls indicated that they would prefer indoor sports during bad weather conditions.

3.6. Benefits of Exercise Participation

3.6.1. Fun and Enjoyment

This subtheme, fun and enjoyment, was identified frequently as a fundamental reason for participant retention in a chronic exercise training programme. Participants suggested fun and enjoyment associated with the programme were essential when engaging with exercise. As one girl stated; "I wouldn't do something if I didn't enjoy it". Opportunities to socialise and exercise with friends were reported to make exercise more attractive. One girl stated, "I enjoy sport when I'm doing it with someone I know". The importance of enjoyment was highlighted, by some girls stating they would still join exercise programmes without their friends if they enjoyed the programme, recognising they could make new friends. Some practical methods to enhance enjoyment of the sessions were alluded to in the exercise programme theme particularly.

3.6.2. Body Image

Some girls expressed continued attendance to an exercise training programme would be associated with improvements in their physical appearance. Muscle toning, burning calories and weight loss were all perceived by some participants to be important benefits of engaging in an exercise programme. If these results were expected or seen during a programme the girls suggested they would feel happier with their looks and body image and thus maintain their engagement throughout the study.

3.6.3. Physical and Psychological Self

Participants identified physiological improvements as a reason to maintain participation in an exercise programme. The benefits associated with improving health, fitness levels and learning new skills were reported to aid participation and retention. When asked why they would enjoy exercise, one girl stated, "knowing that you're getting fit and doing something you enjoy and knowing that you are improving at it". The perception of psychological benefits, including increased self-confidence, self-satisfaction and feeling better were also considered beneficial to retention. Finally, both the mental and physical challenges associated with participating in, and the achievements accompanying completion of an exercise programme were considered worthy incentives to participate in a long-term exercise-based research study.

3.7. Participant Characteristics and Peer Relationships

Positive, supportive and motivational peers within the exercise training programme were reported to improve retention by fostering enjoyment. When other girls are determined, committed and demonstrating buy-in to the research and exercise programme, this was reported to enhance participation and retention consequently. However, peer pressure was reported to deter some participants from continued participation. One girl reported, "I like rounders, just not when people shout at me," while a second stated as a reason for disliking exercise, "if I'm playing a sport with other people I usually get yelled at". Peer engagement was an important factor, in team games particularly, because this can impact on individuals' experiences. When recruiting more active girls to exercise physiology research studies, a mixed group was reported favourably. Commenting on a discussion about girls and boys participating in team sports separately, one girl reported, "the boys I would say play more fairly because they, the boys, like most of the boys like the sport and want to get on with it, whereas the girls don't so most girls that want to do the sport want to be with the boys because actually it's more fair and they are playing by the rules and you're getting stuff done".

Similarly, another girl reported, "Some of the girls want to play but most of the girls don't play so it ruins the game". In contrast the less active girls appeared to prefer a gender split because they perceived the boys were too rough during games and limited the girls' involvement. For example, "If it's like football and it's mixed, then they [the boys] won't pass the ball to you. Basically they won't involve the girls".

3.8. Instructor Characteristics

This theme captures the qualities and personal characteristics of the instructor that the participants perceived to be important for maintaining participant retention. It was suggested that the positive attributes of the instructor, for example approachable, likeable, positive, encouraging and motivating, would enhance exercise retention, for example; "If you have a teacher that demonstrated it to you, then wasn't shouting at you all the time and taking it in a calm voice, girls may approach it [PE] differently because they know it can actually be fun if you are not shouted at".

Knowledge, expertise and qualifications in the activities and their delivery were reported by the participants as valuable qualities to help maintain engagement. Finally, the participants identified the ability to build relationships with each participant to be a key characteristic, "if you got to know the instructors because then it kind of becomes more personal…and they help you achieve, like, and they attend to your individual needs".

4. Discussion

There is a need to address the challenges of recruiting and retaining adolescent girls to chronic exercise training programmes with physiological outcome variables. Qualitative work has great potential to enhance the development of such health related interventions [16]. This qualitative study contributes to the development of exercise physiology research and how such exercise training programmes might be enhanced by identifying important factors, specific to adolescent girls, which influence recruitment and retention to prospective studies. The key themes that emerged provide vital knowledge of the factors that require consideration in terms of recruitment and retention of participants to chronic exercise programmes. These are now discussed with reference to the practical recommendations that emerge from the qualitative results and are shown in Table 1.

Table 1. Chronic exercise training programme table synthesis.

Process	Theme	Subtheme	Recommendations
Recruitment	1. Dynamics of Communication	1.1 Presenter 1.2 Peers	1. Define key terms
	2. Presentation of Content	2.1 Images 2.2 Choice of words and phrases	1. Define key terms 2. Representative images
	3. Motives to Participate	-	2. Images capture motives 4. Understand and monitor the motivations
Retention	4. Barriers	4.1 Logistical Barriers 4.2 Comparative Barriers	5. Address the barriers 6. Participant grouping—size/composition
	5. Exercise Training Programme	5.1 Activity Characteristics 5.2 Group Composition 5.3 Session Details	6. Participant grouping—size/composition 7. Activity variety
Retention	6. Benefits of Participation	6.1 Fun and enjoyment 6.2 Body image 6.3 Physical/psychological self	3. Maximise enjoyment 4. Understand and monitor the motivations 7. Activity variety
	7. Participant Characteristics and Peer Relationships	-	3. Maximise enjoyment 6. Participant grouping size/composition
	8. Instructor Characteristics	-	3. Maximise enjoyment

The first recommendation to improve the recruitment of participants in studies with a chronic exercise training component that emerges from this work is that key terms, such as physical activity, sport and exercise, need to be defined to ensure honest and clear communication of the study expectations. In previous research investigating engagement with intervention studies Jones and Broome [24] explain how adolescent girls wanted to know what would be expected of them during the intervention. The current study supports these findings, but further highlights the importance of defining key terms. While physiological research protocols and equipment are explained regularly, researchers often assume prior knowledge of terms such as physical activity, exercise and sport. Our results suggest exercise-related words in recruitment material are often interpreted differently to academic use. Therefore, this could lead to the misinterpretation of study expectations and potentially hinder recruitment. Communicating the nature of training studies accurately is also crucial for ethical reasons [25].

The second recommendation to emerge from the results is that the images used in recruitment material need to be representative of the exercise training programme but also capture the participants' motives for volunteering. Our results provide an understanding of how images in recruitment material (*i.e.*, posters, presentations, leaflets) can influence adolescent girls' decisions to participate. Consistent with previous research concerning reasons why girls do not like to exercise, for example Women's Sport and Fitness Foundation [26], the girls highlighted their dislike for images showing exercise to be sweaty and hard work. Omitting these photos, however, might portray the exercise programme in an unrealistic manner, contradicting the previous comments about honest communication and raising ethical issues of participant deception. A suitable alternative would be to use images that are representative of the exercise programme, but place a greater emphasis on the girls' motives for participating rather than the negative appearance girls' often associate with physical exertion [27]. For example, picturing girls having fun exercising in groups and engaging with novel activities, might capture the enjoyment and social opportunities associated with participation.

The third recommendation is to maximise enjoyment in every aspect of an exercise training programme for all volunteers. Enjoyment is a largely underplayed factor for initiating involvement and subsequent adherence in research, but its prevalence in all group discussions and the literature suggests this is a critical motive. For instance, Whitehead and Biddle [27] propose that clarity of the enjoyment concept is required to increase physical activity in adolescent girls. Furthermore, in work with older adults the various types of pleasure and enjoyment that can emerge from being active, such as when being with friends while walking, were seen as vital in maintaining a physically active lifestyle [28]. In the present study enjoyment appeared closely related with opportunities to socialise with friends, peers and research staff. This is consistent with the relatedness principle of self-determination theory (SDT), in which connecting with significant others can impact on motivations to participate and engage in research [29]. The efficacy of this recommendation can also be traced to the importance of participating with friends for support and opportunities to make new friends suggested by Jago *et al.* [19,30].

The fourth recommendation that this qualitative research offers to improve recruitment and retention of participants is to understand and monitor individual motivations for participation. Improving body image via exercise training participation was a motive cited commonly by year 9 (grade 8) girls. Physiology research with a chronic exercise training component needs to explicitly factor into the process the issue of body image and the desire to conform to the Western culture ideal of a slender body to be physically attractive when recruiting and seeking to retain participants [31]. Although a familiar motive for initiating participation, if the perceived benefits to body image are not met then a consequent lack of retention might result [27]. The positive and negative impact of body image on exercise participation can be traced to the broader literature in which it has been found that girls are highly concerned about their body image [27,31]. The authors suggest monitoring desired motivations and establishing realistic achievements during chronic exercise training research to sustain the motivation of participants and maintain adherence to the intervention. It is also of ethical importance that researchers are careful not to promote unrealistic body ideals when using exercise interventions.

Additionally, monitoring physiological and psychological improvements from participation can promote retention. Improvements in various physical components of fitness and skill to complete activities can satisfy the basic psychological need for competency. Psychological gains in self-confidence and self-satisfaction are correlated with intrinsic motivation and thus continued participation [32]. Within exercise physiology research it is feasible to monitor both physiological and psychological measures and provide regular feedback to the participants throughout the study. The extrinsic incentives reported are also realistic to address and monitor. Good communication with schools and parents about the educational benefits of participating means days off school are feasible to factor into a study. The geographical location of this study, with high athlete profiles and sporting events, could have encouraged the desire to meet athletes, which might not be as accessible in other locations or not considered a key motivation to participate and should be employed with caution. Previous research has focussed on the ethical issue of providing monetary incentives to young people [33,34]. The findings from this study do not suggest monetary incentives are a necessary motive for recruitment of adolescent girls to chronic exercise training research. Highlighting intrinsic motivations and non-monetary extrinsic motivations to participants should be considered.

The fifth recommendation to improve the recruitment and retention of participants is to address the relevant logistical barriers when planning and developing chronic exercise training programmes and ensuring flexibility within scheduling. The logistical barriers reported by the girls, lack of time, transport and cost of the facilities and programme, are consistent with previous research [32,35]. Maximising the opportunities available for participants to attend study visits would ease scheduling around existing commitments. This recommendation identifies with offering tangible support and a flexible approach suggested by Coday *et al.* [12]. Allowing flexibility also lends itself to affording participants a degree of ownership. This can satisfy the autonomy principle of SDT, facilitating self-motivation and behaviour regulation [29], improving subsequent participation and retention in chronic exercise training research studies.

The sixth recommendation is that participant groups should be relatively small and selection should reflect age, ability and friendship groups. Small groups, of up to 10 participants, were positively suggested to meet the needs for individual attention from the researcher and the building of relationships within the group, satisfying the need for relatedness [29]. The retention of participants in chronic exercise training studies also needs to factor in the process of social comparison. To negate the undesirable impact of upward social comparisons to more able peers the use of homogenous ability groups are suggested. This recommendation extends the suggestion by Barnes and Spray [36], to encourage similar ability comparison in physical education classes, into a physiology research context. Body dissatisfaction concerns, in particular when exercising in front of boys, can be detrimental to adolescent girls participation in physical activity [27,35]. Nevertheless, a group exercise intervention remained preferable to an individual programme. Homogenous ability-based groups of the same gender might alleviate body dissatisfaction concerns. The efficacy of this recommendation can also be traced to the broader literature in which it has been found that less-active girls prefer "girls-only" exercise groups [24,37].

The final recommendation is to ensure chronic exercise interventions within physiology research contain a variety of activities consistent with the girls' preferences. The number of activities reported highlights individual variability and the challenge to maximise engagement of all participants throughout the exercise intervention. These findings support Women's Sport and Fitness Foundation [26] in suggesting a variety of activities can affect retention positively by increasing choice and enjoyment. It also provides a greater chance of promoting self-improvement and achievement of goals during the programme, satisfying the need for competency and consequently promoting intrinsic motivation to retain participation [29].

One opportunity to emerge to enhance recruitment and retention is to incorporate dance into an exercise training programme. Dance was commonly cited as a preferred activity, complementing previous research focussing on the use of dance interventions to promote girls physical activity [19,38]. Burgess *et al.* argue, "aerobic dance can provide a more supportive environment (*i.e.*, non-competitive and non-threatening) and multiple opportunities for adolescent females with low body attitudes and physical self-perceptions to feel better about themselves." [38] (p. 64). These advantages appear to match the suggested motives for volunteering and benefits associated with continued participation, supporting the use of dance within physiology research. Team-based activities were also reported frequently; yet they are associated with varying levels of engagement, intensity and enthusiasm. Exercise physiology research often requires all participants to exercise at a specified intensity, and as such, these activities would require modification to sustain involvement by all. Careful consideration and further research into how to incorporate team based activities into physiology research interventions would be advised.

Researchers need to be ethically aware of the possible dangers that can accompany exercising, for example eating disorders or injury and monitor such matters. Cognisant of the potential detrimental aspects that go with dance, such as creating an ideal body aesthetic and perfectionism [39], dance sessions need to ensure competence and self-satisfaction can be achieved by all participants. Integrating a mixture of activities, a degree of flexibility and autonomy suitable to a range of participants and motivations can be complicated and difficult to design, implement and evaluate [14]. In addition to other constraints such as research funding, facility accessibility and physiological measures, researchers must appreciate there are limits in what can be offered during exercise training programmes. It might be more feasible to introduce novel and greater variety of activities within future exercise physiology research with advancements of non-invasive free-living measures of energy expenditure and physical activity [40]. While replicating adolescent girls' preferred activity more closely, this could consequently add ecological validity to the studies when translating research into practice.

With more physiology research targeting paediatric populations, successful recruitment and maximal adherence within our studies are crucial to improve the credibility of study findings. Implementing this qualitative work with subgroups of adolescent girls (*i.e.*, socio-economic status, family support structure, school type weight status and physical activity level) could be beneficial to extend the proposed recommendations. Children and adolescent's involvement in research, often requires support and commitment from their parents (for example, providing lifts, arranging visits with the researcher and assisting with some measurements). Drews *et al.* [8] and Jago *et al.* [19] investigated parents' views related to health promotion interventions. Extending the current research to explore parental views of the physiology research recruitment process and study retention is also warranted. This would provide a greater understanding of parents' motives and needs for consenting to their child's participation. Finally, whilst physical activity interventions and randomised controlled trials with an exercise arm may align with a number of these themes and recommendations, further research with a specific focus on recruitment to randomised controlled trials is warranted. This could provide important views related to the random allocation to study arms and possible issues of preference effects and resentful demoralisation that we are unable to infer from the present study.

5. Conclusions

In conclusion, based on this qualitative study, careful consideration of the phrases and images used in recruitment material which target enjoyment and personal motivations for participating during the recruitment process would be recommended. Allowing a degree of flexibility, appropriate grouping of participants and offering a variety of activities are suggested to improve retention rates in chronic exercise training studies with adolescent girls. It is hoped this article will prove useful in providing evidence-based recommendations to promote successful recruitment and maintained adherence to well-designed chronic exercise training programmes.

Acknowledgments

We thank all the girls who participated in the study and the school staff for their support. This research was supported by the National Institute for Health Research (NIHR) Diet, Lifestyle & Physical Activity Biomedical Research Unit based at University Hospitals of Leicester and Loughborough University. The views expressed are those of the authors and not necessarily those of the NHS, the NIHR or the Department of Health. We also thank the expert reviewers for their helpful comments during the review process, which allowed us to significantly improve the manuscript.

Author Contributions

Rachel Massie and Keith Tolfrey conceived and designed the study; Rachel Massie performed the data collection; Rachel Massie and Brett Smith analysed the data; Rachel Massie wrote the original draft of the paper. All authors critically reviewed, contributed to and approved the manuscript.

Conflicts of Interest

The authors declare no conflict of interest.

References

1. Pfeiffer, K.A.; Dowda, M.; Dishman, R.K.; Sirard, J.R.; Pate, R.R. Cardiorespiratory fitness in girls: Change from middle to high school. *Med. Sci. Sports Exerc.* **2007**, *39*, 2234–2241.
2. Ortega, F.B.; Ruiz, J.R.; Castillo, M.J.; Sjöström, M. Physical fitness in childhood and adolescence: A powerful marker of health. *Int. J. Obes.* **2008**, *32*, 1–11.
3. Steinbeck, K.; Baur, L.; Cowell, C.; Pietrobelli, A. Clinical research in adolescents: Challenges and opportunities using obesity as a model. *Int. J. Obes.* **2009**, *33*, 2–7.
4. Spigarelli, M. Adolescent participation in research. *J. Adolesc. Health* **2008**, *43*, 1–2.
5. Slater, A.; Tiggemann, M. Gender differences in adolescent sport participation, teasing, self-objectification and body image concerns. *J. Adolesc.* **2011**, *34*, 455–463.
6. Douyon, M.; Chavez, M.; Bunte, D.; Horsburgh, R.; Strunin, L. The GirlStars Program: Challenges to recruitment and retention in a physical activity and health education program for adolescent girls living in public housing. Available online: http://www.cdc.gov/pcd/issues/2010/mar/08_0248.htm (accessed on 25 August 2015).

7. Berger, L.K.; Begun, A.L.; Otto-Salaj, L.L. Participant recruitment in intervention research: Scientific integrity and cost-effective strategies. *Int. J. Soc. Res. Methodol.* **2009**, *12*, 79–92.
8. Drews, K.L.; Harrell, J.S.; Thompson, D.; Mazzuto, S.L.; Ford, E.G.; Carter, M.; Ford, D.A.; Yin, Z.; Jessup, A.N.; Roullet, J.-B. Recruitment and retention strategies and methods in the HEALTHY study. *Int. J. Obes.* **2009**, *33*, S21–S28.
9. Gul, R.B.; Ali, P.A. Clinical trials: The challenge of recruitment and retention of participants. *J. Clin. Nurs.* **2012**, *19*, 227–233.
10. Hulley, S.B.; Cummings, S.R.; Browner, S.W.; Grady, D.G.; Newman, T.B. *Designing Clinical Research*; Lippincott Williams & Wilkins: Philadelphia, PA, USA, 2013.
11. Patel, M.X.; Doku, V.; Tennakoon, L. Challenges in recruitment of research participants. *Adv. Psychiatr. Treat.* **2003**, *9*, 229–238.
12. Coday, M.; Boutlin-Foster, C.; Goldman Sher, T.; Tennant, J.; Greaney, M.L.; Saunders, S.D.; Somes, G.W. Strategies for retaining study participants in behavioural intervention trials: Retention experience of the NIH behaviour change consortium. *Ann. Behav. Med.* **2005**, *29*, 55–65.
13. Withall, J.; Jago, R.; Fox, K.R. Why some do but most don't. Barriers and enablers to engaging low-income groups in physical activity programmes: A mixed methods study. *BMC Public Health* **2011**, *11*, doi:10.1186/1471-2458-11-507.
14. Corder, K.; Atkin, A.J.; Ekelund, U.; Van Sluijs, E.M.F. What do adolescents want in order to be more active? *BMC Public Health* **2013**, *13*, doi:10.1186/1471-2458-13-718.
15. Craig, P.; Dieppe, P.; Macintyre, S.; Michie, S.; Nazareth, I.; Petticrew, M. Developing and evaluating complex interventions: The new Medical Research Council guidance. *Brit. Med. J.* **2008**, *337*, doi:10.1136/bmj.a1655.
16. Lewin, S.; Glenton, C.; Oxman, A.D. Use of qualitative methods alongside randomised controlled trials of complex healthcare interventions: Methodological study. *Brit. Med. J.* **2009**, *339*, doi:10.1136/bmj.b3496.
17. Neumark-Sztainer, D.; Story, M.; Hannah, P.J.; Tharp, T.; Rex, J. Factors associated with changes in physical activity: A cohort study of inactive adolescent girls. *Arch. Pediatr. Adolesc. Med.* **2003**, *157*, 803–810.
18. Sallis, J.F.; Prochaska, J.J.; Taylor, W.C. A review of correlates of physical activity of children and adolescents. *Med. Sci. Sport Exerc.* **2000**, *32*, 963–975.
19. Jago, R.; Davis, L.; McNeill, J.; Sebire, S.J.; Haase, A.; Powell, J.; Cooper, A.R. Adolescent girls' and parents' views on recruiting and retaining girls into an after-school dance intervention: Implications for extra-curricular physical activity provision. *Int. J. Behav. Nutr. Phys. Act.* **2011**, *8*, 1–9.
20. Horner, S.D. Using focus group methods with middle school children. *Res. Nurs. Health* **2000**, *23*, 510–517.
21. Heary, C.M.; Hennessy, E. The use of focus group interviews in paediatric health care research. *J. Pediatr. Psychol.* **2002**, *27*, 47–57.
22. Colucci, E. Focus groups can be fun: The use of activity-oriented questions in focus group discussions. *Qual. Health Res.* **2007**, *17*, 1422–1433.
23. Braun, V.; Clarke, V. Using thematic analysis in psychology. *Qual. Res. Psychol.* **2006**, *3*, 77–101.
24. Jones, F.C.; Broome, M.E. Focus groups with African American adolescents: Enhancing recruitment and retention in intervention studies. *J. Pediatr. Nurs.* **2001**, *16*, 88–96.

25. Winter, E.M.; Cobb, M. Ethics in paediatric research: Principles and processes. In *Paediatric Exercise Science and Medicine*, 2nd ed.; Armstrong, N., Van Mechelen, W., Eds.; Oxford University Press: New York, NY, USA, 2008; pp. 3–12.
26. Women's Sport and Fitness Foundation. Changing the Game, for Girls. 2012. Available online: http://www.bhfactive.org.uk/userfiles/Documents/ChangingTheGameForGirlsl.pdf (accessed on 25 August 2015).
27. Whitehead, S.; Biddle, S. Adolescent girls' perceptions of physical activity: A focus group study. *Eur. Phys. Educ. Rev.* **2008**, *14*, 243–262.
28. Phoenix, C.; Orr, N. Pleasure: A forgotten dimension of physical activity in older age. *Soc. Sci. Med.* **2014**, *115*, 94–102.
29. Ryan, R.M.; Deci, E.L. Intrinsic and extrinsic motivations: Classic definitions and new motivations. *Contemp. Educ. Psychol.* **2000**, *25*, 54–67.
30. Jago, R.; Brockman, R.; Fox, K.R.; Cartwright, K.; Page, A.S.; Thompson, J.L. Friendship groups and physical activity: Qualitative findings on how physical activity is initiated and maintained among 10–11 year old children. *Int. J. Behav. Nutr. Phys. Act.* **2009**, *6*, doi:10.1186/1479-5868-6-4.
31. Grogan, S. *Body Image: Understanding Body Dissatisfaction in Men, Women, and Children*, 2nd ed.; Routledge: London, UK, 2008.
32. Biddle, S.J.H.; Whitehead, S.H.; O'Donovan, T.M.; Nevill, M.E. Correlates of participation in physical activity for adolescent girls: A systematic review of recent literature. *J. Phys. Act. Health* **2005**, *2*, 423–434.
33. Rice, M.; Broome, M.E. Incentives for children in research. *J. Nurs. Scholarsh.* **2004**, *36*, 167–172.
34. Wendler, D.; Rackoff, J.E.; Emanuel, E.J.; Grady, C. The ethics of paying for children's participation in research. *J. Pediatr.* **2002**, *141*, 166–171.
35. Dwyer, J.J.; Allison, K.R.; Goldenberg, E.R.; Fein, A.J.; Yoshida, K.K.; Boutilier, M.A. Adolescent girls' perceived barriers to participation in physical activity. *Adolescence* **2006**, *41*, 75–89.
36. Barnes, J.S.; Spray, C.M. Social comparison in physical education: An examination of the relationship between two frames of reference and engagement, disaffection, and physical self-concept. *Psychol. Schools* **2013**, *50*, 1060–1072.
37. Biddle, S.J.H.; Braithwaite, R.; Pearson, N. The effectiveness of interventions to increase physical activity among young girls: A meta-analysis. *Prev. Med.* **2014**, *62*, 119–131.
38. Burgess, G.; Grogan, S.; Burwitz, L. Effects of a 6-week aerobic dance intervention on body image and physical self-perceptions in adolescent girls. *Body Image* **2006**, *3*, 57–66.
39. Acelus, J.; Witcomb, G.L.; Mitchell, A. Prevalence of eating disorders amongst dancers: A systemic review and meta-analysis. *Eur. Eat. Disord. Rev.* **2014**, *22*, 92–101.
40. Brage, S.; Brage, N.; Franks, P.W.; Ekelund, U.; Wareham, N.J. Reliability and validity of the combined heart rate and movement sensor Actiheart. *Eur. J. Clin. Nutr.* **2005**, *59*, 561–570.

14

Neuromuscular Retraining in Female Adolescent Athletes: Effect on Athletic Performance Indices and Noncontact Anterior Cruciate Ligament Injury Rates

Frank R. Noyes † **and Sue D. Barber-Westin** †,*

Cincinnati Sportsmedicine and Orthopaedic Center and the Noyes Knee Institute, 10663 Montgomery Road, Cincinnati, OH 45242, USA; E-Mail: frnoyes@gmail.com (F.R.N.)

† These authors contributed equally to this work.

* Author to whom correspondence should be addressed; E-Mail: sbwestin@csmref.org

Academic Editor: Eling Douwe de Bruin

Abstract: While many anterior cruciate ligament (ACL) prevention programs have been published, few have achieved significant reductions in injury rates and improvements in athletic performance indices; both of which may increase compliance and motivation of athletes to participate. A supervised neuromuscular retraining program (18 sessions) was developed, aimed at achieving both of these objectives. The changes in neuromuscular indices were measured after training in 1000 female athletes aged 13–18 years, and the noncontact ACL injury rate in 700 of these trained athletes was compared with that of 1120 control athletes. There were significant improvements in the drop-jump test, ($p < 0.0001$, effect size [ES] 0.97), the single-leg triple crossover hop ($p < 0.0001$, ES 0.47), the *t*-test ($p < 0.0001$, ES 0.64), the multi-stage fitness test ($p < 0.0001$, ES 0.57), hamstring strength ($p < 0.0001$), and quadriceps strength ($p < 0.01$). The trained athletes had a significant reduction in the noncontact ACL injury incidence rate compared with the controls (1 ACL injury in 36,724 athlete-exposures [0.03] and 13 ACL injuries in 61,244 exposures [0.21], respectively, $p = 0.03$). The neuromuscular retraining program was effective in reducing noncontact ACL injury rate and improving athletic performance indicators.

Keywords: anterior cruciate ligament; neuromuscular retraining; noncontact ACL injury; female athlete

1. Introduction

It is well known that adolescent female athletes have a 4- to 8-fold higher incidence of sustaining a complete noncontact anterior cruciate ligament (ACL) injury compared with male athletes participating in the same sport or activity [1–3]. A complete ACL injury is indicated by 5 mm or more of increased anteroposterior tibial displacement on an instrumented or clinical Lachman test and a fully positive pivot shift test (grade 2 or 3 on a 0–3 point scale). At least two-thirds of ACL tears are noncontact in nature and occur when an athlete is cutting, pivoting, accelerating, decelerating, or landing from a jump [4–6]. The short- and long-term consequences of ACL injuries in young athletes include high cost of medical treatment, a heightened risk of future reinjuries (to both knee joints), psychological morbidity, lost productivity in work or school, potential for lost scholarship funding, and premature osteoarthritis [7–10]. Over the past 20 years, many ACL injury prevention programs have been developed in an effort to decrease the injury rate in female athletes [11,12]. There is tremendous variation among these programs in regard to the components that comprise the intervention, the duration and intensity of training, supervision and compliance tracking, and when training takes place (pre-season or within-season). Consensus statements from research retreats and committees agree that the ideal ACL-injury prevention program remains unclear in terms of exercise components, amount of supervision required, and timing due to the complex problem of the injury itself [13–16]. Reviews of published programs have suggested that plyometric and strengthening components are important components, and that the favorable effects of training are most pronounced in female soccer players under 18 years of age [17–21].

Investigators from the sixth ACL Research Retreat recommended that ACL injury prevention programs should be evaluated to determine their effect on both noncontact ACL injuries and athletic performance indices [15]. It has been hypothesized that programs that have a positive influence on both injury rate reduction and performance enhancement will have better compliance with training [15]. This is due to the perception that convincing athletes, parents, coaches, and others of the necessity for injury prevention training may be more successful if evidence exists that athletic performance will also benefit. Although several programs have reported ACL injury incidence data, few have undergone a rigorous assessment of their ability to improve athletic performance indices.

A 6-week, 18-session supervised ACL injury prevention program was developed and first described in 1996 [22]. Subsequently, this program was shown to significantly reduce the incidence of noncontact ACL injuries in young female athletes [23]. A group of 366 athletes that completed training had 17,222 athlete-exposures (AE) and 0 noncontact ACL injuries. A control group of 463 athletes that did not undergo training had 23,138 AE and five noncontact ACL injuries (incidence rate, 0.022, $p < 0.05$). Studies in relatively small numbers of athletes that completed this training program (34 volleyball players [24], 57 basketball players [25], 62 soccer players [26]), demonstrated significant improvements in athletic indices such as estimated VO_2max [24–26], agility and sprint tests [26], a sit-up test [24], and vertical jump tests [24,26]. There were also improvements in overall lower limb alignment on landing during a video drop-jump in these athletes [24–26]. As our experience continued to grow with this training program, we wished to determine if these same goals (significant decrease in ACL injury rates and increase in athletic performance indices) would be met in a larger group of athletes.

The goal of this investigation was to determine, in a group of 1000 female adolescent athletes, if significant improvements occurred after training in tests that measured neuromuscular and athletic indices such as lower limb alignment on a drop-jump, distance and limb symmetry on single-leg hop tests, agility, speed, lower limb muscle strength, and estimated VO_2max. The second goal was to determine noncontact ACL injury rates in a subset of 700 of the trained athletes compared with 1120 control athletes matched for age, sport, and body mass index. We hypothesized that this program would significantly improve neuromuscular and athletic performance indicators and significantly decrease the risk of noncontact ACL injuries in female high school athletes.

2. Subjects and Methods

2.1. Subjects

There were 1,000 female athletes (age 13–18 years, height 167 ± 7 cm, weight 59 ± 9 kg, body mass index 21 ± 3) from Cincinnati area high schools and club leagues who volunteered to participate in the training program over an 8-year time period. Initially, researchers and athletic trainers from our Center approached coaches and invited their teams to participate (free of charge) [23]. After the first four years, individual athletes began to request to participate based on observations and discussions with others who had completed team training. All athletes in this study completed one 6-week training session; those who completed more than one session were excluded. From these 1000 athletes, a subgroup of 700 were followed for one season to determine ACL injury incidence rates. These 700 athletes completed training just before the beginning of their sports season and were in high schools in which our athletic trainers worked and were able to track athlete-exposures (AE) on a weekly basis during the subsequent sports season. One AE equaled participation in one practice or game.

Before data collection, all athletes and their parents provided their informed written consent in accordance with the Internal Review Board of the Jewish Hospital of Cincinnati, Ohio for use of human subjects. All procedures were performed in accordance with the 1964 World Medical Association Declaration of Helsinki.

The sports the trained athletes participated in at the time of the study were volleyball (401), basketball (202), soccer (192), lacrosse (30), softball (15), field hockey (8), gymnastics (7), track and field (4), and multiple sports (141). Tanner staging [27,28] was not performed on these subjects. There were 118 subjects aged 13, 353 subjects aged 14, 260 subjects aged 15, 174 subjects aged 16, 83 subjects aged 17, and 12 subjects aged 18. In girls, the mean time to achieve peak height velocity is 11.5 years [29] and the mean time to reach skeletal maturity is 13.3 years [30]. Therefore, it appeared that the majority of athletes had completed expected growth and maturation. No athlete had a history of a serious knee injury or surgery.

An additional 1120 athletes from Cincinnati area high school teams served as controls and were matched to the trained athletes for age (13–18 yr), sport, and body mass index (21 ± 3). These athletes participated in their team practices and games, but did not perform any component of the ACL injury prevention program. Because this was not a randomized study, there was no intention to treat analysis performed.

Exclusionary criteria for training for this investigation were pre-existing multiple ankle sprains, evidence of a lower extremity joint effusion, or a history of a noteworthy knee injury such as a ligament rupture, meniscus tear, or patellar dislocation.

2.2. Study Design

The athletes underwent a series of tests no more than one week before the first training session (pre-test) and no more than one week after the last training session (post-test) in either the laboratory or at the training sites, which were usually indoor high school gymnasiums or soccer fields. Before testing and training, the athletes completed approximately 10 min of supervised dynamic warm-up exercises. Training sessions lasted 1–1.5 h and were held three days a week (Monday, Wednesday, Friday) in the afternoons for six weeks. All 18 training sessions were supervised by certified Sportsmetrics instructors. The entire program was completed just before the athletes' sports season began (*i.e.*, pre-season). Because neuromuscular and athletic performance testing evolved over time, with the addition and deletion of certain tests, not all subjects underwent the same tests reported. In addition, certain agility and speed tests were designated for specific sports and, therefore, were not conducted in all athletes. The number of athletes that completed each test is shown in Table 1.

Table 1. Number of athletes that completed each test.

Test	Number of Athletes
Video drop-jump	912
Single-leg triple crossover hop	280
Single-leg triple hop	223
Vertical jump, no countermovement	807
Vertical jump with countermovement	502
Agility *t*-test	221
37-m sprint	136
18-m sprint	350
Multi-stage fitness test	356
Sit-up test	110
Isokinetic strength test, 300°/s, quadriceps & hamstrings	141

Athlete exposures (AE) were documented for every practice and game the players (trained and control) participated in on a weekly basis. Coaches, athletic trainers, and research assistants assisted with ensuring weekly AE logs were completed. There was a larger number of control athletes than trained athletes due to the voluntary nature of this multi-year study; more athletes declined training than accepted to participate.

All knee injuries were tracked for the one sport season that followed the training. All athletes that sustained knee injuries were examined by the senior author. ACL ruptures were determined clinically according to grade 2–3 Lachman [31] and pivot shift [32] tests and magnetic resonance imaging.

2.3. Video Drop-Jump Test

A video drop-jump test was used to measure overall lower limb alignment in the coronal plane [33]. A camcorder equipped with a memory stick was placed on a stand 102.24 cm in height and positioned approximately 365.76 cm in front of a box (dimensions: 30.48 cm in height, 38.1 cm in width). Velcro circles (2.54 cm) were placed on each of the four corners of the box that faced the camera. The athletes were dressed in fitted, dark shorts and low cut gym shoes. Reflective markers were placed at the greater trochanter and lateral malleolus of both legs and velcro circles were positioned on the center of each patella. The jump-land sequence was demonstrated and the athletes completed two practice trials allowed to ensure they understood the test. No verbal instructions regarding how to land or jump were provided. The athletes were simply instructed to land straight in front of the box to be in the correct angle for the camera to record properly. The athletes performed the jump-land sequence by first jumping off the box, landing, and immediately performing a maximum vertical jump. This sequence was repeated three times.

After completion of the test, all three trials were viewed and the one that best represented each athlete's jumping ability was selected for measurement. Advancing the video frame-by-frame, the following images were captured as still photographs: (1) pre-land, the frame in which the athlete's toes just touched the ground after the jump off of the box; (2) land, the frame in which the athlete was at the deepest point; and (3) take-off, the frame that demonstrated the initial forward and upward movement of the arms and the body as the athlete prepared to go into the maximum vertical jump.

The captured images were imported into a hard drive of a computer and digitized on the screen using commercially available software (Cincinnati Sportsmedicine Research and Education Foundation, Cincinnati, OH). A calibration procedure was done by placing the cursor and clicking in the center of each Velcro marker on each of the four corners of the drop jump box. The anatomic reference points represented by the reflective markers were selected by clicking in a designated sequence the cursor for each image.

The absolute cm of separation distance between the right and left hip and normalized separation distances for the knees and ankles, standardized according to the hip separation distance, were produced using the software. Normalized knee separation distance was calculated as knee separation distance/hip separation distance × 100 and normalized ankle separation distance was calculated as ankle separation distance/hip separation distance × 100. We empirically believe that < 60% knee separation distance represents a distinctly abnormal lower limb valgus alignment position.

The reliability of the drop-jump video test was previously documented [33]. Test-retest trials produced high intraclass correlation coefficients (ICC) for the hip separation distance (pre-land, 0.96; land, 0.94; take-off, 0.94). For the within-test trial, the ICCs for the hip, knee, and ankle separation distance were all ≥0.90. We previously found no correlation between knee and ankle separation distances [33] and, therefore, report only absolute and normalized knee separation distances in this investigation.

2.4. Single-Leg Hop Tests

The first 57 athletes tested completed one single-leg hop test (triple) [34]. Then, because no limb symmetry problems were detected, we added a second hop (triple crossover [34]) in order to potentially detect limb asymmetry in more athletes. A tape measure was secured to the ground for a distance of approximately 6 m. Testing was first performed on either the right or leg, which was selected at random. The athletes stood on the leg to be tested with their toe just behind the starting line. For the triple hop test, three consecutive hops were done going straight ahead on the leg. In the triple crossover hop test, three consecutive hops were done on one leg, crossing diagonally over the measuring tape on each hop. The athletes had to be in control and hold the landing of the third hop for 3 s for the test to be valid. The athletes were allowed to use their arms for balance as required. Two or three practice trials were done for each test on each leg. Then, two hops were done on each limb. For athletes who completed both hops, the triple hop was done first on each leg, followed by the triple crossover hop. The right-left leg limb symmetry index was calculated by dividing the maximum distance hopped (best result) of the right leg by the maximum distance hopped (best result) of the left leg, and then multiplying the result by 100. These tests have excellent reliability, with ICC > 0.85 [35,36].

2.5. Vertical Jump Tests

The athletes' vertical jump was determined using the Vertec Jump Training System (Sports Imports, Columbus, OH). First, the standing reach was measured with the athlete standing with the heels touching the ground. Then, a maximum jump without arm swing or a countermovement maximum jump with arm swing was performed three times and the highest jump obtained recorded. In the first 305 athletes tested, only the maximum jump without arm swing test was performed. In the next 502 athletes, both tests were performed. The ICC using the Vertec is excellent (>0.90 [37,38]).

2.6. Agility t-Test

The *t*-test is a commonly used measure of agility [39–43]. The athletes sprinted from a standing point in a straight line to a cone placed 9-m away. Then, the athletes side-shuffled to their left without crossing their feet to another cone placed 4.5-m away. After touching this cone, they side-shuffled to their right to a third cone placed 9-m away, side-shuffled back to the middle cone, and then ran backwards to the starting position. Two tests were completed, with the best time recorded. The time to complete this test was recorded with a digital stopwatch in one-hundredths of a second. This test has excellent reliability, with ICCs ≥ 0.90 [44,45].

2.7. Sprint Tests

The athletes performed a single maximum sprint, starting from a stationary position with one foot in front of the other. Encouragement was provided throughout the run. The tests were performed (of either 18-m or 37-m in length) with the time recorded to the nearest one hundredth of a second with a digital stopwatch. During the first two years of this study, the 38-m sprint was conducted, followed for the remaining years of the study with the 18-m sprint in accordance with discussions with coaches who wanted to determine sprint speed over the shorter distance. The reliability of sprint tests using a hand-held stopwatch is excellent, with ICCs > 0.90 [46].

2.8. Multi-Stage Fitness Test

A common field test used to estimate maximal oxygen uptake (VO_2max) is the 20-meter multi-stage fitness test (MSFT).[47] The equipment required are the MSFT commercially available audio compact disc (CD) and a CD player. Two cones were used to mark the course. The athletes began with their toes behind the designated starting cone. The second cone was located 20 m away. On command, the athletes ran back and forth between the two cones in time to recorded beeps on the CD. The athletes performed shuttle runs back and forth along the 20-m course, keeping in time with the series of signals (beeps) on the CD by touching the appropriate end cone in time with each audio signal. The frequency of the audible signals was progressively increased until the athletes reached volitional exhaustion and could no longer maintain pace with the audio signals, indicated when three beeps were missed in a row. The level and number of shuttles reached before the athletes were unable to keep up with the audio recording were recorded. The VO_2max of each athlete was estimated using the equation described by Ramsbottom *et al.* [48]: $VO_2max = (5.857 \times \text{speed on the last stage}) — 19.458$. The test-retest reliability of this test is excellent, with ICCs > 0.90 [49,50].

2.9. Sit-up Test

The athletes were placed supine, with the knees bent and feet flat on the floor (held in place by a partner) and arms folded across the chest. On command, full sit-ups were performed by raising up so that the elbows touched the knees and then lowering back down to the floor. The number of repetitions completed in 60 s was recorded. The sit-up test has been reported to have acceptable reliability in normal subjects of 0.84 (ICC) [51].

2.10. Isokinetic Strength Test

Isokinetic knee flexion and extension testing was performed at 300 deg/s (Biodex Medical Systems, Inc., Shirley, NY, USA) [52–56]. The athletes were positioned in the device with appropriate torso, pelvis and thigh straps placed according to the manufacturer's protocol. The pivot point of the arm of the dynamometer was aligned with the lateral epicondyle of the knee, with the knee flexed to 90°. The chair was adjusted for each athlete to allow proper positioning. The range of motion during the test was fixed from 90° to 0°. Gravitational factors were calculated by the dynamometer and automatically compensated for during the tests. The athletes were familiarized with the machine and the test velocity by performing three to four sub-maximal trials. There was a 30-s rest period between the flexion and extension tests. Verbal encouragement was given throughout the tests, as the athletes were told to kick as hard and as fast as possible, but no visual feedback was available. A total of 10 repetitions were completed and the highest peak torque value used for analyses. Mean peak torque values (Nm) were normalized for body-weight (BW) in kg, and were expressed therefore as a ratio (Nm/BW). Acceptable reliability of isokinetic measurements in children and adults have been reported by many investigators [52–56].

2.11. Neuromuscular Retraining Program

The neuromuscular retraining program (Sportsmetrics) has been described in detail elsewhere [11,24–26]. The dynamic warm-up (Table 2), jump/plyometric (Table 3), and flexibility components were the same for all athletes. The philosophy regarding the jump/plyometric component of the program was to emphasis and teach correct jumping and landing techniques. Specific drills and instruction were used to train the athletes to preposition their entire body safely when accelerating into a jump and when decelerating on landing. The exercises progressed from simple jumping drills (to instill correct form) to multi-directional, single-foot hops and plyometrics with an emphasis on quick turnover (to add movements that mimic sports-specific motions such as cutting, pivoting, and change of direction). The jump training was divided into three two-week phases, each of which had a different training focus and exercises. Sports-specific agility, reaction, speed, endurance, and strength drills and exercises were incorporated for approximately 30–45 min for basketball, soccer, volleyball, and lacrosse players. All sessions ended with static stretching of the hamstrings, iliotibial band, quadriceps, hip flexors, gastrocnemius, soleus, deltoid, triceps, biceps, and low back.

Table 2. Dynamic warm-up*.

Exercise	Instructions
Toe walk	Walk on the toes and keep the legs straight. Do not allow the heel to touch the ground.
Heel walk	Walk on the heels and keep the legs straight. Do not allow the toes to touch the ground. Do not lock the knees, but keep them slightly flexed.
Straight leg march	Walk with both legs straight, alternating lifting up each leg as high as possible without compromising form. Keep the knees straight and the posture erect. Do not the lean backward.
Leg cradle	Walk forward and keep the entire body straight and neutrally aligned. Lift one leg off of the ground in front of the body, bending at the knee. Turn the knee outward and grasp the foot with both hands. Hold this position for 3 s, then place the foot back down and repeat with the opposite leg.
Hip rotator walk	Pretend there is an obstacle directly in front of you. Face forward and keep the shoulders and hips square. Extend one leg at the hip and keep the knee bent. Rotate the leg out at the hip and bend the knee to 90°. Rotate and bring the leg up and over the obstacle, then place it back on the ground. Repeat with the opposite leg.
High knee skip	This exercise involves skipping in which one knee is driven up in the air as high as possible, while the other is used to land and hop off the ground. Immediate repeat the skip on the opposite side with each land. Swing the arm opposite of the high knee up in the air to help gain height.
High knees	This exercise involves jogging where, with each step, the knees are driven up as high as possible using short, choppy steps. The shoulders and hips are kept square throughout the exercise.
Glut kicks	This exercise involves jogging where, with each step, the athlete kicks the feet back as if trying to reach the gluts with the heel, using short, choppy steps. The shoulders and hips are kept square throughout the exercise.
Stride out	Begin jogging forward using an exaggerated running form. Drive the knees as high as possible and kick the feet back, as if trying to make a large complete circle with the legs. Stay up on the balls of the feet throughout the exercise.
All-out sprint	Sprint forward as fast as possible, making sure to maintain proper technique and running form.

* The exercises are performed across the width of a court or field, or for approximately 20–30 s. This component will take approximately 10 min to complete.

Table 3. Jump training component.

Jumps	Duration	
Phase I: Technique	Week 1	Week 2
Wall jump	20 s	25 s
Tuck jump	20 s	25 s
Squat jump	10 s	15 s
Barrier jump (side-to-side)	20 s	25 s
Barrier jump (forward-back)	20 s	25 s
180° jump	20 s	25 s
Broad jump (hold 5 s)	5 reps	10 reps
Bounding in place	20 s	25 s
Phase II: Fundamentals	Week 3	Week 4
Wall jump	25 s	30 s
Tuck jump	25 s	30 s
Jump, jump, jump, vertical jump	5 reps	8 reps
Squat jump	15 s	20 s
Single-leg barrier hop side-to-side*	25 s	30 s
Single-leg barrier hop forward-back*	25 s	30 s
Scissors jump	25 s	30 s
Single-leg hop* (hold 5 s)	5 reps	5 reps
Bounding for distance	1 run	2 runs
Phase III: Performance	Week 5	Week 6
Wall jump	25 s	20 s
Jump up, down, 180°, vertical	5 reps	10 reps
Squat jump	25 s	25 s
Mattress jump side-to-side	30 s	30 s
Mattress jump forward-back	30 s	30 s
Single-leg hop, hop, hop, stick*	5 reps	5 reps
Jump into bounding	3 runs	4 runs

* Repeat on both sides for duration or repetitions listed.

2.12. Statistical Analyses

All data were normally distributed (Kolmogorov-Smirnov test). One-tailed paired *t* tests were used to determine whether significant differences existed between pre-train and post-train test results. Chi-square tests were used to determine the difference in the distribution of athletes who had <40%, 40%–60%, 61%–80%, and >80% normalized knee separation distance on landing. Effect sizes (ES) were calculated and interpreted according to Cohen's standards [57] where ≤0.2 was considered small; 0.21–0.79, moderate; and ≥0.8, large. The ACL crude incidence rate ratios were calculated for the trained and control groups per 1000 AE and tested for significance. In addition, Fisher's exact test was conducted to determine whether the proportion of injuries in the trained group was significantly difference from the proportion of injuries in the control group. For all analyses, the level of significance was set at 0.05.

3. Results

3.1. Compliance with Training

All athletes completed at least 14 of the 18 training sessions (mean, 15 ± 1). There were no injuries sustained that caused any athlete to stop training. Because each session was supervised, all athletes completed all jumps and sports-specific drills and exercises.

3.2. Video Drop-Jump

After training, statistically significant improvements and large ES were found in the absolute cm of knee separation distance and in the normalized knee separation distance values (Table 4).

Table 4. Effect of training on video drop-jump test.

	Pre-Train *	Post-Train *	Difference *	*p* Value	Effect Size
Knee separation distance (cm)	20 ± 8 (range, 6–56)	27 ± 8 (range, 9–57)	8 ± 8 (range, −19–41)	<0.0001	0.87
Normalized knee separation distance (%)	47 ± 19 (range, 14–150)	65 ± 18 (range, 21–118)	18 ± 19 (range, −53–92)	<0.0001	0.97

* Values shown are mean ± standard deviation.

Before training, approximately 80% of the athletes had a distinctly abnormal lower limb valgus alignment position on landing (empirically designated as ≤60% normalized knee separation distance). After training, 60% of the athletes displayed a neutral position on landing. The distribution of the athletes before and after training according to four normalized knee separation distance categories is shown in Figure 1. The change in the distribution of athletes in these categories between the pre-train and post-train tests was statistically significant ($p < 0.0001$). An athlete example is shown in Figure 2.

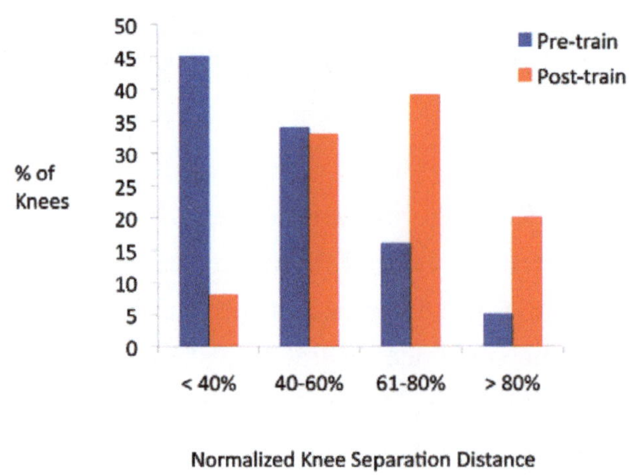

Figure 1. Results of video drop-jump test.

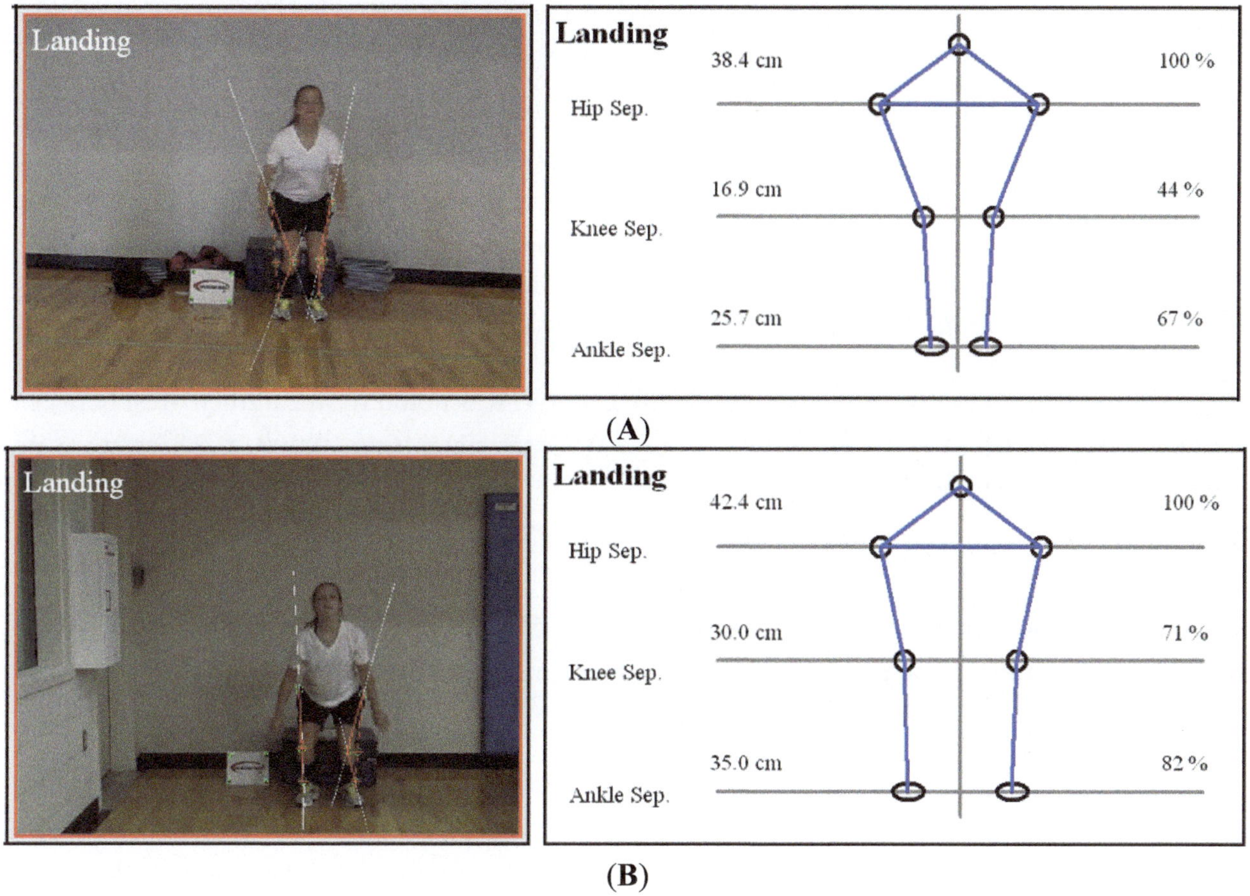

Figure 2. (**A**) Before training, this adolescent female athlete demonstrated a distinctly abnormal lower limb alignment, with a normalized knee separation distance of 44%; (**B**) After training, the athlete markedly improved her lower limb alignment to a normalized knee separation distance of 71%.

3.3. Single-Leg Hop Tests

Statistically significant improvements were found in the mean distances hopped for both single-leg hop tests for the right and left legs (Table 5). The ES were moderate in the triple crossover hop and small in the triple (straight) hop. There was no significant difference in the mean limb symmetry between pre-train and post-train values for both hop tests. Before training, 13% had abnormal symmetry (<85%) in the triple crossover hop, whereas after training, only 2% continued to have abnormal values. In the triple hop test, 8% had abnormal values before training and 2% had these values after training.

Table 5. Effects of training on the single-leg hop tests for the right leg.

Test	Pre-Train (cm)*	Post-Train (cm)*	Difference (cm)*	*p* Value	Effect Size
Triple crossover	360 ± 71 (range, 140–523)	393 ± 69 (range, 185–555)	33 ± 54 (range, −136–261)	<0.0001	0.47
Triple straight	405 ± 96 (range, 117–554)	414 ± 95 (range, 128–602)	9 ± 48 (range, −110–164)	0.003	0.09

* Values shown are mean ± standard deviation.

3.4. Vertical Jump Tests

Statistically significant improvements were noted for the two vertical jump tests; however, the ES were small. The mean difference in the test performed without countermovement was 1.1 ± 5.9 cm and the mean difference in the countermovement test was 1.3 ± 6.5 cm ($p < 0.0001$ for both analyses). Overall, 57% of the athletes showed improvement after training.

3.5. Agility t-Test, Sprints, Multi-Stage Fitness Test, Sit-up Test

A statistically significant improvement and moderate ES (.64) was noted for the agility *t*-test between the pre-train (12.10 ± 1.01 s) and post-train (11.51 ± 0.83 s) values ($p < 0.0001$). There were no significant improvements in the sprint runs.

A statistically significant improvement and moderate ES (0.23) was found in the sit-up test ($p < 0.001$).

A statistically significant improvement and moderate ES (.57) was noted for the MSFT between the pre-train (36.4 ± 5.0 VO_2max) and post-train (39.2 ± 4.8 VO_2max) values ($p < 0.0001$).

3.6. Isokinetic Test

Statistically significant improvements and moderate ES were found for the hamstrings, quadriceps, and hamstrings/quadriceps ratio on the isokinetic strength test on both the dominant (preferred kicking leg) and nondominant sides (Table 6).

Table 6. Effect of training on isokinetic quadriceps and hamstrings strength at 300°/s.

Test	Pre-Train *	Post-Train *	Difference *	*p* Value	Effect Size
Hamstrings Dominant	29 ± 6 (range, 10–45)	33 ± 8 (range, 15–73)	4 ± 7 (range, −9–53)	<0.0001	0.57
Hamstrings Nondominant	27 ± 6 (range, 14–43)	31 ± 7 (range, 9–56)	4 ± 6 (range, −8–32)	<0.0001	0.61
Quadriceps Dominant	35 ± 7 (range, 15–56)	37 ± 8 (range, 17–67)	2 ± 7 (range, −16–32)	0.001	0.27
Quadriceps Nondominant	35 ± 7 (range, 16–57)	38 ± 10 (range, 6–103)	3 ± 9 (range, −17–60)	0.0001	0.35
Ham/Quad Ratio Dominant	83 ± 17 (range, 44–163)	90 ± 24 (range, 54–272)	7 ± 27 (range, −88–206)	0.001	0.34
Ham/Quad Ratio Nondominant	78 ± 18 (range, 38–145)	83 ± 19 (range, 39–191)	5 ± 23 (range, −59–131)	0.006	0.27

* Values shown are mean ± standard deviation.

3.7. Noncontact ACL Injury Rate

The 700 trained athletes had 36,724 AE and the 1120 control athletes had 61,244 AE. There was one noncontact ACL injury in the trained group and 13 in the control group. The difference in the ACL injury incidence rates (per 1000 athlete-exposures) between the trained and control athletes was statistically significant (0.03 and 0.21, respectively, $p = 0.03$).

4. Discussion

The major finding of this investigation is that the ACL neuromuscular retraining program both significantly decreased the incidence of noncontact ACL injuries and improved athletic performance indicators in adolescent female athletes. This study entailed the largest cohort published to date in which athletic performance indices were measured after completion of ACL prevention neuromuscular training. Problems with training compliance have been addressed by others [14,15] and it has been suggested that an incentive to improve these issues is evidence that the program will improve athletic performance indicators. Although other ACL injury prevention training programs have improved certain athletic performance indices such as lower extremity muscle strength [58–63], vertical jump height [64–67], and distance hopped on single-leg tests [65,68,69], none of these programs also significantly reduced the noncontact ACL injury rate.

Since the first publication of a knee ligament injury prevention training program for female high school athletes appeared in the sports medicine literature in 1996 [22], at least 50 have followed that focused on this population [70]. A recent systematic review of all published ACL prevention training programs in female athletes aged 19 or younger found that only three programs (Sportsmetrics [23], Prevent Injury and Enhance Performance Program [PEP] [71], and Knee Injury Prevention [KIPP] [72]) significantly reduced the noncontact ACL injury rate as determined by athlete-exposures [20]. To our knowledge, no study has determined if the KIPP program improves athletic performance indices. An independent investigation of the PEP program demonstrated significant increases in electromyographic muscle peak torque and average power data (hip abduction, hip extension, knee flexion) after eight weeks of training in a group of 11 female high school athletes [73]. There was no significant improvement in jump height. Another study of the PEP program reported no benefit from the program on agility tests or vertical jump height in 31 female adolescent soccer players [74]. Although improvements were reported in sprint times during the first six weeks of training, these improvements reverted back to baseline values by 12 weeks [74].

Several ACL intervention programs have not been successful in significantly reducing noncontact ACL injury rates in adolescent female athletes [75–79]. It is important to note that some programs did reduce the incidence of lower limb injuries [75], acute knee injuries [78], contact knee injuries [78], and contact combined with noncontact ACL injuries [79]. Issues pertaining to poor compliance with training and limited statistical power due to the small number of exposures and noncontact ACL injuries were commonly cited as the reasons for the outcomes of prior investigations. Some investigators concluded that coach-led instruction, with no control on the quality of instruction or progression of exercises, was not the most desirable method in which to conduct training [77,79]. Shultz *et al.* [15] noted the importance of feedback that emphasizes correct form and technique, along with positive motivation of the athlete during training. We believe supervision is a vital component, especially in athletes that demonstrate potentially dangerous landing and cutting techniques that are believed to increase the risk of a noncontact ACL injury, such as low knee and hip flexion angles and landing flatfooted, with the foot far away from the center of body mass [80–83]. During training, athletes were constantly reminded to land softly with high knee flexion when jumping, to decelerate using small quiet steps, and to stop during sprinting drills with as little impact as possible. In addition, exaggerated knee flexion was stressed in order to avoid an extended or hyperextended position. Although not measured in our current study, we and many investigators have noted decreased ground-reaction forces and improved lower extremity alignment on landing and during cutting when these techniques are used that may decrease the risk of lower extremity injury [22,33,84–87].

For this study, we excluded any athlete with a history of a noteworthy knee injury such as a ligament rupture, meniscus tear, or patellar dislocation from training. However, in our practice, we encourage patients who wish to resume high-risk athletics such as soccer and basketball after ACL reconstruction and other major knee operations to complete this neuromuscular retraining program as end-stage rehabilitation. The criteria patients must demonstrate in order to begin training are completion of a running/agility program, completion of a basic plyometric program, negative pivot shift test, $\leq$3 mm increased anteroposterior displacement on the Lachman test, full range of knee motion, $\leq$15% deficit peak torque hamstrings and quadriceps isokinetic test, $\leq$15% deficit in distance hopped on single-leg hop tests, and no pain, swelling, or giving-way with any activity [88].

A limitation of this study is the difference in the number of athletes who completed the various tests before and after training to measure athletic performance indices. Isokinetic testing was conducted initially in all athletes because they were tested in our laboratory. However, over time, it became apparent that testing needed to be performed at the training sites because many athletes were unable to travel to our facility. The sprint tests were designated for soccer and basketball players only. The MSFT was introduced in the fourth year of data collection. Not all athletes completed all 18 training sessions, or completed both pre-train and post-train testing, because of reasons such as illness, time constraints, or schedule conflicts. Even so, the strengths of this study are the large number of athletes that participated in the program, the major training components remained constant throughout the multi-year study period, and there was a sufficient number of AE and noncontact ACL injuries to prevent a type II statistical error.

Many issues and questions remain regarding the gender disparity in noncontact ACL injury rates and others have offered multiple suggestions for future research directions [15,16]. Although it is well appreciated that a gender disparity exists among high school and collegiate male and female athletes, the exact reasons remain unknown. Large-scale, multifactorial studies are required on all potential risk factors for this injury that include anatomical, structural, genetic, hormonal, climate, and equipment. Secondly, it is uncertain if all female athletes should undergo a neuromuscular training program such as the one in this investigation. Once a hierarchy of risk factors is known, the identification of highly sensitive and practical screening tools to target those athletes at greatest risk for injury would be of tremendous benefit.

5. Conclusions

An ACL prevention neuromuscular retraining program was developed and conducted in 1,000 female athletes aged 13–18 years. The program resulted in statistically significant improvements in overall lower limb alignment on a drop-jump test, distance hopped in single-leg hop tests, agility on the *t*-test, estimated VO_2max on the multi-stage fitness test, and isokinetic hamstrings and quadriceps strength. The trained athletes had a significant reduction in the noncontact ACL injury incidence rate compared with the control group. The neuromuscular retraining program was effective in reducing noncontact ACL injury rate and improving athletic performance indicators.

Acknowledgments

We thank Stephanie Smith, Thomas Campbell, Catherine Walsh, Michelle Brock, Jennifer Riccobene, and Cassie Fleckenstein for their assistance with data collected for this study. We also thank Martin Levy for his assistance with the statistical analysis regarding ACL injury rates. This study was funded by the Noyes Knee Institute and the Cincinnati Sportsmedicine Research and Education Foundation, Cincinnati, OH, USA.

Author Contributions

FN designed the major components of the Sportsmetrics program and designed the investigation. SBW and FN collectively determined the tests to conduct, statistically analyzed the test data and the literature published to date, and wrote the manuscript.

Conflicts of Interest

The authors declare no conflict of interest.

References

1. Joseph, A.M.; Collins, C.L.; Henke, N.M.; Yard, E.E.; Fields, S.K.; Comstock, R.D. A multisport epidemiologic comparison of anterior cruciate ligament injuries in high school athletics. *J. Athl. Train.* **2013**, *48*, 810–817.
2. Mountcastle, S.B.; Posner, M.; Kragh, J.F., Jr.; Taylor, D.C. Gender differences in anterior cruciate ligament injury vary with activity: Epidemiology of anterior cruciate ligament injuries in a young, athletic population. *Am. J. Sports Med.* **2007**, *35*, 1635–1642.
3. Hootman, J.M.; Dick, R.; Agel, J. Epidemiology of collegiate injuries for 15 sports: Summary and recommendations for injury prevention initiatives. *J. Athl. Train.* **2007**, *42*, 311–319.
4. Beynnon, B.D.; Johnson, R.J.; Abate, J.A.; Fleming, B.C.; Nichols, C.E. Treatment of anterior cruciate ligament injuries, part i. *Am. J. Sports Med.* **2005**, *33*, 1579–1602.
5. Boden, B.P.; Dean, G.S.; Feagin, J.A., Jr.; Garrett, W.E., Jr. Mechanisms of anterior cruciate ligament injury. *Orthopedics* **2000**, *23*, 573–578.
6. Shimokochi, Y.; Shultz, S.J. Mechanisms of noncontact anterior cruciate ligament injury. *J. Athl. Train.* **2008**, *43*, 396–408.
7. Mather, R.C., 3rd; Koenig, L.; Kocher, M.S.; Dall, T.M.; Gallo, P.; Scott, D.J.; Bach, B.R., Jr.; Spindler, K.P.; Group, M.K. Societal and economic impact of anterior cruciate ligament tears. *J. Bone Joint Surg. Am.* **2013**, *95*, 1751–1759.
8. Hanypsiak, B.T.; Spindler, K.P.; Rothrock, C.R.; Calabrese, G.J.; Richmond, B.; Herrenbruck, T.M.; Parker, R.D. Twelve-year follow-up on anterior cruciate ligament reconstruction: Long-term outcomes of prospectively studied osseous and articular injuries. *Am. J. Sports Med.* **2008**, *36*, 671–677.
9. Ait Si Selmi, T.; Fithian, D.; Neyret, P. The evolution of osteoarthritis in 103 patients with acl reconstruction at 17 years follow-up. *Knee* **2006**, *13*, 353–358.

10. Barber-Westin, S.D.; Noyes, F.R. Consequences of complete acl ruptures. In *Acl Injuries in the Female Athlete: Causes, Impacts, and Conditioning Programs*; Noyes, F.R., Barber-Westin, S.D., Eds.; Springer-Verlag: Berlin Heidelberg, Germany, 2012; pp. 27–53.
11. Noyes, F.R.; Barber-Westin, S.D. Sportsmetrics acl intervention training program: Components, results. In *Acl Injuries in the Female Athlete: Causes, Impacts, and Conditioning Programs*; Noyes, F.R., Barber-Westin, S.D., Eds.; Springer-Verlag: Berlin Heidelberg, Germany, 2012; pp. 275–308.
12. Noyes, F.R.; Barber-Westin, S.D. Acl injury prevention warm-up programs. In *Acl Injuries in the Female Athlete: Causes, Impacts, and Conditioning Programs*; Noyes, F.R., Barber-Westin, S.D., Eds.; Springer-Verlag: Berlin Heidelberg, Germany, 2012; pp. 371–390.
13. Campbell, C.J.; Carson, J.D.; Diaconescu, E.D.; Celebrini, R.; Rizzardo, M.R.; Godbout, V.; Fletcher, J.A.; McCormack, R.; Outerbridge, R.; Taylor, T.; *et al.* Canadian academy of sport and exercise medicine position statement: Neuromuscular training programs can decrease anterior cruciate ligament injuries in youth soccer players. *Clin. J. Sport Med.* **2014**, *24*, 263–267.
14. Postma, W.F.; West, R.V. Anterior cruciate ligament injury-prevention programs. *J. Bone Joint Surg. Am.* **2013**, *95*, 661–669.
15. Shultz, S.J.; Schmitz, R.J.; Benjaminse, A.; Chaudhari, A.M.; Collins, M.; Padua, D.A. Acl research retreat vi: An update on acl injury risk and prevention. *J. Athl. Train.* **2012**, *47*, 591–603.
16. Renstrom, P.; Ljungqvist, A.; Arendt, E.; Beynnon, B.; Fukubayashi, T.; Garrett, W.; Georgoulis, T.; Hewett, T.E.; Johnson, R.; Krosshaug, T.; *et al.* Non-contact acl injuries in female athletes: An international olympic committee current concepts statement. *Br. J. Sports Med.* **2008**, *42*, 394–412.
17. Barber-Westin, S.D.; Noyes, F.R.; Smith, S.T.; Campbell, T.M. Reducing the risk of noncontact anterior cruciate ligament injuries in the female athlete. *Phys. Sportsmed.* **2009**, *37*, 49–61.
18. Gagnier, J.J.; Morgenstern, H.; Chess, L. Interventions designed to prevent anterior cruciate ligament injuries in adolescents and adults: A systematic review and meta-analysis. *Am. J. Sports Med.* **2013**, *41*, 1952–1962.
19. Stojanovic, M.D.; Ostojic, S.M. Preventing acl injuries in team-sport athletes: A systematic review of training interventions. *Res. Sports Med.* **2012**, *20*, 223–238.
20. Noyes, F.R.; Barber-Westin, S.D. Neuromuscular retraining intervention programs: Do they reduce noncontact anterior cruciate ligament injury rates in adolescent female athletes? *Arthroscopy* **2014**, *30*, 245–255.
21. Yoo, J.H.; Lim, B.O.; Ha, M.; Lee, S.W.; Oh, S.J.; Lee, Y.S.; Kim, J.G. A meta-analysis of the effect of neuromuscular training on the prevention of the anterior cruciate ligament injury in female athletes. *Knee Surg. Sports Traumatol. Arthrosc.* **2010**, *18*, 824–830.
22. Hewett, T.E.; Stroupe, A.L.; Nance, T.A.; Noyes, F.R. Plyometric training in female athletes. Decreased impact forces and increased hamstring torques. *Am. J. Sports Med.* **1996**, *24*, 765–773.
23. Hewett, T.E.; Lindenfeld, T.N.; Riccobene, J.V.; Noyes, F.R. The effect of neuromuscular training on the incidence of knee injury in female athletes. A prospective study. *Am. J. Sports Med.* **1999**, *27*, 699–706.
24. Noyes, F.R.; Barber-Westin, S.D.; Smith, S.T.; Campbell, T. A training program to improve neuromuscular indices in female high school volleyball players. *J. Strength Cond. Res.* **2011**, *25*, 2151–2160.

25. Noyes, F.R.; Barber-Westin, S.D.; Smith, S.T.; Campbell, T.; Garrison, T.T. A training program to improve neuromuscular and performance indices in female high school basketball players. *J. Strength Cond. Res.* **2012**, *26*, 709–719.
26. Noyes, F.R.; Barber-Westin, S.D.; Tutalo Smith, S.T.; Campbell, T. A training program to improve neuromuscular and performance indices in female high school soccer players. *J. Strength Cond. Res.* **2013**, *27*, 340–351.
27. Marshall, W.A.; Tanner, J.M. Variations in pattern of pubertal changes in girls. *Arch. Dis. Child.* **1969**, *44*, 291–303.
28. Marshall, W.A.; Tanner, J.M. Variations in the pattern of pubertal changes in boys. *Arch. Dis. Child.* **1970**, *45*, 13–23.
29. Tanner, J.M.; Davies, P.S. Clinical longitudinal standards for height and height velocity for north american children. *J. Pediatr.* **1985**, *107*, 317–329.
30. Anderson, M.; Messner, M.B.; Green, W.T. Distribution of lengths of the normal femur and tibia in children from one to eighteen years of age. *J. Bone Joint Surg. Am.* **1964**, *46*, 1197–1202.
31. Mulligan, E.P.; McGuffie, D.Q.; Coyner, K.; Khazzam, M. The reliability and diagnostic accuracy of assessing the translation endpoint during the lachman test. *Int. J. Sports Phys. Ther.* **2015**, *10*, 52–61.
32. Benjaminse, A.; Gokeler, A.; van der Schans, C.P. Clinical diagnosis of an anterior cruciate ligament rupture: A meta-analysis. *J. Orthop. Sports Phys. Ther.* **2006**, *36*, 267–288.
33. Noyes, F.R.; Barber-Westin, S.D.; Fleckenstein, C.; Walsh, C.; West, J. The drop-jump screening test: Difference in lower limb control by gender and effect of neuromuscular training in female athletes. *Am. J. Sports Med.* **2005**, *33*, 197–207.
34. Noyes, F.R.; Barber, S.D.; Mangine, R.E. Abnormal lower limb symmetry determined by function hop tests after anterior cruciate ligament rupture. *Am. J. Sports Med.* **1991**, *19*, 513–518.
35. Reid, A.; Birmingham, T.B.; Stratford, P.W.; Alcock, G.K.; Giffin, J.R. Hop testing provides a reliable and valid outcome measure during rehabilitation after anterior cruciate ligament reconstruction. *Phys. Ther.* **2007**, *87*, 337–349.
36. Ross, M.D.; Langford, B.; Whelan, P.J. Test-retest reliability of 4 single-leg horizontal hop tests. *J. Strength Cond. Res.* **2002**, *16*, 617–622.
37. Chimera, N.J.; Swanik, K.A.; Swanik, C.B.; Straub, S.J. Effects of plyometric training on muscle-activation strategies and performance in female athletes. *J. Athl. Train.* **2004**, *39*, 24–31.
38. Young, W.; MacDonald, C.; Heggen, T.; Fitzpatrick, J. An evaluation of the specificity, validity and reliability of jumping tests. *J. Sports Med. Phys. Fit.* **1997**, *37*, 240–245.
39. Ben Abdelkrim, N.; Castagna, C.; Jabri, I.; Battikh, T.; el Fazaa, S.; el Ati, J. Activity profile and physiological requirements of junior elite basketball players in relation to aerobic-anaerobic fitness. *J. Strength Cond. Res.* **2010**, *24*, 2330–2342.
40. Delextrat, A.; Cohen, D. Physiological testing of basketball players: Toward a standard evaluation of anaerobic fitness. *J. Strength Cond. Res.* **2008**, *22*, 1066–1072.
41. Delextrat, A.; Cohen, D. Strength, power, speed, and agility of women basketball players according to playing position. *J. Strength Cond. Res.* **2009**, *23*, 1974–1981.
42. Myrick, S. Injury prevention and performance enhancement: A training program for basketball. *Conn. Med.* **2007**, *71*, 5–8.

43. Lidor, R.; Ziv, G. Physical and physiological attributes of female volleyball players—A review. *J. Strength Cond. Res.* **2010**, *24*, 1963–1973.
44. Sassi, R.H.; Dardouri, W.; Yahmed, M.H.; Gmada, N.; Mahfoudhi, M.E.; Gharbi, Z. Relative and absolute reliability of a modified agility *t*-test and its relationship with vertical jump and straight sprint. *J. Strength Cond. Res.* **2009**, *23*, 1644–1651.
45. Pauole, K.; Madole, K.; Garhammer, J.; Lacourse, M.; Rozenek, R. Reliability and validity of the *t*-test as a measure of agility, leg power, and leg speed in college-aged men and women. *J. Strength Cond. Res.* **2000**, *14*, 443–450.
46. Hetzler, R.K.; Stickley, C.D.; Lundquist, K.M.; Kimura, I.F. Reliability and accuracy of handheld stopwatches compared with electronic timing in measuring sprint performance. *J. Strength Cond. Res.* **2008**, *22*, 1969–1976.
47. Leger, L.A.; Lambert, J. A maximal multistage 20-m shuttle run test to predict vo2 max. *Eur. J. Appl. Physiol. Occup. Physiol.* **1982**, *49*, 1–12.
48. Ramsbottom, R.; Brewer, J.; Williams, C. A progressive shuttle run test to estimate maximal oxygen uptake. *Br. J. Sports Med.* **1988**, *22*, 141–144.
49. Gabbett, T.J. A comparison of physiological and anthropometric characteristics among playing positions in junior rugby league players. *Br. J. Sports Med.* **2005**, *39*, 675–680.
50. Williford, H.N.; Scharff-Olson, M.; Duey, W.J.; Pugh, S.; Barksdale, J.M. Physiological status and prediction of cardiovascular fitness in highly trained youth soccer athletes. *J. Strength Cond. Res.* **1999**, *13*, 10–15.
51. Alaranta, H.; Hurri, H.; Heliovaara, M.; Soukka, A.; Harju, R. Non-dynamometric trunk performance tests: Reliability and normative data. *Scand. J. Rehabil. Med.* **1994**, *26*, 211–215.
52. Carvalho, H.M.; Coelho, E.S.M.J.; Ronque, E.R.; Goncalves, R.S.; Philippaerts, R.M.; Malina, R.M. Assessment of reliability in isokinetic testing among adolescent basketball players. *Medicina (Kaunas)* **2011**, *47*, 446–452.
53. De Araujo Ribeiro Alvares, J.B.; Rodrigues, R.; de Azevedo Franke, R.; da Silva, B.G.; Pinto, R.S.; Vaz, M.A.; Baroni, B.M. Inter-machine reliability of the biodex and cybex isokinetic dynamometers for knee flexor/extensor isometric, concentric and eccentric tests. *Phys. Ther. Sport* **2015**, *16*, 59–65.
54. Nuyens, G.; de Weerdt, W.; Spaepen, A.; Janssens, L.; Ketelaer, P.; Bogaerts, K. Reliability of torque measurements during passive isokinetic knee movements in healthy subjects. *Scand J. Rehabil. Med.* **2000**, *32*, 61–65.
55. Tsiros, M.D.; Grimshaw, P.N.; Schield, A.J.; Buckley, J.D. Test-retest reliability of the biodex system 4 isokinetic dynamometer for knee strength assessment in paediatric populations. *J. Allied Health* **2011**, *40*, 115–119.
56. Sole, G.; Hamren, J.; Milosavljevic, S.; Nicholson, H.; Sullivan, S.J. Test-retest reliability of isokinetic knee extension and flexion. *Arch. Phys. Med. Rehabil.* **2007**, *88*, 626–631.
57. Cohen, J. *Statistical Power Analysis for the Behavioral Sciences*; Academic Press: New York, NY, USA, 1977; pp. 19–74.
58. Wilkerson, G.B.; Colston, M.A.; Short, N.I.; Neal, K.L.; Hoewischer, P.E.; Pixley, J.J. Neuromuscular changes in female collegiate athletes resulting from a plyometric jump-training program. *J. Athl. Train.* **2004**, *39*, 17–23.

59. Herman, D.C.; Weinhold, P.S.; Guskiewicz, K.M.; Garrett, W.E.; Yu, B.; Padua, D.A. The effects of strength training on the lower extremity biomechanics of female recreational athletes during a stop-jump task. *Am. J. Sports Med.* **2008**, *36*, 733–740.
60. Herman, D.C.; Onate, J.A.; Weinhold, P.S.; Guskiewicz, K.M.; Garrett, W.E.; Yu, B.; Padua, D.A. The effects of feedback with and without strength training on lower extremity biomechanics. *Am. J. Sports Med.* **2009**, *37*, 1301–1308.
61. Tsang, K.K.; Dipasquale, A.A. Improving the q:H strength ratio in women using plyometric exercises. *J. Strength Cond. Res.* **2011**, *25*, 2740–2745.
62. Wilderman, D.R.; Ross, S.E.; Padua, D.A. Thigh muscle activity, knee motion, and impact force during side-step pivoting in agility-trained female basketball players. *J. Athl. Train.* **2009**, *44*, 14–25.
63. Lephart, S.M.; Abt, J.P.; Ferris, C.M.; Sell, T.C.; Nagai, T.; Myers, J.B.; Irrgang, J.J. Neuromuscular and biomechanical characteristic changes in high school athletes: A plyometric *versus* basic resistance program. *Br. J. Sports Med.* **2005**, *39*, 932–938.
64. Chappell, J.D.; Limpisvasti, O. Effect of a neuromuscular training program on the kinetics and kinematics of jumping tasks. *Am. J. Sports Med.* **2008**, *36*, 1081–1086.
65. Myer, G.D.; Ford, K.R.; Palumbo, J.P.; Hewett, T.E. Neuromuscular training improves performance and lower-extremity biomechanics in female athletes. *J. Strength Cond. Res.* **2005**, *19*, 51–60.
66. Zebis, M.K.; Bencke, J.; Andersen, L.L.; Dossing, S.; Alkjaer, T.; Magnusson, S.P.; Kjaer, M.; Aagaard, P. The effects of neuromuscular training on knee joint motor control during sidecutting in female elite soccer and handball players. *Clin. J. Sport Med.* **2008**, *18*, 329–337.
67. Distefano, L.J.; Padua, D.A.; Blackburn, J.T.; Garrett, W.E.; Guskiewicz, K.M.; Marshall, S.W. Integrated injury prevention program improves balance and vertical jump height in children. *J. Strength Cond. Res.* **2010**, *24*, 332–342.
68. Herrington, L. The effects of 4 weeks of jump training on landing knee valgus and crossover hop performance in female basketball players. *J. Strength Cond. Res.* **2010**, *24*, 3427–3432.
69. Barendrecht, M.; Lezeman, H.C.; Duysens, J.; Smits-Engelsman, B.C. Neuromuscular training improves knee kinematics, in particular in valgus aligned adolescent team handball players of both sexes. *J. Strength Cond. Res.* **2011**, *25*, 575–584.
70. Barber-Westin, S.D.; Noyes, F.R. Effect of intervention programs on reducing the incidence of acl injuries, improving neuromuscular deficiencies, and enhancing athletic performance. In *Acl Injuries in the Female Athlete: Causes, Impacts, and Conditioning Programs*; Noyes, F.R., Barber-Westin, S.D., Eds.; Springer-Verlag: Berline Heidelberg, Germany, 2012; pp. 391–423.
71. Mandelbaum, B.R.; Silvers, H.J.; Watanabe, D.S.; Knarr, J.F.; Thomas, S.D.; Griffin, L.Y.; Kirkendall, D.T.; Garrett, W., Jr. Effectiveness of a neuromuscular and proprioceptive training program in preventing anterior cruciate ligament injuries in female athletes: 2-Year follow-up. *Am. J. Sports Med.* **2005**, *33*, 1003–1010.
72. Labella, C.R.; Huxford, M.R.; Grissom, J.; Kim, K.Y.; Peng, J.; Christoffel, K.K. Effect of neuromuscular warm-up on injuries in female soccer and basketball athletes in urban public high schools: Cluster randomized controlled trial. *Arch. Pediatr. Adolesc. Med.* **2011**, *165*, 1033–1040.

73. Lim, B.O.; Lee, Y.S.; Kim, J.G.; An, K.O.; Yoo, J.; Kwon, Y.H. Effects of sports injury prevention training on the biomechanical risk factors of anterior cruciate ligament injury in high school female basketball players. *Am. J. Sports Med.* **2009**, *37*, 1728–1734.
74. Vescovi, J.D.; VanHeest, J.L. Effects of an anterior cruciate ligament injury prevention program on performance in adolescent female soccer players. *Scand. J. Med. Sci. Sports* **2010**, *20*, 394–402.
75. Olsen, O.E.; Myklebust, G.; Engebretsen, L.; Holme, I.; Bahr, R. Exercises to prevent lower limb injuries in youth sports: Cluster randomised controlled trial. *BMJ* **2005**, *330*, 449.
76. Pfeiffer, R.P.; Shea, K.G.; Roberts, D.; Grandstrand, S.; Bond, L. Lack of effect of a knee ligament injury prevention program on the incidence of noncontact anterior cruciate ligament injury. *J. Bone Joint Surg. Am.* **2006**, *88*, 1769–1774.
77. Steffen, K.; Myklebust, G.; Olsen, O.E.; Holme, I.; Bahr, R. Preventing injuries in female youth football--a cluster-randomized controlled trial. *Scand. J. Med. Sci. Sports* **2008**, *18*, 605–614.
78. Kiani, A.; Hellquist, E.; Ahlqvist, K.; Gedeborg, R.; Michaelsson, K.; Byberg, L. Prevention of soccer-related knee injuries in teenaged girls. *Arch. Intern. Med.* **2010**, *170*, 43–49.
79. Walden, M.; Atroshi, I.; Magnusson, H.; Wagner, P.; Hagglund, M. Prevention of acute knee injuries in adolescent female football players: Cluster randomised controlled trial. *BMJ* **2012**, *344*, e3042.
80. Pollard, C.D.; Sigward, S.M.; Powers, C.M. Limited hip and knee flexion during landing is associated with increased frontal plane knee motion and moments. *Clin. Biomech. (Bristol., Avon.)* **2010**, *25*, 142–146.
81. Ebben, W.P. Analysis of male and female athletes' muscle activation patterns during running, cutting, and jumping. In *Acl Injuries in the Female Athlete: Causes, Impacts, and Conditioning Programs*; Noyes, F.R., Barber-Westin, S.D., Eds.; Springer-Verlag: Berlin Heidelberg, Germany, 2012; pp. 149–168.
82. Miranda, D.L.; Fadale, P.D.; Hulstyn, M.J.; Shalvoy, R.M.; Machan, J.T.; Fleming, B.C. Knee biomechanics during a jump-cut maneuver: Effects of sex and acl surgery. *Med. Sci. Sports Exerc.* **2013**, *45*, 942–951.
83. Hanson, A.M.; Padua, D.A.; Troy Blackburn, J.; Prentice, W.E.; Hirth, C.J. Muscle activation during side-step cutting maneuvers in male and female soccer athletes. *J. Athl. Train.* **2008**, *43*, 133–143.
84. Laughlin, W.A.; Weinhandl, J.T.; Kernozek, T.W.; Cobb, S.C.; Keenan, K.G.; O'Connor, K.M. The effects of single-leg landing technique on acl loading. *J. Biomech.* **2011**, *44*, 1845–1851.
85. Greska, E.K.; Cortes, N.; van Lunen, B.L.; Onate, J.A. A feedback inclusive neuromuscular training program alters frontal plane kinematics. *J. Strength Cond. Res.* **2012**, *26*, 1609–1619.
86. Celebrini, R.G.; Eng, J.J.; Miller, W.C.; Ekegren, C.L.; Johnston, J.D.; MacIntyre, D.L. The effect of a novel movement strategy in decreasing acl risk factors in female adolescent soccer players. *J. Strength Cond. Res.* **2012**, *26*, 3406–3417.
87. Kristianslund, E.; Faul, O.; Bahr, R.; Myklebust, G.; Krosshaug, T. Sidestep cutting technique and knee abduction loading: Implications for acl prevention exercises. *Br. J. Sports Med.* **2014**, *48*, 779–783.

88. Heckmann, T.P.; Noyes, F.R.; Barber-Westin, S.D. Rehabilitation after acl reconstruction. In *Acl Injuries in the Female Athlete: Causes, impacts, and Conditioning Programs*; Noyes, F.R., Barber-Westin, S.D., Eds.; Springer-Verlag: Berlin Heidelberg, Germany, 2013; pp. 427–454.

15

Effects of Respiratory Muscle Warm-up on High-Intensity Exercise Performance

Taylor S. Thurston, Jared W. Coburn, Lee E. Brown, Albert Bartolini, Tori L. Beaudette, Patrick Karg, Kathryn A. McLeland, Jose A. Arevalo, Daniel A. Judelson and Andrew J. Galpin *

Center for Sport Performance, Department of Kinesiology, California State University, Fullerton, CA 92834, USA; E-Mails: taylor.thurston@utah.edu (T.S.T.); Jcoburn@fullerton.edu (J.W.C.); leebrown@fullerton.edu (L.E.B.); abartolini@fullerton.edu (A.B.); TBeaudette@csusb.edu (T.L.B.); pkarg@fullerton.edu (P.K.); k.a.mcleland@gmail.com (K.A.M.); jarevalo@fullerton.edu (J.A.A.); dan.judelson@nike.com (D.A.J.)

* Author to whom correspondence should be addressed; E-Mail: agalpin@fullerton.edu

Academic Editor: Eling de Bruin

Abstract: Exercise performance is partially limited by the functionality of the respiratory musculature. Training these muscles improves steady-state exercise performance. However, less is known about the efficacy of executing a respiratory muscle warm-up (RWU) immediately prior to high-intensity exercise. Our study purpose was to use a practitioner-friendly airflow restriction device to investigate the effects of a high, medium, or low intensity RWU on short, high-intensity exercise and pulmonary, cardiovascular, and metabolic function. Eleven recreationally active, males (24.9 ± 4.2 y, 178.8 ± 9.0 cm, 78.5 ± 10.4 kg, 13.4% ± 4.2% body fat) cycled at 85% peak power to exhaustion (TTE) following four different RWU conditions (separate days, in random order): (1) high; (2) medium; (3) low airflow inspiration restriction, or no RWU. When analyzed as a group, TTE did not improve following any RWU (4.73 ± 0.33 min). However, 10 of the 11 participants improved ≥25 s in one of the three RWU conditions (average = 47.6 ± 13.2 s), which was significantly better than ($p < 0.05$) the control trial (CON). Neither blood lactate nor perceived difficulty was altered by condition. In general, respiratory exchange ratios were significantly lower during the early stages of TTE in all RWU conditions. Our findings suggest RWU efficacy is predicated on identifying optimal inspiration intensity, which clearly differs between individuals.

Keywords: intervals; high-intensity; performance; respiratory; hypoxia; breathing; restriction; hypocapnia; fatigue

1. Introduction

Numerous physiological factors such as pH, temperature, neurological input, and substrate availability limit exercise performance. One particularly understudied aspect is the role of the respiratory musculature. The available literature provides clear evidence that fatigue of this system hampers exercise performance [1–4] by inducing a metaboreflex response, which causes sympathetic outflow and a resulting vasoconstriction/reduced oxygen delivery to working muscles [3,5–9]. Fortunately, functional capacity of the respiratory musculature is modifiable. Intentionally restricting airflow during inhalation, exhalation, or both [10–12] forces the respiratory muscles to increase work output to adequately support airflow and gas exchange needs. Improvements in whole-body performance have been found in a variety of sports [12–15] and general exercise settings [16–18] following these types of respiratory exercise. For example, Romer, McConnell, and Jones (2002) reported that chronic respiratory training significantly improved 20 km and 40 km cycling time trial performance by ~3%–5% [12].

Restrictive airflow breathing activities may also improve acute exercise performance by functioning as a pre-exercise respiratory muscle warm-up (RWU). This is of particular importance when engaging in high-intensity exercise. The respiratory muscles have high aerobic capacities, multiple sources of blood supply, and a unique resilience to vasoconstriction; making them naturally fatigue-resistant to low-moderate exercise intensities. However, they are susceptible to fatigue when exercising at intensities greater than 80% of VO_2max for prolonged periods of time [5]. Volianitis and colleagues (1999) understood this phenomenon and sought to examine whether or not a RWU (which presumably improves function of the respiratory muscles) could sufficiently alter high intensity exercise performance.

This was accomplished by comparing performance during a six-minute maximal rowing test following either a sport-specific warm-up or a RWU. The researchers noted the RWU induced a significant increase in rowing distance of 18 m. On the contrary, Johnson *et al.*, (2014) found no change in 10 km cycling time trial performance following a RWU combined with a sport specific warm-up (compared to a sport specific warm-up alone). Thus, while RWU appears helpful when utilized prior to short duration, high-intensity rowing, its effectiveness may be eliminated when cycling. Further examination of this speculation is important given the popularity of high-intensity cycling among personal trainers, strength and conditioning coaches, and health professionals.

Confusing the matter even more, the intensity (*i.e.*, amount of airflow restriction) and volume of the RWU significantly affect its outcome. Most studies report success when implementing two sets of 30 respiratory cycles at 40% of maximal inspiratory pressure [1–15,18]. Higher intensity restriction actually fatigues the system, while less restriction is insufficient [19]. Measurement of maximal inspiratory pressure typically requires specialized, expensive equipment. Practitioners attempting to implement a RWU are unlikely to possess such devices. However, less expensive RWU devices that allow manipulation of airflow restriction intensity are commercially available, but lack scientific scrutiny. Therefore, the purpose of this study was to utilize one of these practitioner friendly devices to investigate the effects of a high, medium, or low intensity RWU on cycling time to exhaustion and pulmonary, cardiovascular, and metabolic function.

2. Materials and Method

2.1. Study Design

This study was designed to investigate the effectiveness of three different RWU intensities on exercise performance. Day 1 consisted of baseline measurements and familiarization of the RWU protocol. On Days 2–5, participants performed a RWU with either high (HI), medium (MID), or low (LO) amounts of airflow restriction (or no RWU CON) immediately prior to a cycling test to exhaustion (TTE). Each trial (HI, MID, LO, CON) was separated by at least 48 h, and the order of each trial was randomized. Exercise performance and measures of pulmonary, cardiovascular, and metabolic function were collected and analyzed during each of the four trials.

2.2. Study Controls

Trial order was randomized via a Latin Squares design, with each trial occurring at least 48, but no more than 96, h apart. All trials occurred in the morning between 6:00 and 10:00 am, with each trial occurring ±1 h from the first experimental visit for each individual participant. To ensure training status did not change throughout the study, participants kept a training log for the week prior to their first testing session. Activity levels were then mimicked and recorded their throughout the duration of their involvement in the study. Participants were asked to refrain from exercise for the 36 h before testing and were encouraged to sleep ≥8 h the night before each test. Similar measures were taken for dietary intake during the 24 h period that preceded each individual testing session. Participants fasted 12 h prior to each testing session. Nonetheless, three participants were removed from the study because of significant differences in their carbohydrate intake the 24 h prior to one or more of their trials. To ensure sufficient hydration, participants were instructed to drink water the night before (~1000 mL) and the morning of (~500 mL) testing. Hydration status was monitored via urine specific gravity analysis prior to each trial. Recordings of greater than 1.020 resulted in a rescheduling of the exercise trial [20]. No external motivation (e.g., cheering, yelling, music, *etc.*) was provided or allowed during the RWU, pulmonary testing, or the TTE.

2.3. Participants

Fourteen healthy male recreational exercisers enrolled in the study, but three were removed from the final analyses ($n = 11$, Table 1). Participants were excluded prior to beginning any activities of the study if they had any prior experience with RWU (or similar) practices. Inclusion criteria required participants be free from any cardiovascular, metabolic, and pulmonary diseases or illnesses that may affect the pulmonary system, or have any joint, musculoskeletal, and/or neuromuscular injuries or pain that may affect their ability to perform maximal cycling exercise. To ensure adequate levels of aerobic fitness, participants were also required to demonstrate a VO_2max of ≥45 $mL \cdot kg^{1} \cdot min^{-1}$. Prior to participating, all volunteers were informed of the risks and signed a document of informed consent. This document, as well as the study, were approved by The University Institutional Review Board.

Table 1. Participant descriptive information.

Variable	Mean ± SD
Age (y)	24.9 ± 4.2
Height (cm)	178.8 ± 9.0
Mass (kg)	78.5 ± 10.4
Body Fat (%)	13.4 ± 4.2
VO_{2max} ($mL \cdot kg^{-1} \cdot min^{-1}$)	54.8 ± 6.9
Cycling Intensity (W)	274.5 ± 45.8

2.4. Preliminary Testing

During Visit 1, investigators assessed height and mass via stadiometer (SECA, Ontario, CA, USA) and an electronic scale (Healthometer Toledo ES200L, Ohaus, Pine Brook, NJ, USA), respectively. Body fat percentage was calculated via a three site skinfold protocol from the chest, thigh, and abdomen [21]. Participants then performed a cycle ergometer (Ergomedic 839E, Monarch, Stockholm, Sweden) VO_2max test. Expired gasses were measured using a TRUEMAX 2400 metabolic cart (PARVOMEDICS, Sandy, UT, USA), calibrated before each trial. The test required participants to initially cycle at 50 W for five minutes. The test subsequently increased 25 W every minute until the participant was too exhausted to continue, VO_2 plateaued, heart rate (HR) (Polar Electro Inc., FS1 and TS1, Woodbury, NY, USA) failed to increase despite increasing intensity, a respiratory exchange ratio (RER) greater than 1.15 was achieved, or the participant indicated a rating of perceived exertion (RPE) of greater than 18 [22]. Following the VO_2max test, participants were familiarized with the RWU protocol. This consisted of 2 sets of 30 breaths (1 min rest between sets) [19] while the nose was clipped shut and an air flow inhalation restriction device (O_2 Trainer™, Westwood, CA, USA) was placed in the mouth. The device (Figure 1) was set to the highest restriction setting possible during the familiarization for all participants to ensure they were capable of completing the protocol during HI. Participants were instructed to both inhale and exhale with maximum effort per breath.

2.5. Experimental Trials

Visit 2–5 consisted of either a RWU with HI, MID, or LO airflow restriction, or no RWU of any type (CON), followed by TTE. RWU was accomplished by performing 2 sets of 30 repetitions (1 min rest between sets) of maximal breaths at their normal breathing cadence. During CON, participants rested quietly on the cycle and performed no respiratory warm-up. The time between the end of the warm-up and the start of TTE was matched between all four experimental conditions. Participants used the same device for all familiarization and experimental trials. The specific RWU volumes and intra-set rest intervals used here replicated procedure used in previous studies [13–18]. The device was specifically chosen because it is inexpensive, portable, and allows the amount of airflow restriction to be adjusted (range of 3–13 mm), making it a realistic option for practitioners. Moreover, the device includes a three way valve built into the mouthpiece allowing airflow to be restricted during inhalation, yet unrestricted during exhalation. To contribute to this literature regarding optimal inspiratory intensity, we included RWU conditions across the spectrum of airflow inhalation restriction allowed by the device. Linear changes in airflow restriction diameter settings on the device likely translate into exponential changes in flow rate and/or inspiratory pressure. Thus, we chose to perform HI with a 3 mm opening (fitting #13), MID with an 8 mm opening (fitting #7), and LO with a 13 mm opening (fitting #2).

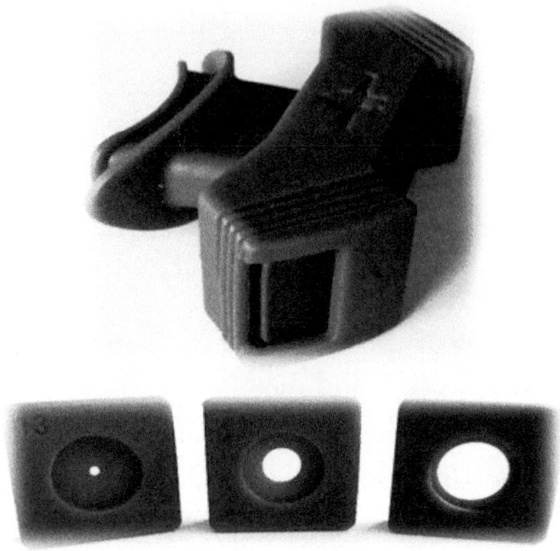

Figure 1. Photo of airflow restriction device used for the respiratory warm-up. Interchangeable caps are placed on one side of the device, restricting inhalation of air to the desired diameter, but allowing unrestricted exhalation. The high restriction (HI) warm-up used the 3 mm opening (fitting #13), the medium restriction (MID) used the 8 mm opening (fitting #7), and the low restriction (LO) used the 13 mm opening (fitting #2).

Upon arrival at the laboratory for all experimental trials, participants were assessed for hydration and training/nutrition logs were examined. After verifying compliance with all pre-study controls, participants were fitted to the cycle ergometer and the metabolic mask was sized to the participant's head and mouth. Personal cycle settings were recorded and reproduced for subsequent trials. After a five minute rest, blood lactate was measured via finger prick of the index finger (Accutrend Lactate Analyzer, Roche Diagnostics, Basel, Switzerland). Participants then performed pulmonary function testing via spirometry (SpiroLab II, SDI Diagnostics, Easton, MA, USA) until three repeatable values were recorded.

Volunteers then performed a five minute warm-up at 50 W on the cycle ergometer. Then, while remaining on the cycle, they performed the appropriate RWU protocol. Another pulmonary function assessment was conducted following the completion of the last set of RWU. This testing, and all pre-TTE preparations (e.g., mask set-up, *etc.*) were completed within two minutes of completing the cycling warm-up. TTE was performed at 85% of the participants adjusted peak wattage (achieved during the VO_2max test). RPE was measured at 1 min intervals using the Borg 6–20 scale. Volume of oxygen exhaled (VO_2), volume of carbon dioxide exhaled (VCO_2), RER, minute ventilation (VE), and HR were recorded using 15 s averages during the TTE. The TTE was terminated when the exerciser failed to maintain ≥60 revolutions per minute for five consecutive seconds [23,24]. Blood lactate was taken immediately after TTE was terminated. Five minutes of rest on the ergometer was given to participants before a post-exercise pulmonary function test was completed.

2.6. Statistical Analyses

Performance during TTE was analyzed by using a 4 (RWU Intensity) × 1 (time) repeated measures analysis of variance (ANOVA). A 4 (RWU Intensity) × 2 (pre and post TTE) repeated ANOVA was used to assess statistical differences among treatments for blood lactate. A 4 (RWU Intensity) × 6 (pre, 1 min, 2 min, 3 min, 4 min, and post TTE) repeated ANOVA was used to assess statistical differences among treatments for RPE. A *t*-test was used to compare the each individual's best performance against CON. Forced vital capacity (FVC), forced expiratory volume in 1 s (FEV_1), forced expiratory volume percentage (FEV1%), forced inspiratory vital capacity (FIVC), and peak expiratory flow (PEF) were analyzed via separate 4 (RWU Intensity) × 3 (baseline, post RWU/pre TTE, and post TTE) repeated ANOVA. Metabolic data were analyzed only to the point of the earliest TTE. Thus, 4 (RWU Intensity) × 13 (time) repeated ANOVA were used to assess statistical differences among treatments for absolute VO_2, VCO_2, RER, VE, and HR. In the presence of a significant F ratio, Tukey's post hoc test was used to analyze pair-wise comparisons. The alpha level was set at 0.05.

3. Results

3.1. Time to Exhaustion

There were no significant differences ($p \geq 0.05$) across conditions for TTE (4.73 ± 0.33 min). However, 10 of the 11 participants displayed a noticeable improvement (≥25 s) in one of the three experimental conditions (HI, MID, or LO) when compared to CON. Five had their best performance during MID (Figure 2), three during LO (Figure 3), and two during HI (Figure 4). The average improvement among these best trials was 47.6 ± 13.2 s, which was significantly different than CON.

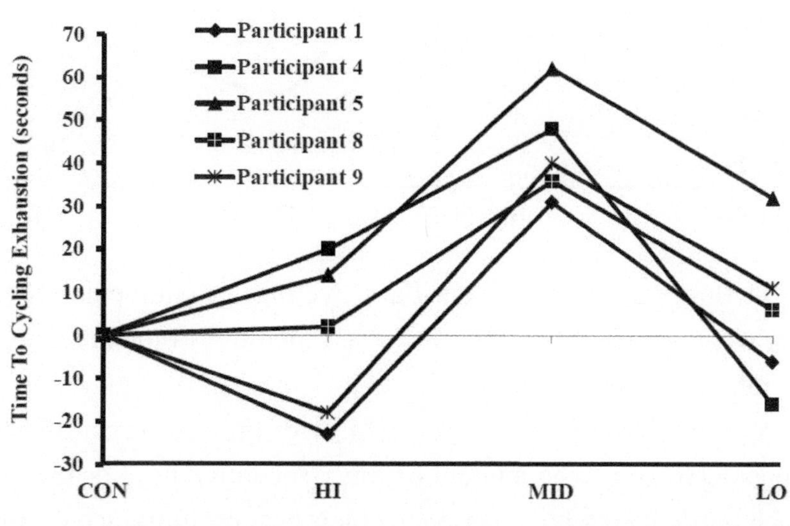

Figure 2. Changes in time to exhaustion during a cycling test immediately following a respiratory warm-up, which consisted of two sets of 30 repeitions of maximal breathes while wearing an air flow inhalation restriction device set at 13 mm (HI), 8 mm (MID), or 3 mm (LO) of restriction. A control trial (CON) was performed with no warm-up. Performance during CON was considered zero. The amount of time (seconds) more or less than CON is plotted above for each participant who experienced their best perfomrance during MID.

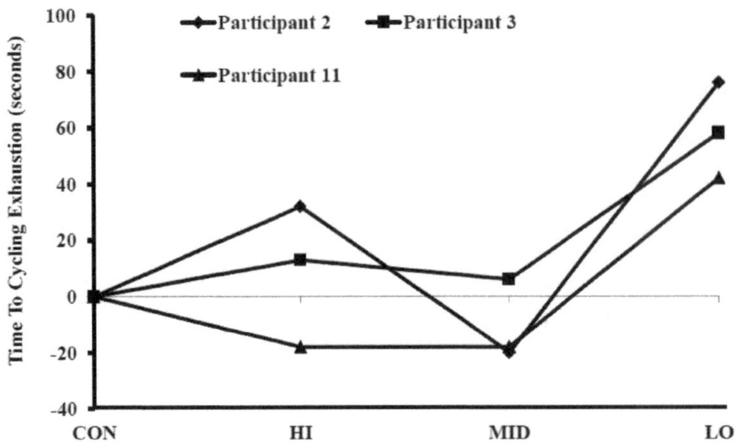

Figure 3. Changes in time to exhaustion during a cycling test immediately following a respiratory warm-up, which consisted of two sets of 30 repeitions of maximal breathes while wearing an air flow inhalation restriction device set at 13 mm (HI), 8 mm (MID), or 3 mm (LO) of restriction. A control trial (CON) was performed with no warm-up. Performance during CON was considered zero. The amount of time (seconds) more or less than CON is plotted above for each participant who experienced their best perfomrance during LO.

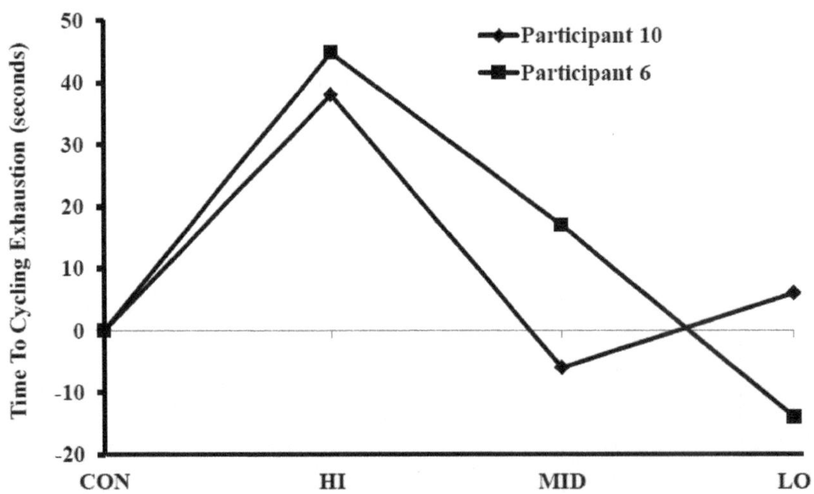

Figure 4. Changes in time to exhaustion during a cycling test immediately following a respiratory warm-up, which consisted of two sets of 30 repeitions of maximal breathes while wearing an air flow inhalation restriction device set at 3 mm (LO), 8 mm (MID, or 13 mm (HI) of restriction. A control trial (CON) was performed with no warm-up. Performance during CON was considered zero. The amount of time (seconds) more or less than CON is plotted above for each participant who experienced their best perfomrance during HI.

3.2. Rating of Perceived Exertion and Lactate

There were significant main effects, but not condition interactions, of time for lactate (Table 2) or RPE (Pre = 7.8 ± 1.4, Post = 20.0 ± 0.0).

Table 2. Lactate before and after a time to exhaustion trial. Data are reported as mean ± SD.

Condition	Pre	Post
HI	1.95 ± 0.56	15.38 ± 4.49
MID	1.91 ± 0.40	15.80 ± 4.03
LOW	2.17 ± 0.82	13.74 ± 4.14
CON	1.88 ± 0.47	14.20 ± 3.70

3.3. Pulmonary Function

No time main effects, condition main effects, or time by condition interactions were reported for FVC, FEV_1, FEV_1%, or FIVC. A significant main effect of time and an interaction by condition existed for PEF. Baseline (10.33 ± 1.54, 10.33 ± 1.48, 10.33 ± 1.49 L/s) and post TTE (10.26 ± 1.47, 10.36 ± 1.70, 10.35 ± 1.61) were not different from each other, but were both significantly greater than post RWU (9.89 ± 1.55, 9.88 ± 1.84, 9.68 ± 1.42) for HI, MID, and CON, respectively. Baseline PEF (10.30 ± 1.68) was significantly greater than both post RWU (9.80 ± 1.81) and post TTE (10.06 ± 1.80) during LO.

3.4. Gas Exchange

A main effect of time was statistically significant for VCO_2, VO_2, RER, and HR. However, interaction effects between condition and time were only significant for VCO_2, RER, and VE, while a trend ($p <$ 0.10) existed for VO_2. Regarding VCO2, CON was significantly greater than MID for all time points up to one minute and 30 s. For time points between 45 s and one minute and 30 s, CON was significantly greater than LOW. Regarding RER, CON was significantly higher than HI, MID, and LO for all time points up to one minute and 30 s, and higher than MID for all time points up to two minutes and 30 s. For VE, CON was significantly greater than LOW and MID, and HI was significantly greater than MID at the one-minute time point.

4. Discussion

The primary findings of this study indicate the effectiveness of the inspiratory RWU is highly contingent upon the intensity (*i.e.*, amount of airflow restriction) being optimized for the individual. If accomplished, the RWU protocol resulted in statistically significant and practically important changes in short-term, cycling to exhaustion performance. Our results also suggest that RWU, regardless of intensity, significantly decreased early stage (of exercise) RER, without altering blood lactate or perceived exertion, or decreasing exercise performance.

4.1. Performance

The interpretation that our RWU provided no performance benefit also holds merit as all conditions (HI, MID, and LO) failed to reach statistical significance. Several potential explanations exist. Firstly, the time between our RWU and the start of our exercise differed from some of the previous research. The current study followed the general methods of previous literature with similar procedures [16,18]. However, we chose to implement a rest interval that was shorter than previous research as it better reflected practices during normal exercise settings. Others have found performance enhancements when engaging in the RWU 30 min before exercise [25,26]. The optimal rest interval between RWU and exercise remains unclear, but our findings, combined with previous research [25,26], suggest longer may be better than shorter. Secondly, the limitations of the RWU device precluded us from controlling and/or quantifying inspiratory pressure or flow rate during the RWU, meaning we could not standardize conditions between or within participants. This directly influenced our grouped performance results.

Most previous research in this area has focused on identifying physiological mechanisms associated with RWU, not necessarily practitioner-friendly applications. This important stage in the research required scientists to control and monitor as many variables as possible [13–18], and led to the prescription of a desired inspiratory pressure of 40% [19]. Our goal was to examine RWU in setting more realistic to practitioners. Thus, we chose to use an inexpensive, commercially available device, knowing it could not be set to an optimal airflow restriction (per participant) *a priori*. We directly examined the loading intensity issue by asking participants to repeat the TTE trial under three different settings (which spanned the ability of the device, and was reasonable to complete the protocol). Finding significant differences among conditions was therefore difficult because of the high deviations in performance between each person's trials. This was particularly evident by the participants who had decreases in performance of ≥18 s (when compared to CON) during HI. These findings support previous research and suggest an optimal range exists for the intensity of a RWU, with too low of an intensity failing to produce benefit and too high of an intensity causing premature respiratory muscle fatigue [19]. However, significant improvements ($p < 0.05$) in performance were noted when the best trial per person was compared to their own CON trial. No clear patterns emerged among participants who performed best at a given RWU intensity. In conclusion: (1) an ideal inspiratory pressure exists; (2) previous research shows significant benefits of respiratory training [13,14,17,18]; and (3) individualized performance benefits of 10 of the 11 participants were more than double the standard deviation (±20 s) better than CON during at least one of the RWU conditions. This collective evidence allows us the confidence to conclude the protocol has the potential to provide practically important benefits to the physical performance test. The viability of a RWU under different circumstances deserves further investigation. For example, our RWU protocol only targeted the inspiratory muscles. Protocols which target the expiratory muscles (or both) may yield different findings.

4.2. Metabolic Function

The RWU significantly altered ventilation and O_2/CO_2, at least during the first two minutes of exercise. Specifically, the decrease in RER appeared to mirror those of VCO_2, but over a slightly longer time point. This was matched by a corresponding increase in VO_2 (trend). These factors could explain the enhanced VE displayed during the first minute of exercise, and combine to suggest the RWU induced arterial hypocapnia. Unfortunately, this speculation cannot be confirmed as measurement of endtidal CO_2 during the RWU was not possible. Previous studies have found hyperventilation-induced hypocapnia increases locomotor vasoconstriction, decreases muscle perfusion, and reduces O_2 delivery [27,28], which should combine to produce a diminution of exercise performance. Yet, here we report performance enhancement. Explanation of this apparent conundrum is not directly possible with the given data as specific examination of the interplay between RWU and hypocapnia requires an entirely different study design and focus. The authors can only speculate that either hypocapnia did not occur, or the RWU offset any potential detriments.

4.3. Blood Lactate and Pulmonary Function

Blood lactate was not different between RWU conditions, meaning it does not explain the changes in performance. Similar conclusions were reported in other related studies [14–16]. As expected, performance enhancements cannot be explained by acute changes in pulmonary function either as it was also generally unresponsive to the RWU, which was expected [4,12,14,29–31]. PEF did show condition specific responses, but the magnitude of change (<8%) indicates a limited clinical relevance [32]. Researchers should consider designing future research in a manner that allows specific evaluation of the pulmonary, metabolic, perceptual, muscular, neurological or other mechanisms responsible for performance enhancements.

5. Conclusions

The current study provides unique insight into the effects of RWU. Our data indicate RWU may enhance short-term, high-intensity exercise performance, but only when performed at an optimal intensity (*i.e.*, airflow restriction). Practitioners should implement with caution as intensity differs between individuals, and too difficult of a RWU hinders exercise performance. Further examination of the relationship between (1) performance-based classifications of optimal airflow restriction and (2) previously established guidelines of 40% maximum inspiratory pressure [19] would provide validation to both approaches and afford coaches/users the ability to effectively incorporate RWU into practice. It is unknown if other warm-up protocols (e.g., different volumes, longer rest between RWU, *etc.*) provide similar benefits. Moreover, the effectiveness of this RWU on exercise of other intensities, durations, or modes (e.g., running, rowing, swimming, *etc.*) is unknown. Researchers should also apply a similar, application-based research approach to study participants from other populations, particularly those with cardiopulmonary abnormalities. Further investigations in this area would benefit both the scientific community and practitioners.

Acknowledgments

The research team would like to thank all the participants for their hard work and effort in this exhausting task.

Author Contributions

Taylor S. Thurston, Jared W. Coburn, Lee E. Brown, Daniel A. Judelson and Andrew J. Galpin conceived and designed the experiments; Taylor S. Thurston, Albert Bartolini, Tori L. Beaudette, Patrick Karg, Kathryn A. McLeland, and Jose A. Arevalo performed the experiments; Taylor S. Thurston, Jared W. Coburn, Lee E. Brown, Daniel A. Judelson, and Andrew J. Galpin analyzed the data; Andrew J. Galpin contributed reagents/materials/analysis tools; Taylor S. Thurston, Jared W. Coburn, Lee E. Brown, Daniel A. Judelson and Andrew J. Galpin wrote the paper.

Conflicts of Interest

The authors declare no conflict of interest.

References

1. Mador, M.J.; Acevedo, F.A. Effect of respiratory muscle fatigue on subsequent exercise performance. *J. Appl. Physiol.* **1991**, *70*, 2059–2065.
2. Verges, S.; Sager, Y.; Erni, C.; Spengler, C.M. Expiratory muscle fatigue impairs exercise performance. *Eur. J. Appl. Physiol.* **2007**, *101*, 225–232.
3. Romer, L.M.; Polkey, M.I. Exercise-induced respiratory muscle fatigue: Implications for performance. *J. Appl. Physiol.* **2008**, *104*, 879–888.
4. Volianitis, S.; McConnell, A.K.; Jones, D.A. Assessment of maximum inspiratory pressure. Prior submaximal respiratory muscle activity ("warm-up") enhances maximum inspiratory activity and attenuates the learning effect of repeated measurement. *Respir. Int. Rev. Thorac. Dis.* **2001**, *68*, 22–27.
5. Dempsey, J.A.; Romer, L.; Rodman, J.; Miller, J.; Smith, C. Consequences of exercise-induced respiratory muscle work. *Respir. Physiol. Neurobiol.* **2006**, *151*, 242–250.
6. Hill, J.M. Discharge of group iv phrenic afferent fibers increases during diaphragmatic fatigue. *Brain Res.* **2000**, *856*, 240–244.
7. Jammes, Y.; Balzamo, E. Changes in afferent and efferent phrenic activities with electrically induced diaphragmatic fatigue. *J. Appl. Physiol.* **1992**, *73*, 894–902.
8. Harms, C.A.; Babcock, M.A.; McClaran, S.R.; Pegelow, D.F.; Nickele, G.A.; Nelson, W.B.; Dempsey, J.A. Respiratory muscle work compromises leg blood flow during maximal exercise. *J. Appl. Physiol.* **1997**, *82*, 1573–1583.
9. Sheel, A.W.; Derchak, P.A.; Morgan, B.J.; Pegelow, D.F.; Jacques, A.J.; Dempsey, J.A. Fatiguing inspiratory muscle work causes reflex reduction in resting leg blood flow in humans. *J. Physiol.* **2001**, *537*, 277–289.
10. Verges, S.; Lenherr, O.; Haner, A.C.; Schulz, C.; Spengler, C.M. Increased fatigue resistance of respiratory muscles during exercise after respiratory muscle endurance training. *Am. J. Physiol. Regul. Integr. Comp. Physiol.* **2007**, *292*, R1246–R1253.
11. Verges, S.; Renggli, A.S.; Notter, D.A.; Spengler, C.M. Effects of different respiratory muscle training regimes on fatigue-related variables during volitional hyperpnoea. *Respir. Physiol. Neurobiol.* **2009**, *169*, 282–290.
12. Romer, L.M.; McConnell, A.K.; Jones, D.A. Inspiratory muscle fatigue in trained cyclists: Effects of inspiratory muscle training. *Med. Sci. Sports Exerc.* **2002**, *34*, 785–792.
13. Volianitis, S.; McConnell, A.K.; Koutedakis, Y.; Jones, D.A. Specific respiratory warm-up improves rowing performance and exertional dyspnea. *Med. Sci. Sports Exerc.* **2001**, *33*, 1189–1193.
14. Wilson, E.E.; McKeever, T.M.; Lobb, C.; Sherriff, T.; Gupta, L.; Hearson, G.; Martin, N.; Lindley, M.R.; Shaw, D.E. Respiratory muscle specific warm-up and elite swimming performance. *Br. J. Sports Med.* **2013**, *48*, 789–791.

15. Lin, H.; Tong, T.K.; Huang, C.; Nie, J.; Lu, K.; Quach, B. Specific inspiratory muscle warm-up enhances badminton footwork performance. *Appl. Physiol. Nutr. Metab. Physiol. Appl. Nutr. Metab.* **2007**, *32*, 1082–1088.
16. Cheng, C.F.; Tong, T.K.; Kuo, Y.C.; Chen, P.H.; Huang, H.W.; Lee, C.L. Inspiratory muscle warm-up attenuates muscle deoxygenation during cycling exercise in women athletes. *Respir. Physiol. Neurobiol.* **2013**, *186*, 296–302.
17. Tong, T.K.; Fu, F.H. Effect of specific inspiratory muscle warm-up on intense intermittent run to exhaustion. *Eur. J. Appl. Physiol.* **2006**, *97*, 673–680.
18. Lomax, M.; Grant, I.; Corbett, J. Inspiratory muscle warm-up and inspiratory muscle training: Separate and combined effects on intermittent running to exhaustion. *J. Sports Sci.* **2011**, *29*, 563–569.
19. Roussos, C.S.; Macklem, P.T. Diaphragmatic fatigue in man. *J. Appl. Physiol. Respir. Environ. Exerc. Physiol.* **1977**, *43*, 189–197.
20. Armstrong, L.E.; Maresh, C.M.; Castellani, J.W.; Bergeron, M.F.; Kenefick, R.W.; LaGasse, K.E.; Riebe, D. Urinary indices of hydration status. *Int. J. Sport Nutr.* **1994**, *4*, 265–279.
21. Jackson, A.S.; Pollock, M.L. Practical assessment of body composition. *Phys. Sports Med.* **1985**, *13*, 76–90.
22. American College of Sports Medicine. *Acsm's Guidelines for Exercise Testing and Prescription*, 7th ed.; Lippincott Williams & Wilkins: Philadelphia, PA, USA, 2006; p. 366.
23. Ghosh, A.K.; Rahaman, A.A.; Singh, R. Combination of sago and soy-protein supplementation during endurance cycling exercise and subsequent high-intensity endurance capacity. *Int. J. Sport Nutr. Exerc. Metab.* **2010**, *20*, 216–223.
24. Ferguson-Stegall, L.; McCleave, E.L.; Ding, Z.; Kammer, L.M.; Wang, B.; Doerner, P.G.; Liu, Y.; Ivy, J.L. The effect of a low carbohydrate beverage with added protein on cycling endurance performance in trained athletes. *J. Strength Cond. Res.* **2010**, *24*, 2577–2586.
25. Volianitis, S.; McConnell, A.K.; Koutedakis, Y.; Jones, D.A. The influence of prior activity upon inspiratory muscle strength in rowers and non-rowers. *Int. J. Sports Med.* **1999**, *20*, 542–547.
26. Johnson, M.A.; Gregson, I.R.; Mills, D.E.; Gonzalez, J.T.; Sharpe, G.R. Inspiratory muscle warm-up does not improve cycling time-trial performance. *Eur. J. Appl. Physiol.* **2014**, *114*, 1821–1830.
27. Chin, L.M.; Heigenhauser, G.J.; Paterson, D.H.; Kowalchuk, J.M. Effect of voluntary hyperventilation with supplemental CO_2 on pulmonary O_2 uptake and leg blood flow kinetics during moderate-intensity exercise. *Exp. Physiol.* **2013**, *98*, 1668–1682.
28. Fan, J.L.; Bourdillon, N.; Kayser, B. Effect of end-tidal CO_2 clamping on cerebrovascular function, oxygenation, and performance during 15-km time trial cycling in severe normobaric hypoxia: The role of cerebral O_2 delivery. *Physiol. Rep.* **2013**, *1*, doi:10.1002/phy2.66.
29. Enright, S.J.; Unnithan, V.B.; Heward, C.; Withnall, L.; Davies, D.H. Effect of high-intensity inspiratory muscle training on lung volumes, diaphragm thickness, and exercise capacity in subjects who are healthy. *Phys. Ther.* **2006**, *86*, 345–354.
30. Kilding, A.E.; Brown, S.; McConnell, A.K. Inspiratory muscle training improves 100 and 200 m swimming performance. *Eur. J. Appl. Physiol.* **2010**, *108*, 505–511.
31. Romer, L.M.; McConnell, A.K. Specificity and reversibility of inspiratory muscle training. *Med. Sci. Sports Exerc.* **2003**, *35*, 237–244.

32. Jain, P.; Kavuru, M.S. A practical guide for peak expiratory flow monitoring in asthma patients. *Clevel. Clin. J. Med.* **1997**, *64*, 195–202.

16

Narratives of Psychosocial Response to Microtrauma Injury among Long-Distance Runners

Hayley C. Russell [1,*] and Diane M. Wiese-Bjornstal [2]

1 Department of Kinesiology, The Pennsylvania State University, Altoona Campus, Altoona, PA 16601, USA

2 School of Kinesiology, University of Minnesota, Twin Cities, Minneapolis, MN 55455, USA; E-Mail: dwiese@umn.edu

* Author to whom correspondence should be addressed; E-Mail: hcr3@psu.edu

Academic Editor: Arno Schmidt-Trucksäss

Abstract: Athletes with microtrauma or overuse injuries resulting from an accumulation of repeated small forces may differ from athletes with macrotrauma or acute injuries in their psychosocial responses because of the unique challenges presented by these insidious-onset and often chronic injuries. Our purpose was to use narrative inquiry to examine the psychosocial experiences and responses of 10 long-distance runners who had experienced microtrauma injuries. Qualitative data analysis of interview data led to a chronological timeline of the injury experience and an assessment of the meaning attributed to these injury experiences using a variation of Mishler's core-narrative approach. Participants reported distinct thoughts, feelings, and behaviors during each phase of the injury—pre-injury, injury onset, and outcome. In the pre-injury period, participants indicated specific running-related goals and attributed their injuries to overtraining or a change in training. During the injury onset phase, participants consistently indicated two themes: self-diagnosis and treatment, and not taking time off. Within the outcome phase of injury, participants acknowledged changed training because of the injury, and lessons learned from their injury experiences. The narratives of microtrauma-injured runners revealed psychosocial distress and behavioral tendencies post-injury that have important implications for runners, coaches, and healthcare professionals.

Keywords: injury; running; chronic injury; sport psychology

1. Introduction

Injuries are relatively common consequence of long-distance running. Researchers have found that 79% of long-distance runners will experience an injury during one year of training [1]. Long-distance runners who experienced a disruption in training due to a sport injury reported a variety of psychosocial symptoms such as depression and anxiety as well as endorsed low self-esteem and feelings of confusion and frustration [2]. Psychosocial refers to thoughts, feelings, and behaviors experienced by injured runners, as well as the social context in which these responses occur. In line with predictions of the integrated model of psychological response to sport injury [3], these findings provide evidence that long-distance runners experience potentially negative and distressing psychosocial responses to the sport injury process. Given the increased interest in long-distance running in the United States and the associated risk for injury, long-distance runners are an important subset of athletes to study to better understand the chronology of events as well as the psychosocial responses to injuries.

Individuals' responses to sport injuries can vary and, according to Wiese-Bjornstal [4], both personal and situational factors affect athletes' cognitive, emotional, and behavioral responses to sport injuries. Injury type is one of the personal factors suggested to influence an individual's responses to sport injury [3]. Injuries are typically categorized as one of two types—macrotrauma or microtrauma. Macrotrauma injuries result from an isolated, sudden impact or force (e.g., strains, sprains, dislocations, and fractures), whereas microtrauma injuries occur as a result of the accrual of repeated small forces over a period of time (e.g., stress fractures, tendinitis) [5]. The majority of evidence suggests that long-distance runners are more prone to microtrauma injuries than macrotrauma injuries. In a systematic review, van Gent and colleagues [6] found that the incidence of lower extremity running injuries was as high as 79.3% during the reporting period for studies reviewed (ranging from one day to 18 months); most of which were microtrauma in nature. Consistent with the integrated model of psychological response to sport injury [3], Flint [5] suggested that due to the differences in the onset of injury, psychosocial responses of individuals incurring microtrauma injuries might differ from those of individuals who experience macrotrauma injuries. For instance, individuals dealing with microtrauma injuries report a period of gradually increasing pain accompanied by decreased athletic performance during onset [5]. Due to the insidious onset and longevity of microtrauma injuries, athletes may experience significant and prolonged emotional distress (e.g., frustration, sadness), whereas the sudden onset of macrotrauma injuries allows athletes to immediately deal with the injury and rehabilitation process [5].

2. Context

Previous research has supported the suggestion by Flint [5] that differences exist in the psychosocial responses to microtrauma injuries and macrotrauma injuries. In particular, Wasley and Lox [7] found that athletes who experienced a microtrauma injury scored more negatively on measures of self-esteem, sought social support less, and reported more avoidance or escape behaviors than athletes who incurred a macrotrauma injury. Although limited by a small sample size and only presenting preliminary results, the findings suggest that the type of injury an athlete experiences may influence the nature of psychosocial response to a sport injury. Concerning social support, Henert [8] found that individuals with microtrauma injuries rated most types of social support as being more important to their overall well-being than individuals with macrotrauma injuries. These studies highlight two key points. First, psychosocial responses to injury differ based on the type of sport injury an individual experiences. Second, athletes report a discrepancy in the value of social support such that individuals with microtrauma injuries identify social support as being more important to overall well-being [8]; however, these individuals tend to seek social support to a lesser degree than individuals who experience a macrotrauma injury [7]. Because of the limited studies examining microtrauma injuries as well as the discrepancy in findings regarding psychosocial responses based on injury type, the current study was exploratory in nature, to better understand the process of psychosocial responses to microtrauma sport injuries.

Due to the complex and multi-dimensional nature of psychosocial responses to sport injuries [3], it is important to understand the full experiences of injured athletes. To date, researchers have primarily examined the psychosocial responses of athletes to sport injuries using quantitative methods or semi-structured interviews [9–12]. Another type of qualitative research that can be used to better understand lived experiences of athletes recovering from a sport injury involves narrative research methods; however, these methods have rarely been used in examining the experience of injured athletes. Narrative research methods are effective in studying an individual's experiences over time [13] and provide "coherence and continuity to one's experience" [14]. Thus, narrative research methods may provide a full picture of the injury and recovery process over time. By using this research method with long-distance runners incurring microtrauma injuries, we gain a fuller understanding of the unique aspects of these types of injuries that have been underrepresented in the psychology of sport injury literature to date.

Narrative research methods have been used to better understand the psychosocial responses of individuals with health-related issues [15] and with individuals recovering from non-sport related injuries [16]. In general, narrative research methods allow individuals to provide more thorough, less researcher-directed discussions of psychosocial responses to health issues or injuries as compared to quantitative research methods using self-report questionnaires or even semi-structured interviews. Thus, narrative research methods may help researchers identify responses that have been overlooked by other methods. With respect to sport injuries, Brock and Kleiber [10] used narrative research methods to examine athletes who suffered career-ending injuries 20 or more years prior to the investigation. The authors found that sport injuries inevitably led to a mild-to-severe change in both identity and self-esteem. Brock and Kleiber found a regular pattern within the stories that the injured athletes shared. Specifically, each athlete's story always included a section on the athlete's emotional response (e.g., feelings of confusion, isolation, anger) that resulted from experiencing a loss associated with the injury. Based on information derived from narrative research methodology in health-related research and sport injury research, we believe that the use of narrative research methodology is a valuable way to gain knowledge of the full experience of athletes who have experienced a microtrauma sport injury.

The use of narrative research methods in the present study fills a gap in research by providing a better understanding of the psychosocial responses (defined as thoughts, feelings, and behaviors) that individuals experience during microtrauma injuries. Thus, the purpose of the current study was to use narrative inquiry and analysis to examine the distinct experiences and responses of long-distance runners who had recently experienced microtrauma injuries. Results are reported for two main research questions:

1. What psychosocial responses do long-distance runners experience surrounding a microtrauma injury?
2. What is the chronology of psychosocial experiences associated with microtrauma injuries in long-distance runners?

3. Method

3.1. Participants

A purposeful sample of runners was chosen. This sample was selected because they were able to provide useful information about the phenomenon of study, specifically, microtrauma running injuries [17]. Participant recruitment continued until data saturation was reached. Ultimately, 10 participants (eight females, two males) between the ages of 19 and 37 years of age ($M_{age} = 25.1$) were recruited from a local running store and a long-distance running group at a large Midwestern university to participate in this study (see Table 1 for demographic and participant injury information). Participants were recruited to participate in this study if they met the following inclusion criteria. Participants must have suffered a microtrauma (defined, for the purposes of the current study, as an injury occurring due to the accrual of repeated small forces over a period of time as a result of long-distance running training) [5] within the 18 months prior to recruitment. Participants' injuries were self-reported. Participants also had to be competitive runners, defined for the purpose of this study as having trained for and were planning to, or had run, in at least one five-kilometer race in the preceding 12 months. Participants varied from novice to experienced runners. Additionally, participants had to be between the ages of 18 and 64 at the time of the interviews. Pseudonyms were used for all participants in order to maintain anonymity and confidentiality.

Table 1. Participant characteristics.

Pseudonym	Gender	Age	Self-Reported Injury
Logan	Male	22	Sciatic nerve; shin splints
Anne	Female	37	Pulled hamstring/illiotibial band; skin pain
Grace	Female	23	Achilles tendonitis; stress fracture
Caroline *	Female	22	Achilles tendonitis; knee patella femoral
Jordan	Female	22	Pain on inner right foot; illiotibial band
Laura	Female	21	Patella subluxation (knee)
Jane	Female	19	Knee pain, Sacroiliac pain
Brad	Male	21	Separated shoulder; tibia stress fracture
Maryn	Female	25	Quadriceps strain; pulled gluteus medius
Kathryn	Female	19	Illiotibial band; blisters
Cynthia	Female	20	Runner's knee (right and left); baby fracture

Note: *No audio or video data. Participant's data not include in data analysis.

3.2. Procedure

Institutional review board (IRB) approval was obtained prior to participant recruitment. In order to recruit individuals to participate in this narrative study, advertisements were posted at a local running store and an advertisement was made to a running group at a local university. Advertisements directed participants to contact the principal investigator (PI), by either phone or email, if s/he was interested in participating in the study. Additionally, the advertisements indicated that participants would receive a gift card for a local running store for participating in the study. Upon initial contact with the PI potential participants were asked questions related to the inclusion criteria for the study to determine if they qualified to participate in the study. If they met the inclusion criteria for the study, participants met with one of the researchers to complete the interview. Once the informed consent had been completed, the participants began the interview. Face-to-face interviews were conducted with all participants. Interviews ranged in time from 11 to 33 min. Participants were asked to tell the story of their injury, including events that took place immediately prior to the injury (henceforth referred to as pre-injury factors), the injury itself, and what happened after the injury. Participants were given this interview prompt verbally and in written form to refer to as they told their story. The only specific questions asked by the interviewers were probes to provide further clarification or elaboration on information provided by the participants. All interviews were video- and audio-recorded. Video recording allows the researchers to observe participant's body language, facial expressions, and other idiosyncrasies associated with the communication of the narrative. In addition, this technique aids the researchers in providing consistency during data analysis and coding, as well as the ability to contribute relevant observational comments, which are critical supporting evidence for the research [17].

3.3. Data Analysis

The interviewers transcribed each interview verbatim. The researchers then examined video transcripts of the interviews to add additional detail to the transcripts (e.g., crying). As per the example provided by Brock and Kleiber [11] in their modified narrative analysis technique, transcripts were prepared by numbering each new topic as the conversation progressed, for example:

> 075: P: Um, I've talked to my roommate a lot. She's one of my best friends and I, you know, through talking to her like, I don't want to, like have a pity party about it.
> 076: so I've just kind of, um, come to the realization that, like, I will finish. Like I will probably have to walk some, like I will…it will tack another hour.

Additionally, two different types of statements from the transcript were transferred to two new transcripts: the core narrative and evaluative commentary. The first transcript, labeled *core narrative* included any statement that contributed to the understanding of the sequence of events relating to the injury. For example statements such as "026: P: Umm I was doing a 5k and it, my leg just all of a sudden started, well, my left butt cheek started hurting it was a throbbing pain, I could literally not run, I would have to walk" were located in the core narrative transcript. The second type of transferred statement was any statement that contributes to the understanding of the sequence of events relating to the injury. This transcript was called the *evaluative commentary*. Statements such as "052: but it lingered on for so long, then it was kind of feelings of what is this and is it ever going to go away" and "053: at times it was feelings of, umm, it was frustration" were located in the evaluative commentary transcript.

Both the core narrative and evaluative commentaries were analyzed for common themes relating to the two primary research questions for this study. Specifically, the core narrative transcripts were analyzed to examine consistency and divergence in the chronology of the experience of athletes with microtrauma injuries. The evaluative commentary and core narrative transcripts were analyzed for common themes relating to the psychosocial response to the injuries as well as the meaning attributed to the injuries. Data analyses were similar to interpretative phenomenological analysis wherein the lived experiences of participants and the meaning attributed to the experiences are examined [18] and following the example provided by Brock and Kleiber [10]. Analyses consisted of the following steps. First, two researchers prepared the core narrative and evaluative commentary transcripts [10] and then reviewed the core narrative transcripts independently. This step involved several thorough readings of the transcripts identifying points of interest [18]. Second, researchers independently identified common statements between participants relating to the psychosocial responses to injury and the chronology of events associated with the injury. Third, researchers clustered common statements into overarching themes. Fourth, researchers compared the independently identified themes for consistency and divergence between researchers. Fifth, transcripts were then re-examined by the researchers to settle any disagreements in emergent themes leading to the final themes relating to the psychosocial responses to injury and the chronology of events. Another researcher then reviewed final themes after reading and re-reading the transcripts and was in agreement with the emergent themes [19].

4. Results

Participants' stories revealed that their experiences with running injuries had a meaningful impact on their lives. Analysis of the narrative data identified psychosocial responses to injury within the participants' stories and a consistent chronology of events and responses associated with injuries. In telling their stories, participants identified common experiences and responses during the pre-injury, injury, and post-injury phases of their injury process

4.1. Research Question 1: Psychosocial Responses

In discussing their injuries, participants revealed consistent psychosocial responses to injury. These themes were consistent cross the injury and recovery process. Overwhelmingly, the participants' responses to their injuries were negative throughout the injury process. Participants noted responses such as being "devastated", "bummed out", and "panicked" by the injury. The psychosocial distress experienced by the participants divided into four overarching sub-themes—frustration, fear, general emotional distress, and social influences.

Frustration. Microtrauma injuries for runners were described as frustrating. This frustration seemed to be due to the uncertainty or ambiguity associated with microtrauma injury. As previously discussed, microtrauma injuries have an insidious onset and can persist for a long period of time, yet may not be perceived as serious as macrotrauma injuries [5]. These characteristics that distinguish microtrauma injuries from macrotrauma injuries seemed to contribute to the frustration experienced by participants.

For example, Anne described the unpredictable nature of microtrauma injuries and perceptions of injury severity as contributing to her frustration.

> "I think a little bit of frustration",

she said in describing her feelings associated with the injury,

> "because every time I would go out running it would hurt and I didn't want it to hurt but it didn't hurt enough to stop necessarily."

Similarly, Grace noted that the unpredictable nature of microtrauma injuries contributed to her frustration, and she said,

> "It like kind of feels like a rubber band, you know. …it reappears just randomly and there wasn't much of a pattern so it would just, it would just get really frustrating."

Even more specific to the nature of microtrauma injuries, Maryn specifically compared the experience with her microtrauma injury to that of a macrotrauma injury in terms of the frustration she experienced. She said,

> "Even though they're [running injuries] not as extreme as tearing your ACL, they're nagging injuries. And they're kind of... sometimes more irritating because they're not concrete. You can't go in and say 'yea, you have an ACL tear, you need to do this, this, and this.' You've got a muscle strain ... you need to just rest".

Generally, the frustration experienced by participants was closely related to the insidious onset, persistent symptoms, and unpredictable nature of microtrauma injuries.

Fear. In addition to frustration, participants also indicated they experienced a great deal of fear associated with their injuries. The theme of fear subdivided into four distinct lower-order themes—fear of not recovering, fear of re-injury, fear of diminished performance, and fear of appearing weak.

Fear of not recovering. In addition to the frustration participants were experiencing in response to the ambiguity in their injury, participants also indicated they feared the uncertainty of the diagnosis and the unpredictability of the recovery, again characteristics that differentiate microtrauma injuries from macrotrauma injuries. Jordan noted experiencing fear about a number of different factors associated with her injury and further demonstrated her fear by identifying some injury-related catastrophic thinking:

> "I really was freaked out about like is this a major foot injury? Am I going to get a stress fracture or something? Like, is this going to prevent me from running the marathon like 5 months later?"

Anne echoed the sentiment of fear of the injury not going away. She said,

> "But it was also like a little bit scared, like what is going on and why is this lingering on for so long and why is my foot still swollen and it was just weird. So, 'cause it usually, nothing's ever lasted that long for me unless it was broken."

Kathryn indicated that the most common emotion she felt during her injury was fear or nervousness as she described it:

> "I think the biggest thing I felt when I had it [the illiotibial (IT) band injury] was nervousness, because I was really scared."

She also indicated that part of her fear was associated with the uncertainty of her injury saying that,

> "I just didn't really know what was happening."

Fear of diminished performance. Most participants in this study were training for a particular race or event when they became injured and feared being unable to meet their goals related to the event, whether they were a specific performance standard or completing the event. For example, Laura was scared of not being able to complete her upcoming marathon:

> "I was like kind of freaking out because I was like, I'm not going to be running so my training, I'm gonna get behind and then I'm not going to be able to run the marathon."

Similarly, Jordan indicated fear in getting behind in her training, stating:

> "I just kind of panicked because, you know, we're over half way done training, the marathon's like a month and a half away."

Through tears, recalling her injury, Jane said,

> "But, it's like I've trained healthy and now, like, the most I've ever run on it is two hours and that was absolutely brutal. And, it's just…I'm just worried that I'm not like physically not going to be able to finish and, that's just absolutely devastating to me right now."

Fear of re-injury. Fear continued to be a prominent theme even after the runners thought they had recovered from their injuries. Overwhelmingly there was a sense of relief among participants once they felt they had recovered from the injury. However, entwined with this sense of relief was also fear and concern over re-injury. Laura indicated that once she considered her knee injury healed, she still worried about injuring it again.

"Sometimes," she said, "like if I'm not really paying attention to like if there's a branch or something and I step on it or a rock and I kind of tweak my leg I just get kind of nervous that it's going to set it off again."

Laura also noted that, despite that her healthcare professional told her it was unnecessary, she continued to wear a brace on her knee out of fear that she would reinjure the knee if she was not wearing the brace. Maryn indicated that the fear of having another injury continued to impact her ability to train even months after the onset of her hip injury

> "When I do my sprint workouts… Um, I don't sprint as hard as I normally would. So, I've learned that I have to take it down and then the next sprint workout I can, I can go more at 100%. So, that first sprint workout is only about 85% because otherwise I'll be right back to where I was again."

Fear of appearing weak. Finally, there was also evidence of fear of appearing weak to others. Participants in this study had many social connections related to running, such as teammates, training partners, coaches, and instructors, and exhibited fears of appearing weak to these important others in their lives. For example, Brad noted fear of being viewed as weak because of his stress fracture. He said,

> "Ah, I just thought that it would be viewed as weakness and that's not the way I wanted people to view/see me as."

Maryn also indicated an awareness of trying not to appear weak to those around her

> "Iinitially it's stressful and the fact that I can't do that, and when you're around a ton of people who are running that day and you can't do what you are supposed to do, it's kind of that you feel as though you're being perceived as being weak."

General psychosocial distress. In addition to frustration and fear, many of the participants in the study indicated that they experienced general emotional distress during the injury phase of their stories. Even though participants had been dealing with their injuries for months and often perceived themselves to be recovered at the time of interviews, in telling their injury stories participants were often visibly emotional—crying, shaking, or becoming flushed. Verbally, participants reported feelings of sadness, devastation, and anger while they were injured. Jordan reported emotional distress over her injury saying,

> "I was like really upset about like almost crying about it, 'cause like this sucks."

While Laura indicated she was

> "like super bummed out"

in response to her injury. For Jane the idea of not being able to complete her upcoming marathon was very upsetting for her:

> "That's just absolutely devastating to me right now."

Moreover, Logan simply said,

> "It sucked because I couldn't run."

Both the body language and the verbal communication by participants indicated a strong degree of psychosocial distress associated with their injury.

Social influence. Participants' psychosocial responses were also influenced by important others in their lives. Participants noted that they elicited or received social support from a number of different sources throughout their injury, including running friends, family, and coaches/instructors. For example, Grace reported receiving social support from her family, indicating:

> "I have a family that is really supportive and so they're praying for me and then they'll just listen",

as well as receiving support from her coaches and teammates. Moreover, Jordan indicated that she received support from her running group, indicating that many of these people had also suffered injuries and thus could relate to what she was experiencing:

> "Like we all support each other," she said, "like we'll text each other like later in the day like, hey, how's your knee feeling now?"

Notably, participants did not necessarily seek out support from healthcare professionals as we might expect considering the amount of distress—both physical and emotional—they were experiencing. This point will be discussed further in the results related to research question 2.

4.2. Research Question 2: Chronology of Experiences

Research question 1 addressed the psychosocial responses to running injuries that persisted throughout the injury experience. In research question 2, we focused more specifically on the chronology of thoughts, feelings, and behaviors that changed systematically as the participants went through the injury process. Thematic analysis of participants' stories revealed consistent patterns of experiences prior to injury, throughout the injury, and at the outcome of the injury. A summary of themes related to research question 2 is available in Figure 1. As per the interview question, participants' experiences with injury fell into three chronological categories—pre-injury, injury onset, and outcome. Within each injury phase participants noted some unique thoughts, feelings, and behaviors associated with their injury.

Pre-injury factors. Pre-injury was defined as the period of time immediately prior to the injury onset when the participant was training for a running event but did not experience symptoms of the injury. Pre-injury factors were characterized by factors prior to injury that influenced the athletes' perceived risk of injury and response to injury.

Injury attributions. It was evident throughout the interviews that participants had carefully considered the question of why they had become injured. Overwhelmingly, participants attributed their injury to one of two factors—overtraining and/or change in running conditions or training. Kathryn, for example, attributed her injury to both overtraining and change in running conditions. Specifically she indicated going from treadmill running to outdoor running and increasing her mileage quickly.

> "It [running] was never outside, it was always on a treadmill for that and then I was way over-doing it, because I'd be like… I'd never, kinda of gradually went up, I just like 'I'm gonna do six miles in the first day'. And that was a bad idea. And I did that for the first two weeks and I was seriously hurting."

Anne also attributed her injury to overtraining, noting:

> "Umm, it's not a big story I guess I was just maybe I was running too much."

Grace and Laura thought that a change in running conditions, specifically weather conditions, was the cause of their injuries. Participants in the study were primarily from the Midwestern United States and interviews were conducted in the spring after a particularly cold and snowy winter. Participants suggested these harsh running conditions and specifically going from fall running, where the trails and sidewalks were free of ice and snow, to slippery winter conditions contributed to their injury risk. For example, Grace indicated that

> "I was just doing a run and I had just like, it was like snowy outside and, um, it was icy so I felt my Achilles."

Laura also attributed her injury to winter running conditions, indicating that

> "the only thing that was kinda like different from my normal running is that we were running in snow so it was kinda slushy so that's kinda how my injury happened."

Goal planning. Another consistent theme in the injury narratives was that participants' experiences with injury seemed to be shaped by the fact they had a goal or deadline by which time they felt they needed their injury to have healed. Specifically, participants overwhelmingly had a race or event that they wanted to complete within the near future. This goal seemed to be influential in participants' emotional responses to injury. For instance, Maryn indicated that her initial response to her quad injury was:

> "stress because I can't afford to take any time off of the running."

Others worried about having their injury get better or at least being able to control their symptoms prior to the time or a race. Specifically, many participants in this study were concerned about being able to complete their first marathon. Participants noted some degree of pressure associated with training for a specific, time-sensitive running goal. Participants indicated these running goals were inflexible and may have contributed to their overtraining or change in training. For example, Logan noted that he chose to run every day rather than taking any rest days because he was trying to complete a marathon in his goal of under three hours. He reported that he thought this contributed to his injury.

Injury onset. The onset category in the chronology of injury experience is considered the period of time during which runners perceive themselves to be injured or have pain that is affecting their running.

Diagnosis and treatment. The next phase of injury stories in this study was the injury phase. Although all injuries in this study were considered microtrauma injuries, which typically have insidious onset, participants usually identified a specific day or run during which the pain became unmanageable or started to negatively impact their running. Once injuries had progressed to this point participants noted that they almost immediately began to try to figure out how to manage the injury. There was a typical pattern of how participants went about treatment of their injuries. The majority of participants did not seek formal medical treatment for their injury. Thus, they typically engaged in self-diagnosis and self-treatment of their injuries. Participants had similar patterns of treating or minimizing physical distress of the injury while being acutely aware of a "goal" or "deadline" by which they needed to be injury-free or at least able to complete a specific running event. Only three of the 10 participants in this study formally visited a healthcare professional to receive a diagnosis or treatment for their injury. More often, participants enlisted information and advice from a number of alternative sources. These sources included healthcare professionals who were friends or family members, coaches or instructors, other runners, and the Internet.

The information participants received from these sources then informed their own treatment plan for their injury. For instance, Jordan said in regard to treating her iliotibial (IT) band injury that she enlisted information from both a running coach and the Internet. She said,

> "I talked to [my coach]… I told him what was going on and, like, umm, I told him I thought it was an IT band issue and he agreed with me and he just said take it easy."

She continued to seek out information about IT band issues, but looked online.

> "I remember that Monday night," she said, "umm, I read online about foam rollers and like how you can foam roll it [IT band] out and a lot of people like who have IT band issues they'll get a foam roller and it like works magic."

This information she received informed her use of a foam roller in treatment of her injury. Additionally, many participants noted engaging in icing, stretching, or physical therapy-type exercises in order to treat their injury or at least minimize the discomfort they were experiencing. Specifically, Laura, who was one of the few participants to see a physical therapist, explained that her physical therapist instructed her on how to tape her knee as well as what exercises to do. This instruction allowed her to care for her injury independently.

Continued training. Despite participants reporting a great deal of discomfort associated with their injuries and that their injuries negatively impacted their running, only one participant out of 10 indicated they took more than a week off from running between the time of their injury and their next running competition. Maryn said that even if she was told by a healthcare professional not to run, she would not take time off from running, specifically noting,

> "Like, if I'm told I can't run, that's just not going to work."

Kathryn indicated that she continued to run despite her injury, saying,

> "I never took more than like one or two days off from running. I tried to stick with it because I figured it would be harder if I just stopped then went back to it."

However, they did note decreasing or changing their running in order to deal with the injury while increasing cross-training activities such as biking or using the elliptical. Logan, in his explanation of why he did not take much time off, said,

> "One day I felt pain so I took a few days off and then I did it, I ran again, and I still felt pain but I could push through it."

Jordan noted modifying her running in order to deal with her injury. Specifically, she said,

> "I haven't felt good since like the injury but like I've really learned how to deal with it and like, umm, on our runs I would just like slow down."

Brad indicated that he was in the taper phase of his marathon training when his injury occurred and therefore he was less concerned about taking time off as compared to during other times in his training.

> "I reduced my mileage," he said, "I originally planned on doing for those two weeks just because I wanted to let it rest and let it recover but I didn't want to just completely stop training so I still ran at least once a week."

Some participants indicated that cross-training aided in minimizing the distress they felt from being injured. Anne said:

> "I think that would have been a big difference would be if I couldn't do anything active, it would have meant a lot more, but I could still do something active with both those injuries so it didn't pull me out of physical activity all together so I think that made a big difference."

Grace noted her coach provided her with workouts that were helpful in dealing with her injury both physically and mentally. Specifically, she said,

> "It's [cross-training workouts developed by her coach] been really helpful to being feeling like I still have a little bit of control of, like maintaining fitness and stuff like. So, doing workouts, that helped me cope with it a little."

Outcome. The outcome phase of the chronology of injury is considered the point at which the runners perceived themselves to have recovered from the injury or the point at which they were at the time of interview. Participants having some change in training as well as learning lessons from the injury characterized this phase.

Change in training. For many participants the outcome phase was short-lived as they often reported a second injury or recurrence of the injury once they thought it had healed. Despite an early reluctance to take time off from training, many participants had made some changes in training in order to cope with their injuries. For example, Jordan said,

> "I haven't felt good since like the injury but like I've really learned how to deal with it and like on our runs I would just like slow down."

Other participants noted they took a substantial break from running after their goal or deadline. Therefore, the outcome phase, for some, was not until after they had completed their goal race and had taken a break from running.

Lessons learned. Additionally, participants reported learning things from their running injury experiences, especially about perseverance as well as preventing injuries in the future. For example, Logan noted that he has developed strategies in his training in order to prevent injuries, specifically he said,

> "I'm more cautious, I would say. I don't go out and do seven miles after seven miles after seven miles anymore."

Brad also learned a lesson about overtraining, indicating the injury

> "kind of taught me that I was maybe overtraining a little bit. I was running prior to that [the injury] and just kept building up on it and at some point I figured something would happen, but I kind of hoped it would be later."

Jane also indicated how important it was to take care of your body. Specifically she said, "Like, I want to be healthy so bad. Um, I definitely respect it [her body] more. Like you have to take care of your body".

In addition to learning how to prevent injuries in the future, participants also shared that they felt they had learned to persevere through difficult times during their injury. Jordan indicated that she learned not to

> "freak out right off the bat, like umm I guess I was really concerned with the outcome, like am I going to be able to reach my goal, like is this going to prevent me from actually doing the marathon, so I was quick to jump to the worst case scenario."

She added that,

> "I don't know, I jumped to conclusions then I realized I need to relax about this so I guess just not panicking and not assuming the worst."

Laura noted that she learned that she could deal with more than she thought, specifically she said,

> "One thing that it [the injury] taught me is like I can push through pain a lot better than I thought I could."

She also said,

> "It also helped me to just work through an obstacle because, I don't know, I hadn't really had a lot of obstacles I've had to work around, especially in exercise."

Jane indicated that

> "I definitely think that I've become tougher."

Upon reflecting on their injury experience when telling their injuries stories, participants generally indicated continued positive feelings about running despite their injuries. Jane, who was training to complete a marathon, reflected that completing the marathon would mean more to her now because of her injury.

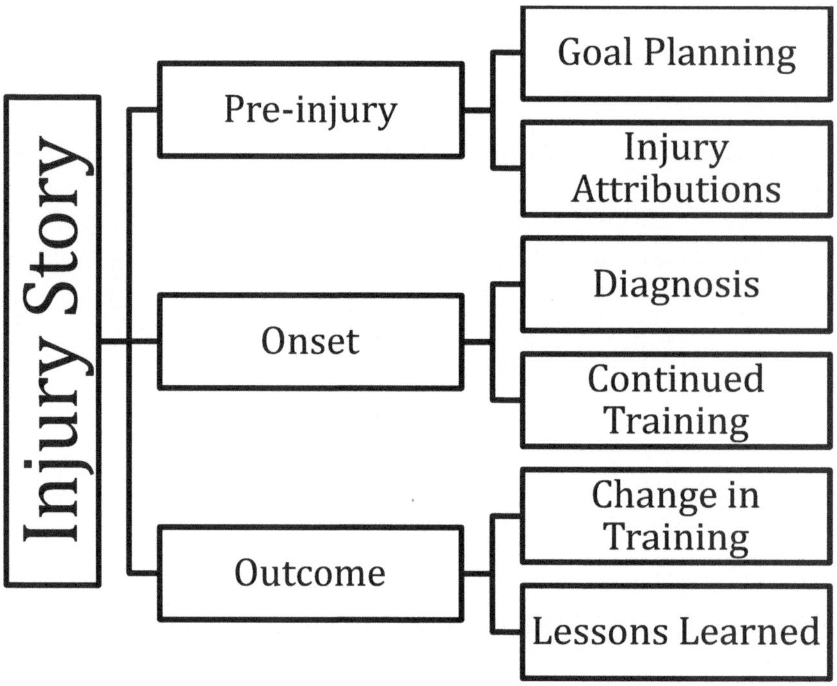

Figure 1. Summary of results related to research question 2, the chronology of responses to microtrauma running injury. The figure denotes that there were three injury phases: pre-injury, onset, and outcome, and each phase had distinct psychosocial responses.

5. Discussion

The purpose of the current study was to use a variation of Mishler's [20] core-narrative approach, as adapted by Brock and Kleiber [10], to examine and better understand the unique experiences and psychosocial responses of adult long-distance runners who had incurred a microtrauma injury. The use of qualitative data analysis of the 10 different interviews led to a consistent chronology of consistent cognitive, affective, and behavioral responses throughout the course of injury. In regard to the chronology of events, participants consistently responded within three distinct phases—pre-injury, injury onset, and outcome—and within each of these time points, certain themes emerged related to psychosocial responses to injury.

Four consistent psychosocial responses were identified throughout the injury process. They included frustration due to uncertainty of the injury and recovery process, fear related to the injury failing to heal, an inability to meet a specific goal, becoming re-injured, and appearing weak, general emotional distress that included descriptors of feeling sad, devastated, and angry, and, finally, social support/social pressure as instigating factors for the onset of the negative psychosocial responses. Unlike the themes related to the chronology of experiences and responses to injury, these psychosocial responses were evident from the onset of injury throughout the recovery and overcoming of the injury.

During the pre-injury period, participants noted the importance of their running goals and discussed how those goals affected their risk of injury and response to injury. They made consistent attributions to overtraining or a change in running conditions as instigating factors for a microtrauma injury. Psychosocial factors during the onset phase included self-diagnosis and treatment for the injury as well as reports of continuing to train through the injury. During the outcome phase, participants reported changing their training as well as learning lessons as a result of their injuries. Specifically, they described they could use the lessons they had learned to get through potential future injuries or other challenges that may occur in life.

In general, findings from the current study add support to the integrated model of psychological response to sport injury [3] and to other previous research findings that athletes incurring sport injuries experience not only the physical consequences of an injury, but also the psychosocial responses surrounding the sport injury [12,21–23]. Findings from the current study provide evidence for a need to study the role of injury type to better understand the psychosocial responses across the time course of the injury process [3]. Furthermore, they confirm the initial hypothesis proposed by Flint [5]: that the progression and longevity of microtrauma injuries contribute to the psychosocial distress experienced by athletes incurring these types of injuries.

The results of this study support some of the findings from the limited research on psychological responses to microtrauma injuries, specifically with respect to social support. Participants in this study reported seeking little social support, especially from healthcare professionals. This is consistent with work by Wasley and Lox [7], who noted that athletes with microtrauma injuries are less likely to seek out social support as compared to athletes with macrotrauma injuries. Injured athletes not seeking medical attention is potentially problematic for both physical and psychosocial well-being. Not seeking formal medical care may lead athletes to make uninformed decisions, thus putting them at risk for sustained injury or additional physical harm. Further, as a number of researchers have identified healthcare professionals as a key source of social support for injured athletes [10,24–26], these athletes who isolate rather than seek assistance are missing out on other opportunities for educational support, such as strategies for the prevention of future injuries. Despite not seeking support from heath care professionals, the results suggest that long-distance runners with microtrauma injuries do rely on social support from other social domains such as friends and family.

The current findings support the notion that long-distance runners who experience a disruption in training due to an injury experience significant psychosocial distress [2] but also provide evidence of variations in psychosocial distress throughout the injury and rehabilitation process. The results of the current study add to the existing literature by indicating that a specific chronology of phases occurs during a microtrauma running injury, each with unique cognitive, affective, and behavioral responses. During each of these phases, athletes incurring a microtrauma injury experienced distinct yet consistent psychosocial responses. This finding is crucial for helping coaches and healthcare professionals become aware of expected responses to a microtrauma injury and to become more aware of when these responses will occur depending on the phase of the injury process. By utilizing a narrative research methodology, we were able to provide a clearer picture of the complexity of psychosocial responses to sport injuries.

The findings from this exploratory study provide important information for athletes, coaches, and practitioners. For example, the majority of participants reported that they engaged in some form of self-diagnosis rather than seeing a healthcare professional. Therefore, coaches need to be aware of this proclivity of athletes and, therefore, encourage a formal diagnosis and provide athletes experiencing microtrauma injuries with the available resources to attain professional care. Likewise, healthcare professionals aware of this tendency are encouraged to provide information through various sources regarding symptoms, treatment, and alternative activities to help these individuals deal with injuries on their own. Additionally, both coaches and healthcare professionals working with athletes who have experienced a microtrauma injury must be aware that either the nature of the injury or characteristics of the individual athlete may decrease the likelihood that s/he will take time off when injured. Compared to macrotrauma injuries that are usually visible (e.g., broken foot) and require individuals to take time off from training, microtrauma injuries are often invisible (e.g., Achilles tendonitis) and, therefore, may lead an athlete to conclude that nothing is wrong if the injury cannot be seen. Given this penchant for continued exercise and training of individuals with microtrauma injuries, both coaches and healthcare professionals need to provide athletes with alternative activities that will help them continue to meet their training and competition goals.

Limitations

Despite the additions to the literature of this study, a number of limitations exist. First, several of the participants were novices training over several months for their first competitive long-distance run as part of a coached group. Many runners felt significant internal and external pressures to achieve the final goal of competing in the targeted run, and this may have cause them to think, feel, or behave differently than if they were training on their own. Nonetheless, the use of participants from a long-distance running group helped to identify the consistent theme that individuals often feel pressure to recover from an injury or to compete while injured in order to meet a specific goal. Additionally, this sample may be different from a more general running population because of their willingness to participate in interviews about their injury. Other injured runners who did not volunteer for our study may have had different psychosocial responses to injuries, therefore the results cannot be generalized to all runners.

Second, the study sample was limited to long-distance runners with microtrauma injuries. Although the findings from the current study provide an understanding of the injury and recovery process associated with microtrauma injuries, the patterns that emerged cannot be generalized to all athletes who experience microtrauma injuries. Moreover, the participants' injuries were self-reported and self-diagnosed, so we cannot definitively determine the diagnoses or severity of each injury. However, the findings from the current study begin to provide a better understanding of the injury and recovery process and will be important to compare with future studies that may look at the injury and recovery process of individuals sustaining microtrauma injuries from training and competing in different types of sports.

Lastly, due to the nature of qualitative studies and the use of narrative research methodology in the current study, specific causal inferences cannot be gleaned from the study's findings. Although we have made inferences throughout the paper that the participants' responses and experiences were related to microtrauma injuries, since we did not interview participants with macrotrauma injuries, we cannot definitively assert that this is the case. Regardless, the findings from the study do provide an important platform of the structure of physical and psychosocial responses to microtrauma sport injuries.

6. Future Directions

Findings from the current study provide an important starting point for researchers and practitioners to better understand the sport injury process for individuals who experience a microtrauma injury. Future research could strengthen the findings from this study by conducting qualitative research studies using narrative research methodology with individuals incurring microtrauma injuries from a variety of sports. This would allow for researchers to better understand the pattern of responses to microtrauma injuries and determine whether injury type does differentiate athletes' responses to injury or if response to injury has more to do with the type of sport an individual engages in. Additionally, future research using qualitative methods could compare the responses to injuries for athletes from the same sport but who differ in injury type to help better determine unique or similar responses. Lastly, once qualitative research has further confirmed that differences in response style exist depending on the type of injury an individual incurs, quantitative research could be used to solidify that athletes with microtrauma injuries score differently on measures of various psychosocial responses than athletes experiencing macrotrauma injuries.

7. Conclusions

The use of a narrative research methodology to study the physical and psychosocial responses of long-distance runners incurring microtrauma injuries provided a clearer picture of the complete injury process and the changes in both physical and psychosocial responses that occur at the different phases of the injury process. The findings provide further support for the integrated model of psychological response to sport injury [3] and, specifically, the importance of better understanding the role of injury type as a factor moderating the psychosocial responses of injured athletes. Rather than limiting participants to predetermined responses, the use of narrative research methodology provided the opportunity to identify unique responses to the injury process. For example, this study highlighted unique cognitive responses to injury, such as fear of taking time off from training, affective responses like frustration about the injury type, and behavioral responses like avoidance of formal medical care, that may have been missed using more structured or constrained methods of inquiry. To understand the dynamic complexities of the physical and psychosocial responses to injury, it is crucial that future research employ a variety of research techniques to test various aspects of the integrated model of psychological response to sport injury [3], as well as other models of responses to sport injuries. Additionally, it is crucial for future research to address the potentially unique psychosocial responses and needs of athletes with differing injury characteristics in order to provide the best care and support for all injured athletes.

Acknowledgments

We thank Reed H. Steele and Ayanna N. Franklin for their important and significant contributions to this project.

Author Contributions

Hayley Russell and Diane Wiese-Bjornstal designed this study. HR collected and analyzed the data. HR and DWB wrote manuscript.

Conflicts of Interest

The authors declare no conflict of interest.

References

1. Lun, V.; Meeuwisse, W.H.; Stergiou, P.; Stefanyshyn, D. Relation between running injury and static lower limb alignment in recreational runners. *Brit. J. Sport Med.* **2004**, *38*, 576–580. doi:10.1136/bjsm.2003.005488.
2. Chan, C.S.; Grossman, H.Y. Psychological effects of running loss on consistent runners. *Percept. Motor Skill.* **1988**, *66*, 875–883. doi:10.2466/pms.1988.66.3.875.
3. Wiese-Bjornstal, D.M.; Smith, A.M.; Shaffer S.M.; Morrey, M.A. An integrated model of response to sport injury: Psychological and sociological dynamics. *J. Appl. Sport Psychol.* **1998**, *10*, 46–69. doi:10.1080/10413209808406377.
4. Wiese-Bjornstal, D.M. Psychology and socioculture affect injury risk, response, and recovery in high-intensity athletes: A consensus statement. *Scand. J. Med. Sci. Sports* **2010**, *20*, 103–111. doi:10.1111/j.1600-0838.2010.01195.x.
5. Flint, F.A. Integrating sport psychology and sports medicine in research: The dilemmas. *J. Appl. Sport Psychol.* **1998**, *10*, 83–102. doi:10.1080/10413209808406379.
6. Van Gent, R.N.; Siem, D.; van Middelkoop, M.; van Os, A.G.; Bierma-Zeinstra, S.M.A.; Koes, B.W. Incidence and determinants of lower extremity running injuries in long distance runners: A systematic review. *Brit. J. Sport Med.* **2007**, *41*, 469–480. doi:10.1136/bjsm.2006.033548.
7. Wasley, D.; Lox, C.L. Self-esteem and coping responses of athletes with acute versus chronic injuries. *Percept. Motor Skill* **1998**, *86*, 1402. doi:10.2466/pms.1998.86.3c.1402.
8. Henert, S.E. Exploring Injured Athletes' Ratings of Social Support and Use of Coping Strategies as a Function of Injury Type and Gender over the Course of Rehabilitation, Ph.D. dissertation. University of Minnesota, Minneapolis, MN, USA, 2000. ProQuest (AAT 9966232).
9. Bianco, T. Social support and recovery from sport injury: Elite skiers share their experiences. *Res. Q. Exercise Sport* **2001**, *72*, 376–388. doi:10.1080/02701367.2001.10608974.
10. Brock, S.C.; Kleiber, D.A. Narrative in medicine: The stories of elite college athletes' career-ending injuries. *Qual. Health Res.* **1994**, *4*, 411–430.
11. Podlog, L.; Eklund, R.C. High level athletes' perceptions of success in returning to sport following injury. *Psychol. Sport Exercise* **2009**, *10*, 535–544. doi:10.1016/j.psychsport.2009.02.003.

12. Tracey, J. The emotional response to the injury and rehabilitation process. *J. Appl. Sport Psychol.* **2003**, *15*, 279–293. doi:10.1080/104132003902137924.
13. Bleakley, A. Stories as data, data as stories: Making sense of narrative inquiry in clinical education. *Med. Educ.* **2005**, *39*, 534–540. doi:10.1111/j.1365-2929.2005.02126.x.
14. Lieblich, A.; Tuval-Mashiach, R.; Zilber, T. *Narrative Research: Reading, Analysis, and Interpretation*; Sage Publications, Inc.: Thousand Oaks, CA, USA, 1998.
15. Bailey, P. The dyspnea-anxiety-dyspnea cycle—COPD patients' stories of breathlessness: "It's scary/When you can't breathe." *Qual. Health Res.* **2004**, *14*, 760–778. doi:10.1177/1049732304265973.
16. Borkan, J.M.; Quirk, M.; Sullivan, M. Finding meaning after the fall: Injury narratives from elderly hip fracture patients. *Soc. Sci. Med.* **1991**, *33*, 947–957. doi:10.1016/0277-9536(91)90265-E.
17. Patton, M.Q. *Qualitative Research and Evaluation Methods*; Sage Publications, Inc.: Thousand Oaks, CA, USA, 2002.
18. Eatough, V.; Smith, J. Interpretative phenomenological anaylsis. In *The Sage Handbook for Qualitative Research in Psychology*; Willig, C., Stainton, W., Eds.; Sage Publications, Inc.: Throusand Oaks, CA, USA, 2008.
19. Tesch, R. *Qualitative Research Analysis Types and Software Tools*; Falmer Press: New York, NY, USA, 1990.
20. Mishler, E.G. The analysis of interview-narratives. In *Narrative Psychology: The Storied Nature of Human Conduct*; Sarbin, T.R., Ed.; Praeger: New York, NY, USA, 1986; pp. 233–255.
21. Jevon, S.M.; Johnston, L.H. The perceived knowledge and attitudes of governing body chartered physiotherapists towards the psychological aspects of rehabilitation. *Phys. Ther. Sport* **2003**, *4*, 74–81.
22. McDonald, S.A.; Hardy, C.J. Affective response patterns of the injured athlete: An exploratory analysis. *Sport Psychol.* **1990**, *4*, 261–274.
23. Walker, N.; Thatcher, J.; Lavallee, D. Psychological responses to injury in competitive sport: A critical review. *J. R. Soc. Promo. Health* **2007**, *127*, 174–180. doi:10.1177/1466424007079494.
24. Mann, B.J.; William, G.A.; Indelicato, P.A.; O'Neill, D.F.; George, S.Z. A survey of sports medicine physicians regarding psychological issues in patient-athletes. *Am. J. Sport Med.* **2007**, *35*, 2140–2147. doi:10.1177/0363546507304140.
25. Russell, H.; Tracey, J. What do injured athletes want from their health care professionals? *Int. J. Athl. Ther. Train.* **2011**, *16*, 18–21.
26. Tracey, J. Inside the clinic: Health professionals' role in their clients' psychological rehabilitation. *J. Sport Rehabil.* **2008**, *17*, 413–431.

17

An Overview of the Running Performance of Athletes with Lower-Limb Amputation at the Paralympic Games 2004–2012

Hossein Hassani [1,2,*], Mansi Ghodsi [1], Mehran Shadi [1], Siamak Noroozi [3] and Bryce Dyer [3]

[1] The Statistical Research Centre, Business School, Bournemouth University, Bournemouth BH8 8EB, UK; E-Mails: mghodsi@bournemouth.ac.uk (M.G.); mshadi@bournemouth.ac.uk (M.S.)

[2] Institute for International Energy Studies (IIES), 65 Sayeh St., Vali-e-Asr Ave., Tehran 1967743 711, Iran

[3] School of Design, Engineering and Computing, Bournemouth University, Poole House P124, Talbot Campus, Fern Barrow, Poole, Bournemouth BH12 5BB, UK; E-Mails: snoroozi@bournemouth.ac.uk (S.N.); brdyer@bournemouth.ac.uk (B.D.)

* Author to whom correspondence should be addressed; E-Mail: hhassani@bournemouth.ac.uk;

Academic Editor: Eling Douwe de Bruin

Abstract: This paper analyses the performances of lower-limb amputees in the 100, 200 and 400 m running events from the 2004, 2008 and 2012 Paralympic Games. In this paper, four hypotheses are pursued. In the first, it investigates whether the running performance of lower-limb amputees over three consecutive Paralympic Games has changed. In the second, it asks whether a bi-lateral amputee has a competitive advantage over a uni-lateral amputee. In the third, the effect of blade classification has been considered and we attempt to see whether amputees in various classifications have different level of performance. Finally, it is considered whether the final round of competition obtains different levels of performance in comparison to the qualification heats. Based on the outcomes of these investigations, it is proposed that future amputee-based running events should be undertaken with separate and not combined events for the T42, T43 and T44 classifications at the Paralympic Games.

Keywords: running; paralympic games; bi-lateral amputee; athletes

1. Introduction

Athletes who possess some level of disability have participated in competitive sports for over a century. However it was not until after the Second World War that the first formalised sports event for the disabled people took place. This was initially based in Stoke Mandeville in the UK and eventually directly influenced what has subsequently become known as the Paralympic Games from 1960 [1]. These games currently take place every four years [2] at the same venue as the Olympic Games. Athletics forms a key part of the Paralympic Games programme and attracts the largest number of spectators [3]. Structured competition involving running with a lower-limb amputation has taken place consistently since 1976 [4].

If an amputee with a lower-limb amputation wishes to compete in running competition within the Paralympic Games, they are assessed for their physical functionality [5] and then typically allocated into one of three race classifications [6]. These event classifications are defined as:

T42: a single (uni-lateral) above knee (trans-femoral) amputee or athlete with other impairments that is comparable to a single above knee amputation.

T43: double (bi-lateral) below knee (trans-tibial) amputees and other athletes with impairments that are comparable to a double below knee amputation.

T44: an athlete with a below knee lower limb impairment/s that meets minimum disability criteria for: lower limb deficiency; impaired lower limb; impaired lower limb muscle power; or leg length difference.

It should be noted that during the Paralympic Games that have been analysed in this study, the T43 category has been combined with the T44 category in the male running events. This has been mainly been due to the low participation numbers in the T43 category. The governing body has traditionally decided to combine this classification with the T44 category. This combined category is still referred to as 'T44' as it comprises more of these types of athletes.

Competing when using running specific lower-limb prostheses has not been without some level of controversy. For example, in 2008 it was proposed that a lower-limb bi-lateral amputee could have a performance advantage when compared to their able-bodied equivalent due to some level of performance enhancement from their prostheses [7]. Additionally, due to fundamental functional differences, it was proposed that the T43 and T44 should be separated in competition—despite this not currently being the case [4]. As a result, the aim of this paper is to address and reinforce some of the issues that may surround the diversity of athletes that will compete in the typical classifications at the Paralympic Games in recent editions. Four hypotheses are posed:

(1) The performance of athletes with an amputation within the current format of athlete classification has changed from 2004 to 2012.
(2) The number of prosthetic limbs being used by an athlete has an impact on race results when running specific prostheses are used.
(3) The athletes in different classifications will have the same level of performance.
(4) The final round of running competition at the Paralympic Games in each classification has the same level of performance as their qualification rounds.

2. Methodology

The race results from the 100, 200 and 400 m form the basis of a statistical analysis of the 2012 (London), 2008 (Beijing) and the 2004 (Athens) Paralympics Games. These results are located within the public domain and are extracted from the official website of the sport's governing body [8]. This data includes the name, ranking and country of representation, as well as the performance of each athlete. The number of prosthetic lower-limbs that each athlete may have used was derived from the athlete's biography and/or online photographic evidence [8]. The raw data is included in Appendix 1 and 2. While Appendix 1, gives some detailed information for 2012 results, the Appendix 2, represents the information for 2004 and 2008 Paralympic Games in the running event.

As the main purpose of this report is about identifying the differences between two or more groups, the ANOVA test was used as the best statistical tool to address the four hypotheses. The homogeneity test (whether different groups have the same level of variation between them or not) and normality are the two key assumptions when using the ANOVA test [9]. After creating the data sets for each research question, both the normality and homogeneity tests were undertaken. If both of these two key assumptions were satisfied *within* and *between* groups, the ANOVA test was then used in order to address each research hypotheses. If any of these assumptions were not then satisfied, the Kruskal-Wallis test was used instead of ANOVA. The Kruska-Wallis test is a non-parametric test which is not sensitive to normality [10].

3. Analysis

3.1. Hypothesis 1: The Performance of Athletes with an Amputation within the Current Format of Athlete Classification Has Changed from 2004 to 2012.

The answer to this question is primarily addressed in Table 1. In Table 1, the first column ("category") clarifies which specific category analysis was undertaken. The second column ("N") represents the whole sample size and the numbers in parentheses represent the sample size in each year (2004, 2008 and 2012). The third and fourth columns illustrate the p value of homogeneity and normality tests in each group. The fifth and sixed columns represent the results of p value for ANOVA or Kruskal-Wallis test (where relevant).

Table 1. A comparison on the performance of amputees in 100 m in 2004, 2008, and 2012.

Category	N	Homogeneity	Normality	ANOVA	Kruskal-Wallis
100 m-T42	31(20,5,6)	0.97	1.18×10^{-5}	-	0.46
100 m-T44	67(28,19,20)	0.21	0.04	-	0.36
100 m-all	98(48,24,26)	0.05, 0.05, 0.24	0.74	0.49	-
200 m-T44	64(26,18,20)	0.48	0.21, 0.01	-	0.69
200 m-all	80(35,18,27)	0.24	0.01	-	0.18
400 m-T44	41(19,6,16)	0.04	0.96, 0.64, 0.43	-	0.08

In Table 1, the p value of the ANOVA and Kruskal-Wallis tests are all above 5%. Therefore, we can conclude that with adopting a 95% confidence interval, no statistical difference was identified between these three groups (2004, 2008 and 2012). This means that the posed hypothesis was incorrect and based upon the statistical analysis here, it is proposed that the running performance of the amputees from 2004 till 2012 did not change significantly.

3.2. Hypothesis 2: The Number of Prosthetic Limbs Being Used by an Athlete Has an Impact on Race Results

The race-based data was categorized in three different groups. The first group comprises amputees who use just one prosthetic limb. The second group contains amputees who use two prosthetic limbs and the third comprises those who run without prosthetic limbs at all (but due to their functionality, compete in the same classification). In order to detect any differences in the mean completion time of the event, either the ANOVA or the Kruskal-Wallis Test were then applied as appropriate.

In Table 2, the Kruskal-Wallis test did not identify any significant difference regarding the effect of the number of blades with a 5% significance level in either the 100 or 200 m. However, in the 400 and 200 m T44 event, the test identified a significant difference between three groups at a 5% significance level. Alternatively, this finding could also be interpreted as when the distance of the competition gets longer (400 m), the number of prostheses used ultimately affects the results of the event. In order to answer which group in particular has any advantage when compared to other groups, further analysis is required. In order to address this issue, the Tukey *post hoc* test was applied. Tables 3 and 4 represents the results of this test for 400 m and 200 m-T44.

Table 2. The effect of number of blades.

Category	*N*	Homogeneity	Normality	Kruskal-Wallis
100 m-T42-All	31(3,25,3)	0.19	1.88×10^{-5}	0.48
100 m-T44-All	66(13,49,4)	0.28	0.01, 0.25	0.06
200 m-T42-All	15(2,11,2)	0.06	0.66	0.79
200 m-T44-All	64(14,47,3)	0.63	0.03, 0.00	0.01
400 m-T44-all	41(11,27,3)	0.70	0.80, 0.41	0.00

Table 3. Tukey *post hoc* test for 200 m-T44.

Category		Mean Difference	Std. Error	Sig.
1 blade	2 blade	1.57 *	0.38	0.00
	0 blade	−0.03	0.74	0.99
2 blade	1 blade	−1.57 *	0.38	0.00
	0 blade	−1.60	0.80	0.12
0 blade	1 blade	0.03	0.74	0.99
	2 blade	1.60	0.80	0.12

* indicates 5% significance level.

As the sample size in the group possessing no prosthetic limbs is so small (2), we cannot make any robust conclusions from it and instead focus on the results of the other groups. In Table 5 it is demonstrated that there is a statistically significant difference between the results of people who run with 1 blade or 2 blades ($p = 0.00$). Based on the descriptive data for these two groups (22.7 s for 2 blade and 24.27 s for 1 blades), it is proposed that those who are bi-lateral lower-limb amputees have a competitive advantage compared to those who are uni-lateral. It is worth noting that although the normality test in this category was calculated as negative (and that we cannot use *post hoc* test in this case), at least applying that test gives an indication as to where any difference is. Table 4 represents the results of Tukey Post Hoc Test for 400 m competition.

Table 4. Tukey *post hoc* test for 400 m.

Category		Mean difference	Std. error	Sig.
0 blade	1 blade	−0.38	1.35	0.96
	2 blade	3.28	1.45	0.07
1 blade	0 blade	0.38	1.35	0.96
	2 blade	3.65 *	0.80	0.00
2 blade	0 blade	−3.28	1.45	0.07
	1 blade	−3.65 *	0.80	0.00

* indicates 5% significance level.

Table 5. Effect of classification.

Category	*N*	Homogeneity	Normality	Kruskal-Wallis
100 m				
T42/Final-T44/Final	41(18,23)	0.44	0.26, 0.04	6.06×10^{-7}
T42/All-T44/All	99(32,67)	0.36	0.00, 0.02	6.06×10^{-7}
200 m				
T42/Final-T44/Final	37(15,22)	0.17	0.85, 0.11	0.00
T42/all-T44/all	79(15,64)	0.18	0.85, 0.01	2.52×10^{-7}

The results of the Tukey *post hoc* Test indicate a statistically significant difference between the groups who use two blades when compared to the two other groups. By considering the mean time of the race completion by these groups (50.86 s for 2 prostheses, 54.51 s for 1 prostheses and 54.14 s for no prostheses) it is proposed that historically, when racing over 400 m, runners who have used two prosthetic lower-limbs may have had an advantage compared to other groups who had only one (or none).

The results of this analysis supports the posed hypotheses and indicates that, from a statistical perspective, bi-lateral amputees participating in the T44 events in either the 200 m and the 400 m distances, demonstrate better running performance when compared to other types of T44 participants (such as the T43 classification). This finding is supported by published research when evaluating such athletes *physiologically* [11] or as a *mechanical system* [12]. In a study commissioned by the sport's governing body (the IAAF), a bilateral amputee world record holder utilized 25% less energy compared to able-bodied athletes when running at the same speed over the 400 m distance [11]. It was also proposed that when a sinusoidal input is matched to an energy storage and return prostheses, it can make the prostheses susceptible to resonance. Theoretically, if this impulse could be synchronised with the frequency of a humans running effort, it could result in the storage (and then recovery) of a substantial amount of energy in the system therefore offering a degree of performance enhancement [13].

3.3. Hypothesis 3: Athletes Racing in Different Classifications Will Have the Same Level of Performance

The length of any amputated residual limb (such as above-knee or below-knee) could be considered as a factor which could affect the results of competition in running exercise. As it was mentioned earlier, in order to have a fair competition in Paralympic games, athletes are placed in different classifications based upon their functionality. This section of the paper compares the results of athletes who participate in the T42 category with those who participate in the T44 classification. The results are illustrated in Tables 5 and 6.

As in all cases p value is below 5%, there is a statistically significant difference between the T42 and T44 classifications. The descriptive analysis related to these two classifications is shown in Table 6.

Table 6. Descriptive data for T42 and T44.

Category	T42 mean (s)	T44 mean (s)
100 m		
T42/Final-T44/Final	13.05	11.52
T42/All-T44/All	13.15	11.84
200 m		
T42/Final-T44/Final	26.58	23.30
T42/all-T44/all	26.58	23.93

It is proposed that the posed hypothesis was correct and that the T44 category may have had an advantage in running-based competition when compared to T42.

3.4. Hypothesis 4: The Final Round of Running Competition at the Paralympic Games in Each Classification Has the Same Level of Performance as Their Qualification Rounds

During each Paralympic Games, athletes qualify for a final round based upon successful qualification from a heat or semi-final which had preceded it. However, it is not known how much effort an athlete applies in their heat to ensure qualification for the final. The data of each race classification type is separated into two groups. The first group is the data related to the qualification round and the second group is related to the final round. After the normality and homogeneity tests have been calculated, the p value of Kruskal-Wallis or ANOVA are then also calculated to see whether any difference exists between these rounds. The results of this are shown in Table 7.

Table 7. Effect of final round.

Category	*N*	Homogeneity	Normality	Kruskal-Wallis test
100 m-T42	20(12,8)	0.026	0.001	0.231
100 m-T44	28(20,8)	0.103	0.023	0.001
100 m-all	48(31,17)	0.411	0.000	0.216
200 m-T42	26(18,8)	0.468	0.484, 0.023	0.133
200 m-all	35(18,7)	0.048	0.484, 0.294	0.176
400 m-T44	19(11,8)	0.839	0.978, 0.833	0.247

In all six categories (except the 100 m-T44), the P value of the Kruskal-Wallis test or ANOVA is above 5%. As a result it is proposed that when adopting a 95% confidence interval, the posed hypothesis was correct as these two tests did not identify any significant difference between the qualification rounds and the final rounds performances. This means that although the result in the final is paramount, there is generally no different in the relative result of the same athletes in the qualification rounds. However, due to the limitations of the design of current athletics tracks comprising typically 8–12 lanes, the existing process of qualification is warranted (despite the end result being similar) if overall participation levels of each qualification in the sport are intended to be maximised by the sport's governing body.

4. Conclusions

A statistical analysis of the results from three consecutive Paralympic Games from 2004 to 2012 do not show any significant change in the general performance of athletes. It was identified that the performance of athletes in the qualification heat did not change substantially when the same athletes ran again in the final. The statistical analyses in this research suggested that athletes with below-knee amputation consistently outperformed those with above-knee amputation. Finally, the results in this study demonstrate that in long running competition, bi-lateral lower-limb amputees have an advantage compared to uni-lateral lower-limb amputees. On the basis of the statistical analyses in this study, it is proposed that future Paralympic Games should be undertaken with separate events for the T42, T43 and T44 classifications and not hold combined events as they have done in the past.

Acknowledgments

The authors thank the reviewers for their thorough review and highly appreciate the comments and suggestions, which significantly contributed to improving the quality of the paper.

Conflicts of Interest

The authors declare no conflict of interest.

Appendix

Appendix 1

Table A1-1. 100 m/First Round/Heat 1/T42/London 2012.

Rank	Athlete(s)	Country	Results (s)	Specification
1	Popow, Heinrich	GER	12.43	1 leg
2	Reardon, Scott	AUS	12.45	1 leg
3	Whitehead, Richard	GBR	12.97	2 leg
4	Vance, Shaquille	USA	13.17	1 leg
5	Sveinsson, Helgi	ISL	15.64	1 leg
6	Pilgrim, Jamol Allan	ANT	15.76	1 leg

Table A1-2. 100 m/First Round/Heat 2/T42/London 2012.

Rank	Athlete(s)	Country	Results (s)	Specification
1	Czyz, Wojtek	GER	12.53	1leg
2	Connor, Earle	CAN	12.56	1 leg
3	Kayitare, Clavel	FRA	12.59	0 leg
4	Yamamoto, Atsushi	JPN	12.87	1 leg
5	Jorgensen, Daniel	DEN	13.21	1 leg
6	Garcia-Tolson, Rudy	USA	13.77	2 leg

Table A1-3. 100 m/Final round/T42/London 2012.

Rank	Athlete(s)	Country	Results (s)	Specification
1	Popow, Heinrich	GER	12.4	1 leg
2	Reardon, Scott	AUS	12.43	1 leg
3	Czyz, Wojtek	GER	12.52	1 leg
4	Connor, Earle	CAN	12.65	1 leg
5	Kayitare, Clavel	FRA	12.73	0 leg
6	Yamamoto, Atsushi	JPN	12.92	1 leg
7	Whitehead, Richard	GBR	12.99	2 leg
8	Vance, Shaquille	USA	13.03	1 leg

Table A1-4. 100 m/First Round/Heat 1/T44/London 2012.

Rank	Athlete(s)	Country	Results (s)	Specification
1	Peacock, Jonnie	GBR	11.08	1 leg
2	Singleton, Jerome	USA	11.46	1 leg
3	Oliveira, Alan Fonteles Cardoso	BRA	11.56	2 leg
4	Fernandes, Marcio Miguel Da Costa	CPV	12.16	1 leg
5	Behre, David	GER	12.27	2 leg
6	Scendoni, Riccardo	ITA	12.45	1 leg
7	Jia, Tianlei	CHN	12.49	1 leg

Table A1-5. 100 m/First Round/Heat 2/T44/London 2012.

Rank	Athlete(s)	Country	Results (s)	Specification
1	Pistorius, Oscar	RSA	11.18	2 leg
2	Leeper, Blake	USA	11.34	2 leg
3	Liu, Zhiming	CHN	11.84	0 leg
4	Rehm, Markus	GER	11.92	1 leg
5	Alaize, Jean-Baptiste	FRA	12.11	1 leg
6	Prokopyev, Ivan	RUS	12.21	2 leg
7	Mayer, Robert	AUT	12.61	1 leg

Table A1-6. 100 m/First Round/Heat 3/T44/London 2012.

Rank	Athlete(s)	Country	Results (s)	Specification
1	Fourie, Arnu	RSA	11.29	1 leg
2	Browne, Richard	USA	11.33	1 leg
3	McQueen, Alister	CAN	12.02	1 leg
4	Bausch, Christoph	SUI	12.09	1 leg
5	Oliveira, Andre	BRA	12.35	2 leg
6	Haruta, Jun	JPN	12.69	1 leg

Table A1-7. 100 m/Final round/T44/London 2012.

Rank	Athlete(s)	Country	Results (s)	Specification
1	Peacock, Jonnie	GBR	10.9	1 leg
2	Browne, Richard	USA	11.03	1 leg
3	Fourie, Arnu	RSA	11.08	1 leg
4	Pistorius, Oscar	RSA	11.17	2 leg
5	Leeper, Blake	USA	11.21	2 leg
6	Singleton, Jerome	USA	11.25	1 leg
7	Oliveira, Alan Fonteles Cardoso	BRA	11.33	2 leg
8	Liu, Zhiming	CHN	11.97	0 leg

Table A1-8. 200 m/T42/London 2012.

Rank	Athlete(s)	Country	Results (s)	Specification
1	Whitehead, Richard	GBR	24.38	2 leg
2	Vance, Shaquille	USA	25.55	1 leg
3	Popow, Heinrich	GER	25.9	1 leg
4	Reardon, Scott	AUS	26.03	1 leg
5	Czyz, Wojtek	GER	26.07	1 leg
6	Kayitare, Clavel	FRA	26.22	0 leg
7	Jorgensen, Daniel	DEN	26.46	1 leg
8	Yamamoto, Atsushi	JPN	26.76	1 leg
9	Garcia-Tolson, Rudy	USA	26.97	2 leg

Table A1-9. 200 m/First Round/Heat 1/T44/London 2012.

Rank	Athlete(s)	Country	Results (s)	Specification
1	Oliveira, Alan Fonteles Cardoso	BRA	21.88	2 leg
2	Singleton, Jerome	USA	23.23	1 leg
3	McQueen, Alister	CAN	24.25	1 leg
4	Prokopyev, Ivan	RUS	24.26	2 leg
5	Alaize, Jean-Baptiste	FRA	24.42	2 leg
6	Swift, Jack	AUS	24.88	1 leg

Table A1-10. 200 m/First Round/Heat 2/T44/London 2012.

Rank	Athlete(s)	Country	Results (s)	Specification
1	Leeper, Blake	USA	22.23	2 leg
2	Fourie, Arnu	RSA	22.57	1 leg
3	Behre, David	GER	23.65	1 leg
4	Bausch, Christoph	SUR	24.22	1 leg
5	Mayer, Robert	AUT	24.67	1 leg
6	Jia, Tianlei	CHN	25.62	1 leg

Table A1-11. 200 m/First Round/Heat 3/T44/London 2012.

Rank	Athlete(s)	Country	Results (s)	Specification
1	Pistorius, Oscar	RSA	21.3	2 leg
2	Bizzell, Jim Bob	USA	23.64	1 leg
3	Sato, Keita	JPN	24.34	1 leg
4	Scendoni, Riccardo	ITA	24.51	1 leg
5	Fernandes, Marcio Miguel Da Costa	CPV	24.84	1 leg
6	Pituwala Kankanange, Dumeera Maduranga Alwis	SRI	26.23	0 leg

Table A1-12. 200 m/Final Round/T44/London 2012.

Rank	Athlete(s)	Country	Results (s)	Specification
1	Oliveira, Alan Fonteles Cardoso	BRA	21.45	2 leg
2	Pistorius, Oscar	RSA	21.52	2 leg
3	Leeper, Blake	USA	22.46	2 leg
4	Fourie, Arnu	RSA	22.49	1 leg
5	Singleton, Jerome	USA	23.58	1 leg
6	Bausch, Christoph	SUI	23.7	1 leg
7	Behre, David	GER	23.71	1 leg
8	Bizzell, Jim Bob	USA	28.19	1 leg

Table A1-13. 400 m/First Round/Heat 1/T44/London 2012.

Rank	Athlete(s)	Country	Results (s)	Specification
1	Leeper, Blake	USA	50.63	2 leg
2	Oliveira, Alan Fonteles Cardoso	BRA	53.02	2 leg
3	Liu, Zhiming	CHN	54.82	0 leg
4	Scendoni, Riccardo	ITA	55.88	1 leg
5	Swift, Jack	AUS	55.94	1 leg
6	Benitez Sandoval, Josue	MEX	59.79	1 leg

Table A1-14. 400 m/First Round/Heat 2/T44/London 2012.

Rank	Athlete(s)	Country	Results (s)	Specification
1	Pistorius, Oscar	RSA	48.31	2 leg
2	Behre, David	GER	51.37	2 leg
3	Prince, David	USA	52.29	1 leg
4	Wallace, Jarryd	USA	53.51	1 leg
5	Prokopyev, Ivan Sato, Keita	RUS	53.86	2 leg

Table A1-15. 400 m/Final Round/T44/London 2012.

Rank	Athlete(s)	Country	Results (s)	Specification
1	Pistorius, Oscar	RSA	46.68	2 leg
2	Leeper, Blake	USA	50.14	2 leg
3	Prince, David	USA	50.61	1 leg
4	Oliveira, Alan Fonteles Cardoso	BRA	51.59	2 leg
5	Behre, David	GER	51.65	2 leg
6	Wallace, Jarryd	USA	53.9	1 leg
7	Prokopyev, Ivan	RUS	54.74	2 leg
8	Liu, Zhiming	CHN	55.91	0 leg

Appendix 2

The numbers in parenthesis in second column, indicates the number of bilateral, unilateral, and those who run on natural leg (but considered as an amputee).

Table A2-1. 100 m Descriptive data for 2008 Beijing.

Category	N	Mean	Median	s.d	Min	Max	S-W
T42/Final	6(0,6,0)	13.11	13.08	0.53	12.32	13.68	0.717
T44/Heat 1	6(0,5,1)	11.9	11.96	0.25	11.49	12.12	0.299
T44/Heat 2	6(1,4,1)	12.15	12.04	0.83	11.16	13.45	0.801
T44/Final	8(1,7,0)	11.64	11.56	0.41	11.17	12.25	0.676

Table A2-2. 200 m Descriptive data for 2008 Beijing.

Category	N	Mean	Median	s.d	Min	Max	S-W
T44/Heat 1	5(1,4,0)	24.81	24.17	2.01	23.22	28.32	0.025
T44/Heat 2	5(1,3,1)	24.09	24.22	0.93	22.71	24.95	0.495
T44/Final	8(2,5,1)	23.36	23.47	0.93	21.67	24.61	0.939

Table A2-3. 400 m Descriptive data for 2008 Beijing.

Category	N	Mean	Median	s.d	Min	Max	S-W
T44/Final	6(1,4,1)	52.43	52.42	3.099	47.49	55.76	0.644

Table A2-4. 100 m Descriptive data for 2004 Athens.

Category	N	Mean	Median	s.d	Min	Max	S-W
T42/Final	6(0,5,1)	13.41	13.04	1.085	12.51	15.5	0.052
T44/Heat 1	5(0,5,0)	12.41	12.57	0.73	11.23	12.95	0.115
T44/Heat 2	6(1,5,0)	11.88	11.93	0.515	11.2	12.52	0.74
T44/Final	8(1,7,0)	11.7	11.695	0.561	11.08	12.58	0.36

Table A2-5. 200 m Descriptive data for 2004 Athens.

Category	N	Mean	Median	s.d	Min	Max	S-W
T42/Final	6(0,5,1)	27.12	27.1	0.677	26.18	28.1	0.959
T44/Heat 1	6(1,5,0)	24.71	24.51	1.079	23.42	26.55	0.759
T44/Heat 2	6(0,6,0)	24.81	24.48	1.053	23.5	26.18	0.427
T44/Final	8(1,7,0)	23.15	23.2	0.659	21.97	23.87	0.427

Table A2-6. 400 m Descriptive data for 2004 Athens.

Category	N	Mean	Median	s.d	Min	Max	S-W
T44/Heat 1	5(0,5,0)	55.38	55.67	1.236	53.58	56.7	0.794
T44/Heat 2	4(0,4,0)	55.36	54.31	2.229	54.12	58.7	0.006
T44/Final	7(0,7,0)	53.76	53.98	1.295	51.24	55.02	0.268

References

1. Gold, J.R.; Gold, M.M. Access for all: The rise of the Paralympic Games. *J. R. Soc. Promot. Health* **2007**, *127*, 133–141.
2. Sainsbury, T. *Paralympics, Past, Present and Future*; Centre d'Estudis Olímpics (UAB): Bellaterra, Spain, 2004.
3. International Paralympic Committee (IPC). *A Plan of IPC Athletics for the Period 2013–2016*; Athletics Strategic Plan: Bonn, Germany, 2015.
4. Dyer, B. An Insight into the Acceptable Use & Assessment of Lower-Limb Running Prostheses in Disability Sport. Ph.D. Thesis, Bournemouth University, Poole, UK, 2013.
5. Tweedy, S.M.; Vanlandewijck, Y.C. International Paralympic Committee position stand—Background and scientific principles of classification in Paralympic sport. *Br. J. Sports Med.* **2011**, *45*, 259–269.
6. IPC Athletics. In *Classification Rules and Regulations*; International Paralympic Committee: Bonn, Germany, 2011.
7. Zettler, P. *Is It Cheating to Use Cheetahs? The Implications of Technologically Innovative Prostheses for Sports Value and Rules*; Stanford Law School: Stanford, CA, USA, 2009.
8. Official Website of the Paralympic Movement. Available online: http://www.paralympic.org (accessed on 14 June 2015).
9. Zahayu, Y.; Suhaida, A.; Shapirah, S. Comparing the performance of modified F_t statistic with ANOVA and Kruskal-Wallis Test. *Appl. Math. Inf. Sci.* **2013**, *7*, 403–408.
10. Guo, S.; Zhong, S.; Zhang, A. Privacy-preserving kruskal-wallis test. *Comput. Methods Program Biomed.* **2013**, *112*, 135–145
11. Bruggemann, G.-P.; Arampatzis, A.; Emrich, F.; Potthast, P. Biomechanics of double transtibial amputee sprinting using dedicated sprinting prostheses. *Sports Technol.* **2008**, *1*, 220.
12. Noroozi, S.; Sewell, P.; Rahman, A.G.A.; Vinney, J.; Zhi Chao, O.; Dyer, B.T.J. Performance enhancement of bi-lateral lower-limb amputees in the latter phases of running events: An initial investigation. *Proc. IMechE Part P: J. Sports Eng. Technol.* **2013**, *227*, 105–115.

13. Hassani, H.; Ghodsi, M.; Shadi, M.; Noroozi, S.; Dyer, B. A Statistical perspective on running with prosthetic lower-limbs: An advantage or disadvantage? *Sports* **2014**, *2*, 76–84.

18

A Comparison between Learning Style Preferences, Gender, Sport and Achievement in Elite Team Sport Athletes

Andrea Braakhuis [1,*], Tea Williams [1], Elizabeth Fusco [2], Shawn Hueglin [2] and Alex Popple [3]

[1] Discipline of Nutrition/Dietetics, Faculty of Medical and Health Sciences, The University of Auckland, Private Bag 92019, Auckland, 1142, New Zealand; E-Mail: twil830@aucklanduni.ac.nz

[2] United States Olympic Committee, 2800 Olympic Parkway, Chula Vista, CA 91915, USA; E-Mails: Liz.fusco.nutr@gmail.com (E.F.); Shawn.Hueglin@usoc.org (S.H.)

[3] High Performance Sport New Zealand, Avantidrome, Hanlin Road, Cambridge 3283, New Zealand; E-Mail: Alex.Popple@hpsnz.org.nz

* Author to whom correspondence should be addressed; E-Mail: a.braakhuis@auckland.ac.nz

Academic Editor: Eling de Bruin

Abstract: Athletes have preferences for the way in which they internalize and process information, whether that is visual, aural, by-doing (kinesthetic), reading or a mixture of preferences. Health professionals that interact with athletes rarely consider the individual learning style prior to any communication or education, despite mounting evidence for the benefits of learning-style tailored education. The aim of this study was to characterize athletes with regards to their preferred learning style. Athletes (n = 93) from 24 sports and various sport achievement levels completed a questionnaire, including the visual (V), auditory (A), reading/writing (R), kinesthetic (K)/(VARK) Questionnaire for Athletes. Questionnaire outcomes were analysed by X^2 analysis on SPSS. The main findings were: (1) very few athletes have a visual learning-style preference; (2) there was a significant relationship between gender and VARK preference ($X^2 = 13.84$, $p = 0.003$); (3) and between athletic status and VARK preference ($X^2 = 9.2$, $p = 0.025$); (4) there was a trivial association between individual/ team sport athletes and assessed VARK preference ($X^2 = 3.95$, $p = 0.265$). Our findings show significant variation in learning-style preference between males and females, and those of different athletic status. Health professionals should be aware of the inadequacy of visual information presentation when working with athletes. Furthermore, health professionals working with elite and female athletes should be comfortable using a mixture of learning styles (multi-modal).

Keywords: sports; athletic performance; counseling; education

1. Introduction

In today's sport obsessed society, the modern day athlete is reliant on the advice and support of a health professional team. Health professionals typically play a role in supporting athletes by providing advice on injury prevention, rehabilitation, mental skills and nutrition education. While the majority of research has focused on building the knowledge base of health professionals working with athletes, very little has been done on how to educate health professionals on how they advise athletes. Research has shown athletes have preferences for the ways in which they receive information [1]. The visual (V), auditory (A), reading/writing (R), kinesthetic (K)/(VARK) questionnaire for athletes identifies their preferred mode(s) of presentation of information this mode governs how athletes interpret, process, and understand information. Learners with a visual preference prefer charts, graphs and flow charts among other forms of visual stimuli that could have otherwise been presented in words. Aural learners take in new information by aural and oral methods (hearing and speaking). People with an aural learning preference like to have new ideas explained to them and to discuss topics with others; they can also take in complex and detailed instructions easily. The read/ write mode of learning involves information displayed as text and written words. People with a strong preference for this style of learning find they prefer to use lists, notes, essays and other forms of text-based stimuli to take on and process new forms of information. Kinesthetic learners prefer using experiences and practices rather than conceptual or abstract learning. This type of learner uses their senses to interact with the world around them and enjoys practical opportunities and hands-on approaches to learning new information [1]. An additional category is a mixture of learning styles, called multi-modal (MM).

Gaining insight into athletes preferred mode(s) can (a) help provide healthcare instruction tailored to athletes individual learning preferences to better understand information and improve self-care [1]; (b) overcome the predisposition for health professionals to treat all athletes in a similar way; and (c) be used as a catalyst to encourage health professionals to move from their preferred mode(s) to others [2].

At present the VARK questionnaire for athletes has been used by coaches to tailor coaching instruction to support understanding by athletes by matching perceptual preference with instructional method [3]. It has also been heavily utilized in the teaching environment, where particular learning styles relate to better outcomes outside the classroom [4]. Athletes interacting with the healthcare system are constantly taking in and applying new information; it is therefore, vital that health care professionals adopt learning-style based instruction to maximize the efficiency of their care. To date, health professionals have not incorporated an assessment of an athlete's learning style into rehabilitation or injury management programmes; doing so would likely result in benefits. Current clinical research indicates that education is a pivotal component in effective multi-disciplinary treatment programmes as it enables patients to better understand their condition and acquire adequate skills to perform self-care [2].

The aim of this study is to examine the relationship between assessed sensory modality preferences and athlete status, gender, and sport, using the VARK athlete questionnaire. The outcomes of the research will serve as a valuable tool to health professionals alike to facilitate effective communication and improve health outcomes for athletes.

2. Materials and Methods

Athletes (n = 93) from a variety of sports and sport achievement level completed a questionnaire, including the VARK inventory previously validated for use with athletes [4]. Athletes were from New Zealand and the United States. Athletes were first asked if they wished to participate in the study via a health professional or research assistant and were administered with a participant information sheet detailing the purposes and aims of the study. Athletes and health professionals completed consent forms. For athletes within an elite team, approval from the National Sporting Body was obtained.

All experimental procedures were approved by The University of Auckland Ethics Committee, reference number 9399. Experimental procedures performed in the United States of America were approved by the San Diego State University Division of Research Affairs—Human Research Protection Program. Protocol number 1212087.

2.1. Questionnaire

The Questionnaire was composed of two sections. The first section asked athletes to identify their name (for the purpose of providing learning style feedback), gender, highest level of sport competition in the last 2 years (international, national, regional, recreational), sport and age, as well as whether they play an individual or team sport. The second component of the questionnaire was composed of the 13 questions from Fleming's VARK inventory for athletes, which was used to determine each athlete's assessed sensory modality preference [5]. A selected question from Fleming's VARK inventory for athletes, is described as "(1) You are about to give directions to an athlete who is standing with you. The athlete is new to town and needs to get to the athletic complex. The athlete has a bike. I would: (a) draw a map on paper, (b) tell him/her the directions, (c) write down the directions (without a map), (d) bike with them to the complex."

Copyright for the use of the VARK inventory was send via email and approval granted for the use of the paper version only. Copyright of the athlete VARK questionnaire is held by Julia Dunn (Whitman College, Walla Walla, WA, USA) and Neil Fleming (Christchurch, New Zealand). Neil Fleming holds the copyright of the original version of VARK from which the Athlete's version was developed. Athletes with fewer than 10 responses in the VARK questionnaire were not included in the analysis in accordance with Flemings [6] scoring system for the VARK questionnaire. The sensory modality preference will be assessed using the "stepping stone" scoring criteria outlined by Fleming [6] to determine whether the athlete is unimodal (V, A, R, K) or multi-modal (MM). A multimodal preference occurs when a person has a strong preference for 2 or more of the VARK modes [6].

2.2. Analysis

For the completed questionnaires obtained via the health professional, the athletes' names were replaced with a numeric code, and the results from each questionnaire were manually input into SPSS for analysis.

Statistical associations among athlete status, gender, and age were made with assessed sensory modality preference, respectively, using Pearson Chi-Square analyses (X^2). Where cell counts were below five the Fisher's exact test (X^2) was used to assess statistical associations. Statistical significance was set at $p < 0.05$. All tests were 2-tailed. For this investigation athletes were grouped into Elite (International & National athletes) and Recreational (Regional & Recreational athletes) in order to assess any association between athlete status and assessed VARK preference. Furthermore, we chose to omit the one participant with a V preference in our analysis as the cell counts for a V preference were too low to conduct an accurate statistical significance test. This is justified as the V modality occurs in less than 1% of athletes [1], and is therefore unlikely to be relevant to this investigation. Data are expressed as either means ± SD, percentages or whole counts.

3. Results

A total of 93 athletes completed the questionnaire; ranging in ages from 16 to 53 years old (see Table 1). Participating athletes were recruited in both New Zealand and the United States of America. In total 106 athletes were approached with 18 athletes choosing not to participate in the study, or failing to return a completed questionnaire or consent form. The response rate was 88%.

Table 1. Characteristics of the Athlete Respondents ($n = 93$).

Variable	Mean (SD)
Age (years)	24 (8)
Gender	
Male	44
Female	49
Athlete Status	
International	49
National	8
Regional	15
Recreational	21
Individual *vs.* Team Sport	
Individual	47
Team	46
Elite/Amateur Status	
Elite	57
Amateur	36
VARK Preference	
V	1
A	16
R	10
K	35
MM	31

Twenty-four sports were represented in the study cohort (see Table 2).

Table 2. Sports Represented in the Athlete Respondents

Sport	No. of Athletes
Football	6
Rugby Union	3
Netball	8
Surfing	1
Hockey	14
Tennis	1
Triathlon	3
Lacrosse	1
Mountain Biking	3
Skiing	1
Rowing	1
Swimming	8
Cycling	1
Water polo	1
Squash	2
Running	1
Kayak	6
Archery	1
BMX Cycling	9
Track & Field	8
Rugby Sevens	11
Gymnastics	2
Touch Rugby	1
Tag Football	1

Assessed Sensory Modality Preferences

Using the VARK questionnaire for Athletes, the majority of athletes had a Kinesthetic learning style, followed by Multimodal, Aural, Read-write and then Visual (see Figure 1). These results indicate a strong preference for Kinesthetic and Multimodal learning amongst the athlete cohort. Overall, 62% of the study participants were unimodal learners, with the remaining 38% being multimodal learners.

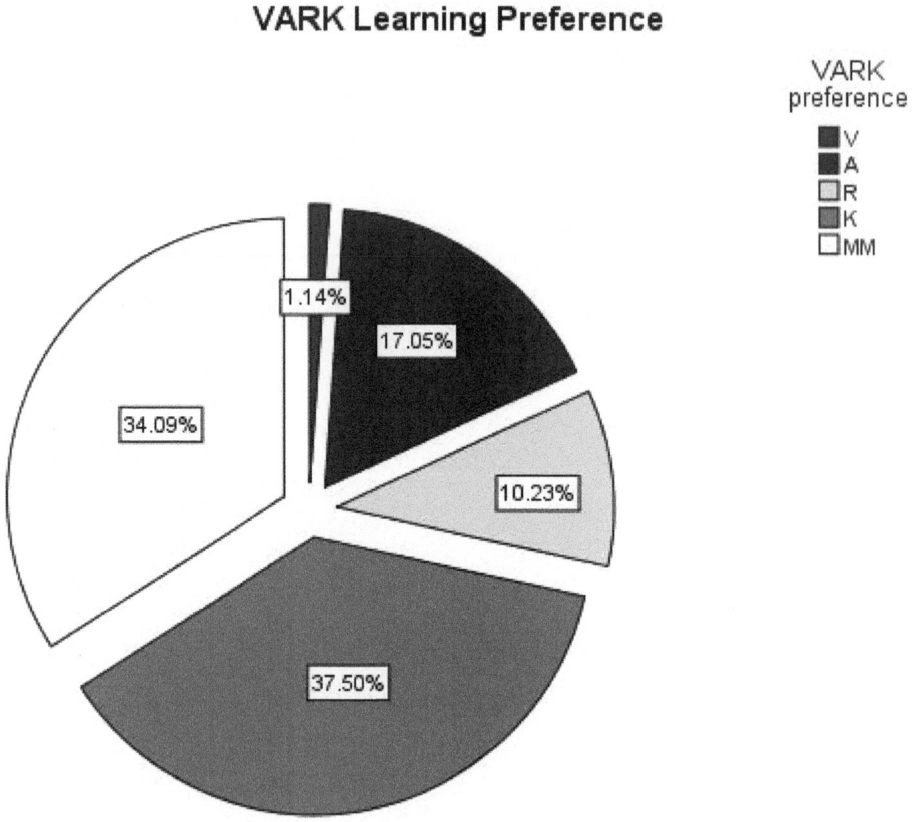

Figure 1. Athlete learning style preference by percent. Data presented as 5-part model. MM = Multimodal; V = Visual; A = Aural; R = Read/Write; K = Kinesthetic.

The X^2 analysis between gender and assessed sensory modality preference indicated a difference in learning style between men and women. Male athletes were found to prefer K learning (39%) followed by A (32%), MM (21%), R (8%). On the other hand, 46% of female athletes showed a preference for MM learning followed by K (37%), R (13%), A (4%). The association between gender and assessed sensory modality preference reached statistical significance with a Fisher's exact test (Table 3).

We also examined the relationship between assessed sensory modality and athlete status. Amongst international athletes 46% were MM learners followed by K (27%), R (16%) and A (11%). National athletes showed a strong preference for A (33%) and K (33%) followed by R (17%) and A (17%). Regional athletes were mostly K (73%) followed by A (20%) and MM (7%). MM (36%) and K (36%) learning styles were the most prevalent amongst recreational athletes with 23% having an A preference and the final 5% having an R modality preference. The association between athletic status and VARK preference reached statistical significance with a Fisher's exact test. This result may have been influenced by the relatively low count of national athletes (see Table 3).

Associations between athletic status and VARK preference were also present when international and national athletes were combined to make the "elite" group and regional and recreational combined to make the "amateur" group. Elite athletes were shown to have a strong preference for MM (39%) learning followed by K (27%), R (18%) and A (16%). In contrast, over half (56%) of the amateur athletes had a K preference with 25% having a MM preference, followed by A (19%) and R (0%). The association between elite and amateur athletes and their perceived learning style also reached statistical significance (see Table 3).

Table 3. VARK Learning Preference *vs.* Gender, Individual/Team Sport and Athletic Status ($n = 92$).

Variable	VARK Preference				Total
	A	R	K	MM	
Gender [a]					
Male	14	4	17	9	44
Female	2	6	18	22	48
Athletic Status [b]					
International	6	8	13	21	48
National	2	2	3	1	8
Regional	3	0	11	1	15
Recreational	5	0	8	8	21
Athletic status (combined) [c]					
Elite	8	10	16	22	56
Amateur	8	0	19	9	36
Individual/team sport [d]					
Individual	9	8	14	15	46
Team	7	2	21	16	46

Notes: Values are whole counts. [a] $X^2 = 15.1$, $p = 0.001$; [b] $X^2 = 20.4$, $p = 0.006$; [c] $X^2 = 13.3$, $p = 0.003$; [d] $X^2 = 5.3$, $p = 0.158$; Note: cell counts below 5, were analysed using Fisher's exact test.

Finally we assessed if there was a possible association between individual and team sport athletes and VARK preference. Team sport athletes were 46% K learners followed by MM (35%), A (15%) and R (4%). In comparison, MM (33%) was the most popular preference amongst individual sport athletes followed by K (30%), A (20%) and R (17%). This association fell short of statistical significance with a Pearson Chi-Square (see Table 3).

4. Discussion

The main conclusions of the study were that (a) there were very few athletes with a visual learning style preference; (b) there was a significant relationship between gender and assessed VARK preference; (c) there was a significant relationship between athletic status and assessed VARK preference; and (d) there was a lack of significance between individual/team sport athletes and assessed VARK preference.

The overall distribution of learning style preferences in this investigation differed significantly from those found by Fleming [7]. The respondents in our study showed a 33% MM preference compared with 65% found by Fleming [7] ($n = 145{,}358$). We found a K preference to be much higher in our study (38%) compared to Fleming's [7] (12%); our study also indicated a much higher A preference (17% in our investigation compared with 7%). There was a smaller difference between R preference (11% in our study compared with 14%) and our V preference (1%) was analogous to Fleming's (3%) [7]. The reason for the disparity in preferences between our investigation and Flemings is not clear. Our investigation found only one respondent with a unimodal V preference amongst the entire study cohort, our finding is consistent with Dunn [1] who reports that less than 1% of the athlete population is comprised of visual learners. This result suggests that health professionals working with athletes should move from traditional visual means of information presentation, such as instructional charts and books, when working with athletes. It is, however, difficult to promote a complete move away from visual methods as many multimodal preferences include the visual mode.

Another important trend identified in our investigation was the association between elite and amateur athletic status and assessed VARK preference. Our study found elite and recreational athletes to be significantly different in VARK preference. Dunn [1] notes that learning style preferences vary among athletes of different levels of sporting competition which is consistent with our findings. Interestingly, we found elite athletes to report a much broader spectrum of learning styles when compared to those of recreational status. Health professionals who are multi-modal learners themselves may be at an advantage when working with an elite athlete group; given MM learners are able to navigate the different learning styles with ease. Also, health professionals should attempt to incorporate different styles of educating athletes. For example, distributing nutrition advice and supplying a menu plan to every athlete without regard for learning preference is likely to be an unsuccessful approach to initiate behavior change. Instead, we might suggest a health professional assess an athlete's learning style and tailor instruction likewise, so the R learner receives a meal plan and a K participates in a cooking class, by way of example.

Another important finding from our investigation was the trend between gender and assessed VARK preference in which male and female athletes showed significantly different modality preferences. Males had a much higher preference for A learning, compared to females, while females were more likely to be multimodal learners. Our findings contrast from those in other studies where a multimodal modality was the most popular preference for both sexes; however, these studies differ from ours in that they used students rather than athletes as well as using the standard VARK questionnaire as opposed to the athlete's version used in our investigation [8–10]. Our results, however, are similar to those reported by Dunn [1] in that males had a higher preference for A learning (32.5% *vs.* 4.3% for females). This significant finding suggests that health professionals working with male athletes should adopt some methods of aural information presentation, such as conducting verbal discussion or recording the consultation so the athlete can listen to the information again in the future; it is fortunate in this case that much of health professional–athlete communication is verbally orientated.

Limitations

Throughout the process of the investigation, it became evident that many of the athlete participants saw the VARK inventory for athletes to be outdated with respect to current technology. For example, one question asks athletes how they would give directions to another athlete, many of our respondents indicated to us that they would use a smartphone in this situation. However, this was not an option in the questionnaire. The authors would recommend a revised version of the VARK inventory for athletes which acknowledge modern technological advancements. A further limitation of the study is that we chose not to examine the learning styles of health professionals interacting with athletes. While the main aim of the study was to profile the learning styles of different classes of athletes the authors feel that insight into the modality preferences of the health professionals involved would help to provide more effective implementation strategies.

5. Conclusions

As far as we are aware, this is the first independent study used to characterize athletes' learning preferences as a way to educate health professionals on appropriate methods of education. While further research is required for a more comprehensive understanding of the interaction between athletes and health professionals it is evident from our investigation that a trend exists between gender and athletic status and VARK learning style preferences. Therefore, these findings merit real life implementation. The findings from our investigation present the exciting opportunity for a paradigm shift in the way that athletes interact and communicate with health care professionals. Furthermore, this study should serve as a platform for further research in this field; the authors would recommend a simultaneous investigation into both athletes' and health professionals' learning style in order to gain better insight into how communication between the two parties and how such communication could be enhanced.

Acknowledgments

The authors would like to thank Avinesh Pillai from the University of Auckland, Department of Statistics, for his statistical advice, as well as the University of Auckland School of Medicine Foundation for funding technical support for the investigation.

Author Contributions

Andrea Braakhuis and Shawn Hueglin conceived and designed the research; Andrea Braakhuis, Shawn Hueglin, Elizabeth Fusco, Tea Williams, and Alex Popple performed the experiments; Tea Williams and Andrea Braakhuis analyzed the data; Andrea Braakhuis, Liz Fusco and Tea Williams wrote the paper.

Conflicts of Interest

The authors declare no conflict of interest.

References

1. Dunn, J.L. Using learning preferences to improve coaching and athletic performance. *J. Phys. Educ. Recreat. Dance* **2009**, *80*, 30–37.
2. Boyde, M.; Tuckett, A.; Peters, R.; Thompson, D.R.; Turner, C.; Stewart, S. Learning style and learning needs of heart failure patients (The Need2Know-HF patient study). *Eur. J. Cardiovasc. Nurs.* **2009**, *8*, 316–322.
3. Fuelscher, I.T.; Ball, K.; MacMahon, C. Perspectives on learning styles in motor and sport skills. *Front. Psychiatr.* **2012**, *69*, 1–3.
4. Leite, W.L.; Svinicki, M.; Shi, Y. Attempted validation of the scores of the VARK: Learning styles inventory with multitrait-multimethod confirmatory factor analysis models. *Educ. Psychol. Meas.* **2009**, doi:10.1177/0013164409344507.

5. Fleming, N. The VARK Questionnaire—For Athletes. In *VARK—A Guide to Learning Styles*; 2011. Available online: http://www.vark-learn.com/english/page.asp?p=athletes (accessed on 5 November 2013).
6. Fleming, N.; Bonwell, C. *How Do I Learn Best?: A Student's Guide to Improved Learning: VARK, Visual aural Read/Write Kinesthetic*, 1st ed.; Published by Fleming & Bonwell: Christchurch, New Zealand, 2001.
7. Fleming, N. Research & Statistics. *VARK—A Guide to Learning Styles.* Available online: http://www.vark-learn.com/english/page.asp?p=research. 2012 (accessed on 3 March 2014).
8. Choudhary, R.; Dullo, P.; Tandon, R.V. Gender differences in learning style preferences of first year Medical students. *Pak. J. Physiol.* **2011**, *7*, 42–45.
9. Slater, J.A.; Lujan, H.L.; DiCarlo, S. Does gender influence learning style preferences of first-year medical students? *Adv. Physiol. Educ.* **2007**, *31*, 336–342.
10. Wehrwein, E.A.; Lujan, H.L.; DiCarlo, S.E. Gender differences in learning style preferences among undergraduate physiology students. *Adv. Physiol. Educ.* **2007**, *31*, 153–157.

19

Reliability of the Single-Visit Field Test of Critical Speed in Trained and Untrained Adolescents

Alfred Nimmerichter [1,*], Mathias Steindl [1,†] and Craig Anthony Williams [2,†]

[1] Faculty of Sport and Exercise Sciences, University of Applied Sciences Wiener Neustadt, Johannes Gutenberg Str. 3, Wiener Neustadt A-2700, Austria; E-Mail: nachwuchs@floorball.at

[2] Children's Health and Exercise Research Centre, Sport and Health Sciences, University of Exeter, St Luke's Campus, Heavitree Road, Exeter EX1 2LU, Devon, UK;
E-Mail: c.a.williams@exeter.ac.uk

† These authors contributed equally to this work.

* Author to whom correspondence should be addressed; E-Mail: nimmerichter@fhwn.ac.at

Academic Editor: Eling de Bruin

Abstract: Recent studies in adults have shown that the critical intensity during running and cycling estimated from three prediction trials interspersed by 30 min is valid and reliable. To establish the reliability of the single-visit field test to determine critical speed (CS) and the distance above critical speed (D′) in adolescents, 29 trained and 14 untrained participants (mean ± SD age: 17.5 ± 0.5 years) performed three tests on a 400-m outdoor track separated by 48 h. Each test consisted of three distances selected to result in finishing times between 2 and 15 min that must be completed as fast as possible. CS and D′ were modeled using the linear 1/time model (Speed = D′(1/t) + CS). While the coefficient of variation (CV) of CS was between 2.4% and 4.3%, the CV of D′ was 9.3% to 13.6%. Also the intraclass correlation coefficient ranged from 0.919 to 0.983 for CS and from 0.325 to 0.828 for D′. The results show that the single-visit field test provides reliable estimates of CS but not D′ in trained and untrained adolescents.

Keywords: critical power; field test; youth athletes; test-retest reliability

1. Introduction

Critical power (CP), which represents the asymptote of a participant's power-duration curve, separates the boundaries of the heavy and very heavy intensity domains and has been broadly associated with maximal lactate steady state [1]. According to the theory of Monod and Scherrer [2], CP represents the maximal power that can be sustained indefinitely. While this has been shown not to be the case, CP has been proposed as an important parameter of aerobic function [3]. The two component CP model assumes that the CP is representative of the maximal rate at which ATP turnover is supplied aerobically, whilst the curvature constant of the hyperbolic curve, represents a finite anaerobic energy store within the muscle, signified as W′ (indicative of work that can be performed above CP) [4]. During an exercise period undertaken above CP, exhaustion will occur when the W′ is depleted, and the rate is determined by how much a participant is exercising above his or her CP, represented by the equation

$$\text{Time to exhaustion} = W'/(P - CP) \tag{1}$$

where P represents power.

To date most studies examining CP have been conducted using cycle ergometers but the CP concept is easily translated to running or swimming, termed critical velocity or critical speed, as a vector or scalar quantity, respectively. For clarity, critical speed (CS) will be used throughout the paper. Based on Equation (1), the time to exhaustion for an acquired speed can be predicted during exercise above CS. Furthermore, if the aim is to require a participant to complete a known amount of work or distance in a training session, the theoretical time to complete this work can be calculated from:

$$\text{Time to exhaustion} = (D - D')/CS \tag{2}$$

where D and D′ represent the distance and distance above CS, respectively.

CP or CS is strongly associated with $\dot{V}O_{2max}$ [5,6] and endurance performance [7,8] indicating the validity to measure aerobic function. In comparison with adults, where CP has been identified as the highest sustainable exercise intensity above which a loss of intramuscular metabolic (e.g., phosphocreatine, pH) and systemic (e.g., $\dot{V}O_2$, blood lactate) homeostasis occurs [9], physiological responses during exercise at CP in young people are limited [6,10]. Williams *et al.* [6] reported non steady-state responses in $\dot{V}O_2$ and blood lactate during cycling at CP and 10% above CP and concluded, that CP does not represent a sustainable exercise intensity in adolescents. In accordance, Barker *et al.* [10] showed increases in $\dot{V}O_2$ and blood lactate over time, accompanied by reduced time to exhaustion during cycling 10% above CP. At an intensity 10% below CP, all participants completed 30 min of exercise and a steady-state in $\dot{V}O_2$ and blood lactate profile was identified [10].

There is a useful and practical application of CS in the prediction and monitoring of young athletes' aerobic fitness and performances. Additionally, coaches would be able to manipulate the time or intensity of training in order to affect the stimulus of training. This practical application of CS can be observed most commonly in swimming, where the calculation of CS is frequently utilized for youth training and performance [7,11–13]. Application can also be found, although infrequent, in other sports e.g., running [14].

Before a wider uptake by coaches and sports science support staff for the CS method to assess aerobic function in a field setting can be undertaken, it is important to determine the reliability of the method.

While the critical speed estimated from the single-visit field test has been shown to be reliable and valid in adults [15,16], the reliability in children and adolescents remains to be shown. Therefore, the aim of this study was to establish the reliability of CS and D′ obtained from the single-visit field test in trained and untrained adolescents.

2. Method

2.1. Participants

A total number of 43 adolescents (19 males) volunteered to participate in this study. According to an interview with the participants and their parents, the group was divided into trained and untrained subjects. Twenty nine participants (15 males) (mean ± SD age: 17.7 ± 0.5 years; stature: 170.7 ± 6.1 cm; body mass: 63.4 ± 8.9 kg) had a training volume of at least 6 $h{\cdot}week^{-1}$ (range: 6–18 $h{\cdot}week^{-1}$) and were classified as trained. All were members of local sport clubs and participated in a variety of sports (football (seven), gymnastics (five), triathlon and tennis (four), volleyball (three), swimming and judo (two), dancing and climbing (one)). The remaining 14 participants (four males) (mean ± SD age: 17.4 ± 0.6 years; stature: 169.9 ± 6.1 cm; body mass: 63.3 ± 14.8 kg) participated in less than 3 $h{\cdot}week^{-1}$ of physical activity (school sports), and therefore were classified as untrained. After being briefed as to the risks of the research, informed written parental consent and the participants' assent were provided before entering the study, which was conducted in accordance with the ethical principles of the Declaration of Helsinki and approved by the University's institutional review board.

2.2. Study Design

At the first visit body mass and stature were measured using an electronic scale and stadiometer (Seca 813 and 213, Seca, Hamburg, Germany). The study involved three testing sessions, separated by 48 h, for each participant on a 400 m outdoor track. During each session, the participants were asked to complete three fixed distances in the shortest possible time (*i.e.*, as fast as possible) using a 30 min recovery between the runs [15,16]. All sessions were performed at sea level, at approximately the same time of the day (±2 h) and the temperature and humidity were 22–25° C and 40%–45%, respectively. The wind speed was less than 2.0 $m{\cdot}s^{-1}$ during all tests [17]. Prior to each session, a standardized warm-up of 5 min jogging followed by a series of five 30 s runs with increasing speed, was completed. The participants were asked to refrain from strenuous exercise in the 24 h before the tests.

2.3. Determination of Critical Speed

The three fixed-distance runs were conducted in the following order: 500 m, 1200 m and 2000 m for the trained and 400 m, 1000 m and 1600 m for the untrained participants. These distances were estimated to result in finishing times between 2 and 15 min [4] and based on previous experience. The participants started in 30 s intervals and were strongly verbally encouraged throughout the tests. All runs were hand-timed and recorded to the nearest second and no information on elapsed time was provided. Linear regression was used to calculate CS and D′ using the 1/time model (Speed = D′(1/t) + CS). The model was chosen as it provides the better parameter estimates of CS compared with the linear distance-time model (standard error: 0.12 ± 0.09 m·s^{-1}, 95% confidence interval: 0.09 to 0.13 m·s^{-1}; r^2 = 0.96 ± 0.06; 95% CI: 0.95 to 0.97).

2.4. Statistical Analyses

The parameter estimates of the linear 1/time model were resolved with the software Graph Pad Prism 6.0 (Graph Pad, La Jolla, CA, USA). Statistical analyses were performed with the software package SPSS Statistics 22 (IBM Corporation, Armonk, NY, USA). Descriptive data are summarized as mean ± standard deviation (SD). The assumption of normality was verified using the Shapiro-Wilk statistic. A two-way analysis of variance was used to compare CS and D′ across the three tests and between the groups (trained *vs.* untrained). Significant main effects were followed up with pairwise comparisons employing the Bonferroni procedure for multiple testing [18]. The reliability of CS and D′ was assessed with the 95% limits of agreement (LoA) [19] and the intraclass correlation coefficient (ICC). In addition, the within-subject variation was calculated as a coefficient of variation (CV) derived from log-transformed data [20]. All measures of reliability are reported with 95% confidence intervals (95% CI). The level of significance was set at $p < 0.05$.

3. Results

3.1. Critical Speed

The CS was significantly higher in the trained than the untrained participants ($F_{1,41}$ = 18.9; $p < 0.001$). There was a significant difference in CS across the three tests in the untrained participants (2.47 ± 0.37 m·s^{-1}, 2.60 ± 0.37 m·s^{-1} and 2.43 ± 0.37 m·s^{-1}; $F_{2,12} = 47.5$; $p < 0.001$). The post-hoc test revealed that CS estimated from the second test was significantly higher compared to the first test ($p = 0.02$) and the third test ($p < 0.001$). No significant differences in CS across the three tests were observed in the trained participants (3.20 ± 0.48 m·s^{-1}, 3.15 ± 0.55 m·s^{-1} and 3.17 ± 0.54 m·s^{-1}; $F_{2,27} = 1.4$; $p = 0.27$).

The bias in the trained participants was -0.04 ± 0.14 m·s^{-1} (−1.6% ± 4.4%; 95% LoA −0.32 to 0.23 m·s^{-1}) for tests 2-1 and 0.01 ± 0.10 m·s^{-1} (0.5% ± 3.3%; −0.19 to 0.22 m·s^{-1}) for tests 3-2 (Figure 1). In the untrained participants the bias was 0.13 ± 0.15 m·s^{-1} (5.3% ± 6.0%; −0.17 to 0.43 m·s^{-1}) and −0.18 ± 0.08 m·s^{-1} (−7.2% ± 3.3%; −0.34 to −0.01 m·s^{-1}) for tests 2-1 and for tests 3-2, respectively (Figure 1). The ICC was 0.963 (95% CI 0.923 to 0.983) for tests 2-1 and 0.982 (0.962 to 0.992) for tests 3-2 in the trained and 0.919 (0.758 to 0.974) for tests 2-1 and 0.960 (0.874 to 0.987) for tests 3-2 in the untrained participants. The within-subject variation, expressed as a coefficient of variation, was 3.2% (2.6% to 4.4%) for tests 2-1 and 2.4% (1.9% to 3.3%) for tests 3-2 in the trained and 4.3% (3.1% to 7.1%) for tests 2-1 and 2.6% (1.9% to 4.3%) for tests 3-2 in the untrained participants.

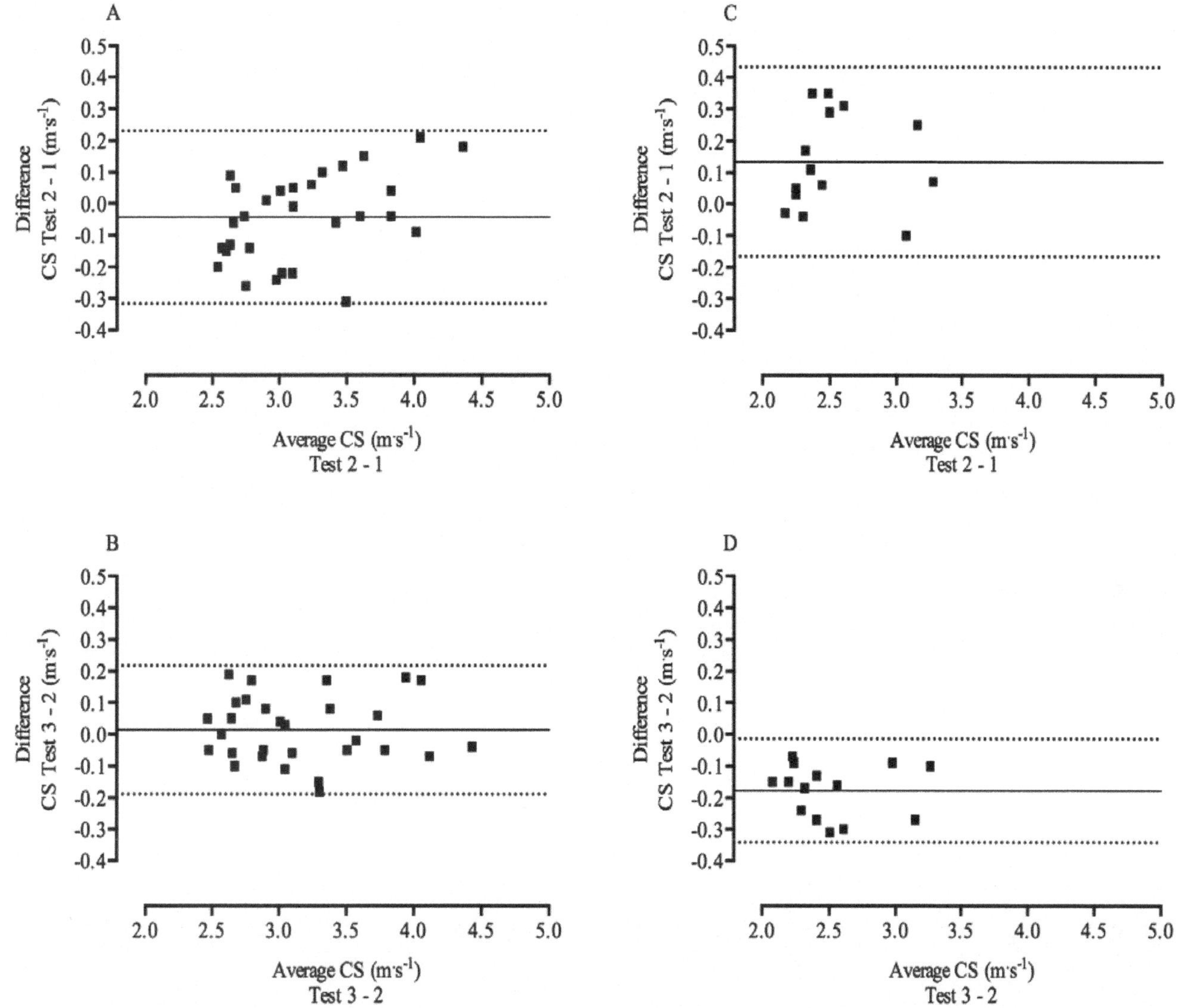

Figure 1. Bland-Altman plots of the mean differences in critical speed between tests 2-1 (**A**) and 3-2 (**B**) for the trained and the untrained adolescents (**C**,**D**). Solid and dotted lines represent the bias and 95% limits of agreement, respectively.

3.2. Distance above Critical Speed

No significant differences between the trained than the untrained participants were found for D′ ($F_{1,41}$ = 1.2; p = 0.28). There was a significant difference in D′ across all three tests in the untrained participants (163 ± 22 m, 134 ± 23 m and 148 ± 20 m; $F_{2,12}$ = 11.4; p = 0.002). No significant differences in D′ across the three tests were observed in the trained participants (135 ± 27 m, 139 ± 28 m and 143 ± 35 m; $F_{2,27}$ = 1.9; p = 0.17).

The bias in the trained participants was 4.3 ± 16.8 m (3.1 ± 12.5%; 95% LoA −28.6 to 37.2 m) for tests 2-1 and 4.4 ± 20.5 m (2.2 ± 15.2%; −35.8 to 44.5 m) for tests 3-2 (Figure 2). In the untrained participants the bias was −29.2 ± 22.3 m (−20.1 ± 17.7%; −73.0 to 14.6 m) and 14.3 ± 19.6 m (10.8% ± 15.0%; −24.1 to 52.7 m) for tests 2-1 and for tests 3-2, respectively (Figure 2). The ICC was 0.818 (95% CI 0.645 to 0.911) for tests 2-1 and 0.796 (0.606 to 0.900) for tests 3-2 in the trained and 0.325 (−0.248 to 0.730) for tests 2-1 and 0.565 (0.050 to 0.843) for tests 3-2 in the untrained participants. The CV was 9.3% (7.7% to 13.4%) for tests 2-1 and 11.4% (9.5% to 16.7%) for tests 3-2 in the trained and 13.6% (10.4% to 24.6%) for tests 2-1 and 11.3% (8.5% to 19.9%) for tests 3-2 in the untrained participants.

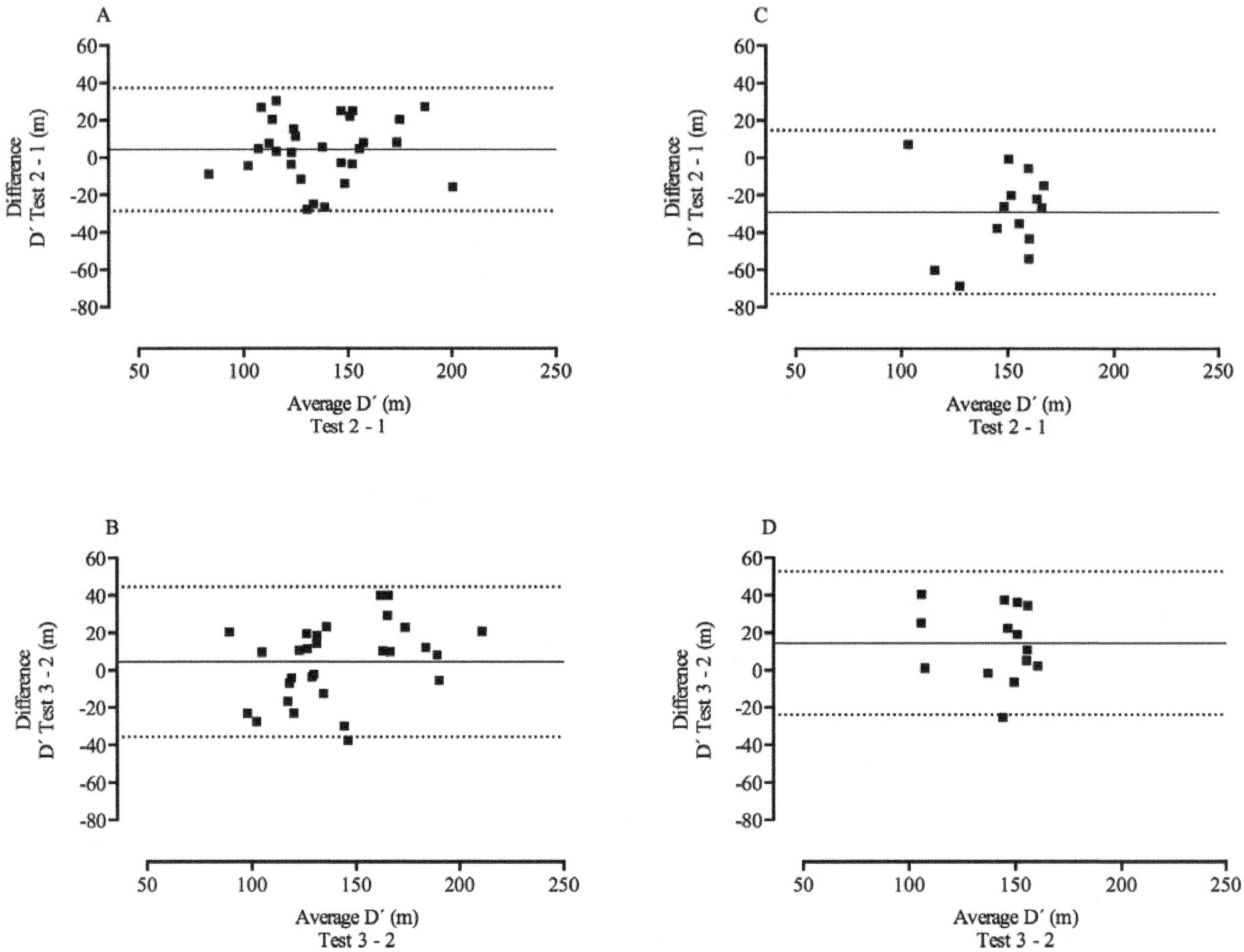

Figure 2. Bland-Altman plots of the mean differences in the distance above critical speed between tests 2-1 (**A**) and 3-2 (**B**) for the trained and the untrained adolescents (**C**,**D**). Solid and dotted lines represent the bias and 95% limits of agreement, respectively.

4. Discussion

The present study investigated the reliability of the single-visit field test of critical speed (CS) in trained and untrained adolescents. The main findings were that the estimates of CS but not the distance above CS (D′) were reproducible in both groups. Specifically, the coefficients of variation (CV) were between 2.4% and 4.3% and the ICC ranged from 0.919 to 0.982 for CS indicating that this test can be used reliably to estimate CS. This was however not found for D′ where the CV was above 9% and the ICC was lower than 0.818.

It was also observed that trained adolescents were more stable than their untrained counterparts when performing maximal-effort trials as requested in the present study. Unsurprisingly, the young trained athletes had significantly higher estimates of CS (mean difference 0.67 $m \cdot s^{-1}$; $p < 0.001$), but more importantly there was no significant difference across the three tests ($p = 0.27$). In contrast, the untrained participants performed significantly better during the second compared with the first ($p = 0.02$) and the third test ($p < 0.001$). These results suggest, that at least one familiarization session appeared to be required for the attainment of a stable estimate of CS [21]. In addition, the Bland-Altman plots revealed mean differences between the second and the first test (0.13 $m{\cdot}s^{-1}$ or 5.3%) as well as between the second and the third test (0.18 $m{\cdot}s^{-1}$ or 7.2%), indicating that although the untrained subjects were able to perform significantly better in the second test compared to the first test, performance dropped back in the third test. We do not believe environmental conditions such as temperature or wind had affected our findings as these were controlled. It is more likely that motivational factors such as goal-orientation, self-perception and willpower could explain the inconsistency in untrained adolescents [22]. It has been shown that males are more ego-oriented than females in outperforming each other [23] and therefore there might also be a gender bias as the trained athletes consisted of 15 boys and 14 girls while the group of untrained participants consisted of four boys and 10 girls. An additional explanation for the inconsistency found in untrained athletes might be the order of the prediction trials. While some studies started with the longest trial [15,16], others started with the shortest trial or randomly applied the trials [24,25]. Starting with the shortest trial in the present study, could have affected the untrained athletes due to inexperience with maximal efforts and this in turn might impact consistency.

The Bland-Altman plots also showed smaller ranges of the 95% LoA (*i.e.*, 1.96 × SD of the bias) between the third and second test compared with the second and first test in both groups, indicating that both groups had a higher consistency after the familiarization trial. This effect was however, much larger in the untrained athletes where the 95% LoA changed from ±0.29 $m{\cdot}s^{-1}$ (±11.8%) to ±0.16 $m{\cdot}s^{-1}$ (±6.5%) compared with the trained participants (±0.27 $m{\cdot}s^{-1}$ or ±8.6% to ±0.19 $m{\cdot}s^{-1}$ or ±6.5%). Assuming a negligible bias in the trained participants this shows that CS may not differ by more than 6.5% between any two tests due to measurement error. This small measurement error in both groups was corroborated by ICCs > 0.960 between the second and third test. With 95% CI between 0.758 and 0.992, the CS demonstrated a good to excellent degree of reproducibility [26]. This was also reflected by the CV, which was ~2.5% in both groups.

Our results are in accordance with previous studies that investigated the reliability of the single-visit protocol during running [15] and cycling [24] in trained adults. For example, Galbraith *et al.* [15] reported CVs of 2.0% (1.4% to 3.8%) and 1.3% (0.9% to 2.4%) for tests 2-1 and 3-2, respectively. In addition, the 95% LoA improved from ±0.27 $m{\cdot}s^{-1}$ or ±5.7% to ±0.18 $m{\cdot}s^{-1}$ or ±3.8%. These observations show that even highly trained distance runners ($\dot{V}O_{2max}$ 69.1 ± 4.2 $mL{\cdot}min^{-1}{\cdot}kg^{-1}$) should use a familiarization trial to improve the reliability of the single-visit field test before its use to monitor performance.

To place the present study into context with other studies on reliability measures in children and adolescents, it appears that the single-visit field test is among those with the highest reliability. To assess the reliability of anaerobic power in 12 to 14 year old rowers, two modified 30-s Wingate anaerobic tests were completed interspersed by a 15-min active recovery period [27]. The authors reported CVs of 2.9% (2.6% to 3.4%) for mean power and 2.4% (2.1% to 2.8%) for peak power. These were accompanied by very high ICCs (0.994 to 0.996). In another study, the same authors investigated the same test in a more heterogeneous group of 12 to 18 year old rowers with the retest performed 5–7 days after the first test [28]. It was shown, that CVs for mean and peak power were 6.7% (5.8 to 7.9%) and

7.3% (6.3% to 8.6%), respectively and the ICCs ranged from 0.973 to 0.982. Dore *et al.* [21] compared the reliability of cycling peak power obtained from the Wingate anaerobic test between pre-pubertal children and young adults. Again the CV changed from 4.7% and 3.0% in children and adults, respectively to less than 3.0% in both groups.

Only a few studies have reported the reliability of field test measures of aerobic fitness in children and adolescents [29–31]. Castagna *et al.* [31] evaluated a popular field test for aerobic fitness in football in Italy. The peak speed during a progressive 45-s run with 15 s passive recovery was used as a reflection of aerobic fitness. In comparison with our results, the CV and ICC were 3.75% (2.85% to 5.62%) and 0.92 (0.78 to 0.97), respectively. The Yo-Yo Intermittent Recovery Test Level 1 is frequently used to assess aerobic fitness in football players [32]. Recently the reliability of the test was evaluated in young football players and it was found, that the test was less reliable in younger age groups (U13 and U15) with CVs of 17.3% (90% CI 14.5% to 21.7%) and 16.7% (13.9% to 21.2%), compared with the U17 category (7.9%; 5.8 to 12.6%) [30]. In a follow-up study, where a third familiarization trial was included, the same authors reported CVs of 7.1% (90% CI 5.6 to 9.5%), 3.1% (2.3 to 4.8%) and 3.0% (1.8% to 8.6%) between the second and third test across the age categories U15, U17 and U19, respectively [29].

From a practical perspective, the results of the present study are important for coaches and physical education teachers involved in the fitness evaluation of young people. First, the concept of critical speed is a non-invasive approach to determine the highest rate of oxygen utilisation matched by oxygen delivery (*i.e.*, "anaerobic threshold") [33,34]. Second, the single-visit field test protocol allows the determination of CS independently from any laboratory equipment within a training session or physical education class. Third, based on the reliability data presented here, meaningful changes in performance could be detected. For example, in a young adolescent athlete with a CS of 3.17 $m \cdot s^{-1}$ and the reported CV of 2.4%, any change in performance of 0.08 $m \cdot s^{-1}$ (0.27 $km \cdot h^{-1}$) would be detected as meaningful. Using the upper limit of the 95% CI of 3.3 and 4.3% these meaningful changes are 0.10 $m \cdot s^{-1}$ (0.38 $km \cdot h^{-1}$) and 0.11 $m \cdot s^{-1}$ (0.39 $km \cdot h^{-1}$) in the trained and untrained participants, respectively.

Finally, our study revealed that the distance above critical speed (D′) is less reliable than CS, which is in agreement with previous studies [15,16,24,25]. On average, the CV ranged from 9.3% to 13.6% and the 95% CI from 7.7% to 24.6%, indicating a limited reliability and thus practical relevance. The reasons for this remain unclear but previous studies excluded residual fatigue, standing start during cycling, duration of the prediction trials and familiarization as possible factors [16,25].

5. Conclusions

In conclusion the present study showed that the single-visit field test to estimate critical speed is a reliable test for assessing physical fitness in trained and untrained adolescents. We also recommend planning at least one familiarization trial to use the estimated critical speed as a valid performance measure. The non-invasive and time saving protocol is of particular practical value for practitioners, such as coaches or physical education teachers and the test is sensitive enough to detect meaningful changes of ~0.3 to 0.4 $km \cdot h^{-1}$. It should also be noted that the distance above critical speed is currently not reliable enough to be used as a valid measure.

Acknowledgments

We would like to thank the participants for their efforts in this study.

Author Contributions

Alfred Nimmerichter and Mathias Steindl designed and conceived the study. Mathias Steindl collected the data. Alfred Nimmerichter, Mathias Steindl and Craig Anthony Williams analyzed the data. Alfred Nimmerichter and Craig Anthony Williams wrote the original draft of the paper. All authors reviewed and approved the manuscript.

Conflicts of Interest

The authors declare no conflict of interest.

References

1. Poole, D.C.; Ward, S.A.; Gardner, G.W.; Whipp, B.J. Metabolic and respiratory profile of the upper limit for prolonged exercise in man. *Ergonomics* **1988**, *31*, 1265–1279.
2. Monod, H.; Scherrer, J. The work capacity of a synergic muscular group. *Ergonomics* **1965**, *8*, 329–338.
3. Jones, A.M.; Carter, H. The effect of endurance training on parameters of aerobic fitness. *Sports Med.* **2000**, *29*, 373–386.
4. Hill, D.W. The critical power concept. A review. *Sports Med.* **1993**, *16*, 237–254.
5. Leclair, E.; Borel, B.; Thevenet, D.; Baquet, G.; Mucci, P.; Berthoin, S. Assessment of child-specific aerobic fitness and anaerobic capacity by the use of the power-time relationships constants. *Pediatr. Exerc. Sci.* **2010**, *22*, 454–466.
6. Williams, C.A.; Dekerle, J.; McGawley, K.; Berthoin, S.; Carter, H. Critical power in adolescent boys and girls—An exploratory study. *Appl. Physiol. Nutr. MeTab.* **2008**, *33*, 1105–1111.
7. Vitor Fde, M.; Bohme, M.T. Performance of young male swimmers in the 100-meters front crawl. *Pediatr. Exerc. Sci.* **2010**, *22*, 278–287.
8. Hill, D.W.; Steward, R.P.; Lane, C.J. Application of the critical power concept to young swimmers. *Pediatr. Exerc. Sci.* **1995**, *7*, 281–293.
9. Jones, A.M.; Wilkerson, D.P.; DiMenna, F.; Fulford, J.; Poole, D.C. Muscle metabolic responses to exercise above and below the "critical power" assessed using 31p-mrs. *Am. J. Physiol. Regul. Integr. Comp. Physiol.* **2008**, *294*, R585–R593.
10. Barker, A.R.; Bond, B.; Toman, C.; Williams, C.A.; Armstrong, N. Critical power in adolescents: Physiological bases and assessment using all-out exercise. *Eur. J. Appl. Physiol.* **2012**, *112*, 1359–1370.
11. Machado, M.V.; Júnior, O.A.; Marques, A.C.; Colantonio, E.; Cyrino, E.S.; de Mello, M.T. Effect of 12 weeks of training on critical velocity and maximal lactate steady state in swimmers. *Eur. J. Sport Sci.* **2011**, *11*, 165–170.
12. Toubekis, A.G.; Vasilaki, A.; Douda, H.; Gourgoulis, V.; Tokmakidis, S. Physiological responses during interval training at relative to critical velocity intensity in young swimmers. *J. Sci. Med. Sport* **2011**, *14*, 363–368.

13. Barbosa, T.M.; Costa, M.; Marinho, D.A.; Coelho, J.; Moreira, M.; Silva, A.J. Modeling the links between young swimmers' performance: Energetic and biomechanic profiles. *Pediatr. Exerc. Sci.* **2010**, *22*, 379–391.
14. Browne, R.A.V.; Sales, M.M.; Sotero, R.D.C.; Asano, R.Y.; de Moraes, J.F.V.N.; Barros, J.D.F.; Campbell, C.S.G.; Simões, H.G. Critical velocity estimates lactate minimum velocity in youth runners. *Mot. Rev. Educ. Fis.* **2015**, *21*, 1–7.
15. Galbraith, A.; Hopker, J.G.; Jobson, S.A.; Passfield, L. A novel field test to determine critical speed. *J. Sports Med. Doping Stuides* **2011**, *1*, 1–4.
16. Galbraith, A.; Hopker, J.; Lelliott, S.; Diddams, L.; Passfield, L. A single-visit field test of critical speed. *Int. J. Sports Physiol. Perform.* **2014**, *9*, 931–935.
17. Jones, A.M.; Doust, J.H. A 1% treadmill grade most accurately reflects the energetic cost of outdoor running. *J. Sports Sci.* **1996**, *14*, 321–327.
18. Bender, R.; Lange, S. Adjusting for multiple testing—When and how? *J. Clin. Epidemiol.* **2001**, *54*, 343–349.
19. Bland, J.M.; Altman, D.G. Statistical methods for assessing agreement between two methods of clinical measurement. *Lancet* **1986**, *1*, 307–310.
20. Hopkins, W.G. Measures of reliability in sports medicine and science. *Sports Med.* **2000**, *30*, 1–15.
21. Doré, E.; Duché, P.; Rouffet, D.; Ratel, S.; Bedu, M.; van Praagh, E. Measurement error in short-term power testing in young people. *J. Sports Sci.* **2003**, *21*, 135–142.
22. Le Bars, H.; Gernigon, C.; Ninot, G. Personal and contextual determinants of elite young athletes' persistence or dropping out over time. *Scand. J. Med. Sci. Sports* **2009**, *19*, 274–285.
23. Moreno Murcia, J.A.; Cervello Gimeno, E.; Gonzalez-Cutre Coll, D. Relationships among goal orientations, motivational climate and flow in adolescent athletes: Differences by gender. *Span. J. Psychol.* **2008**, *11*, 181–191.
24. Karsten, B.; Jobson, S.A.; Hopker, J.; Stevens, L.; Beedie, C. Validity and reliability of critical power field testing. *Eur. J. Appl. Physiol.* **2015**, *115*, 197–204.
25. Triska, C.; Tschan, H.; Tazreiter, G.; Nimmerichter, A. Critical power in laboratory and field conditions using single-visit maximal effort trials. *Int. J. Sports Med.* **2015**, *36*, 1063–1068.
26. Indrayan, A. Clinical agreement in quantitative measurements: Limits of disagreement and the intraclass correlation. In *Methods of Clinical Epidemiology*; Doi, S.A.R., Williams, G.M., Eds.; Springer-Verlag: Berlin, Germany, Heidelberg, Germany, 2013; pp. 17–27.
27. Mikulic, P.; Ruzic, L.; Markovic, G. Evaluation of specific anaerobic power in 12–14-year-old male rowers. *J. Sci. Med. Sport* **2009**, *12*, 662–666.
28. Mikulic, P.; Emersic, D.; Markovic, G. Reliability and discriminative ability of a modified wingate rowing test in 12- to 18-year-old rowers. *J. Sports Sci.* **2010**, *28*, 1409–1414.
29. Deprez, D.; Fransen, J.; Lenoir, M.; Philippaerts, R.; Vaeyens, R. The yo-yo intermittent recovery test level 1 is reliable in young high-level soccer players. *Biol. Sport* **2015**, *32*, 65–70.
30. Deprez, D.; Coutts, A.J.; Lenoir, M.; Fransen, J.; Pion, J.; Philippaerts, R.; Vaeyens, R. Reliability and validity of the yo-yo intermittent recovery test level 1 in young soccer players. *J. Sports Sci.* **2014**, *32*, 903–910.
31. Castagna, C.; Iellamo, F.; Impellizzeri, F.M.; Manzi, V. Validity and reliability of the 45–15 test for aerobic fitness in young soccer players. *Int. J. Sports Physiol. Perform.* **2014**, *9*, 525–531.

32. Bangsbo, J.; Iaia, F.M.; Krustrup, P. The yo-yo intermittent recovery test : A useful tool for evaluation of physical performance in intermittent sports. *Sports Med.* **2008**, *38*, 37–51.
33. Vanhatalo, A.; Jones, A.M.; Burnley, M. Application of critical power in sport. *Int. J. Sports Physiol. Perform.* **2011**, *6*, 128–136.
34. Jones, A.M.; Vanhatalo, A.; Burnley, M.; Morton, R.H.; Poole, D.C. Critical power: Implications for determination of VO_{2max} and exercise tolerance. *Med. Sci. Sports Exerc.* **2010**, *42*, 1876–1890.

20

Angle Specific Analysis of Side-to-Side Asymmetry in the Shoulder Rotators

Cassio V. Ruas [1,*], Ronei S. Pinto [1,†], Eduardo L. Cadore [1,†] and Lee E. Brown [2]

[1] Physical Education School, Federal University of Rio Grande do Sul, Brazil, Felizardo Street, 750—Jardim Botânico, Porto Alegre/RS 90690-200, Brazil; E-Mails: ronei.pinto@ufrgs.br (R.S.P.); cadoreeduardo@gmail.com (E.L.C.)

[2] Department of Kinesiology, KHS 233 800 N. State College Blvd., California State University, Fullerton 92831, CA, USA; E-Mail: leebrown@fullerton.edu

† These authors contributed equally to this work.

* Author to whom correspondence should be addressed; E-Mail: cassiovruas@gmail.com

Academic Editor: Eling de Bruin

Abstract: Although side-to-side asymmetry of the shoulder rotators calculated by independent peak torque (IPT) has been used for interpretation of injury risks in athletes, it may not measure strength through the entire range of motion (ROM) tested. The aim of this study was to compare side-to-side asymmetry of the shoulder rotators between independent peak torque (IPT) and ten-degree angle specific torque (AST). Twenty healthy adult males (24.65 ± 2.4 years) performed concentric and eccentric internal rotation (IR) and external rotation (ER) of the preferred and non-preferred arms on an isokinetic dynamometer at 60°/s through 150° of total ROM. The total ROM was divided into 14 ten-degree angles of the physiological ROM from −90° of ER to 60° of IR. Concentric and eccentric IR IPT (10.5% ± 8.7% and 12.1% ± 7.2%) and ER IPT (13.6% ± 9.8% and 8.7% ± 5.6%) were significantly less than AST at several angles ($p < 0.05$). IPT might lead to erroneous interpretations of side-to-side asymmetry in the shoulder rotators and does not represent the entire ROM tested. This information could be used to prescribe strength exercises to enhance overhead performance and reduce risk of shoulder injuries.

Keywords: angle specific torque; independent peak torque; strength imbalance; injury prevention; performance enhancement

1. Introduction

The shoulder rotator muscles are important for coordinated performance of overhead activities, such as pitching in baseball, swinging a racket in tennis or pushing against the water in swimming [1–3]. Forceful and repetitive actions in overhead sports have been associated with an increased susceptibility of shoulder rotator injuries [3,4], strength differences between external (antagonists) and internal rotator (agonists) muscles [1,3–5], and side-to-side differences between upper-limbs [2,5]. Typical shoulder strength asymmetry has been reported as an upper-limb dominance of 5%–10% measured by independent peak torque (IPT) in nonathletic and recreational-level athletes [5]. However, these IPT measurements fail to reproduce the functionality of muscles during sporting activities, because torque is not calculated through the entire range of motion (ROM), or at corresponding angles [1,6,7].

2. Context

A previous investigation has demonstrated that this can lead to misinterpretation of strength imbalance of the shoulder rotators [1]. In addition, a few studies have opted to use 5°, 10°, 15° or end of ROM angle specific torque (AST) intervals for a more accurate estimation of unilateral dynamic muscle balance of the knee or shoulder joints [1,3,4,6–9]. Dehail *et al.* [7] demonstrated there was a significant progressive decline of flexion/extension and abduction/adduction AST strength ratios as the shoulder progressed to flexion and abduction, respectively. Yildiz *et al.* [4], found that although internal rotator eccentric strength of the preferred side was greater than the non-preferred side at the end of the ROM, only the internal rotator concentric strength was greater than the non-preferred side at the beginning of the ROM. Although IPT evaluations may be more sensitive to assess muscle strength balance changes after strength rehabilitation programs [10], AST analysis has been shown to be a more appropriate tool to precisely locate potential muscle imbalances present at specific joint angles [1,6,7]. This information may be used for the prescription of strength exercises of the weak angles.

Although AST analysis has been used to measure unilateral imbalance, there is a lack of information using this approach to measure side-to-side asymmetry of the shoulder rotators. Thus, the aim of this study was to compare side-to-side asymmetry of the internal and external shoulder rotators between traditional IPT and ten-degree AST methods.

3. Method

3.1. Participants

Twenty healthy adult males (age 24.6 ± 2.4 years, body mass 81.6 ± 15.5 kg, height 175.3 ± 8.0 cm) volunteered to participate in this study. All of them participated in recreational activities (e.g., basketball, jogging, resistance training) at least once a week, and had no history of shoulder injuries in the previous six months prior to testing. Their body mass was measured using a digital scale (Model # ES200L, Ohaus,

Pine Brook, NJ, USA), and height using a wall-mounted stadiometer (Seca Stadiometer, ON, Canada). All participants read and signed an informed consent form prior to participation. The study was approved by the University Institutional Review Board (HSR#130126), and the rights of the subjects were protected.

3.2. Experimental Design

Prior to testing, participants were asked about their preferred arm when throwing an object (dominance) [2]. To examine their torque capabilities, concentric isokinetic tests were performed for the internal and external shoulder rotators of the preferred and non-preferred arms. Side-to-side torque asymmetry was calculated based on these results.

3.3. Experimental Procedures

Maximal internal and external rotator concentric and eccentric strength was measured on a Biodex System 3 isokinetic dynamometer (Biodex Medical Systems, Shirley, NY, USA). Participants laid supine on the dynamometer with straps across their chest and hips to avoid additional movement. Participants grasped the lever arm of the machine and their tested arm was positioned at 90° of shoulder abduction and 90° of elbow flexion with their forearm in a neutral position in the coronal plane for alignment with the dynamometer's axis of rotation [1,11]. This position was considered 0°. Both preferred and non-preferred arms were tested.

Shoulder rotator strength was measured through 150° of total ROM, from 90° ER (−90°) to 60° IR of physiologic ROM. This ROM was chosen as it was uncomfortable for subjects to perform maximal strength beyond these limits in a pilot study. Prior to testing, participants performed a warm up of 5 submaximal repetitions at 180°/s and 3 maximal repetitions at the test speed of 60°/s for familiarization purposes. Testing consisted of 5 reciprocal concentric/concentric and 5 eccentric/eccentric maximal repetitions, with 3 min rest between modes. Preferred and non-preferred arms were assessed in random order. Participants were asked to push and pull as hard and fast as possible and verbal encouragement was provided during the test.

3.4. Outcome Measures

Maximal concentric and eccentric internal rotation (IR) and external rotation (ER) independent peak torque (IPT) were measured, as well as the angles of IPT (AIPT).

All data were collected and analyzed using custom LabVIEW Software (version 2013, National Instruments, Austin, TX, USA) and was divided into 14 ten-degree AST from −90° ER to 60° IR of physiological ROM. Side-to-side asymmetry of the shoulder rotators for both IPT and AST were calculated as the percentage differences between the peak torque of the preferred and non-preferred arms.

3.5. Statistical Analyses

Four (IR and ER) 1 × 14 repeated measures ANOVAs were used to compare concentric and eccentric percentage differences between IPT and AST between arms. The effect size for each significant difference was calculated by using means (M) and standard deviations (SD) between variables to identify the magnitude and direction of the differences ($d = M_{AST} - M_{IPT}/SD_{IPT}$), in which values <0.35 were considered trivial, 0.35–0.80 small, 0.80–1.50 moderate, and >1.50 large for recreationally trained subjects [12]. All analyses were performed with SPSS version 20 (Statistical Package for Social Sciences, Chicago, IL, USA). An *a-priori* alpha level of 0.05 determined statistical significance.

4. Results

Means of concentric and eccentric IPT and AIPT of IR and ER of the preferred and non-preferred arms are presented in Table 1. Means of concentric and eccentric ten-to-ten-degree absolute AST of internal rotation (IR) and external rotation (ER) of the preferred and non-preferred arms (Table 2).

Table 1. Means ± SD of concentric and eccentric independent peak torque (IPT) and angles of independent peak torque (AIPT) of internal rotation (IR) and external rotation (ER) of the preferred and non-preferred arms.

Action	Concentric				Eccentric			
	IPT (N.m)		AIPT (°)		IPT (N.m)		AIPT (°)	
	Preferred	Non-preferred	Preferred	Non-preferred	Preferred	Non-preferred	Preferred	Non-preferred
IR	46.5 ± 16.6	44.3 ± 14.1	−35.6 ± 34.6	−33.2 ± 40.2	58.1 ± 21.0	56.9 ± 17.2	−40.9 ± 24.5	−16.3 ± 29.7
ER	42.7 ± 13.7	39.9 ± 12.1	0.7 ± 35.4	0.7 ± 31.8	52.5 ± 13.8	53.6 ± 15.1	−30.8 ± 10.8	−26.6 ± 13.9

Table 2. Means ± SD of concentric and eccentric absolute ten-to-ten-degree angle specific torque (AST) of internal rotation (IR) and external rotation (ER) of the preferred and non-preferred arms.

Angle (°)	Concentric		Eccentric	
	AST (N.m)		AST (N.m)	
	Preferred	Non-Preferred	Preferred	Non-Preferred
IR-80	38.2 ± 18.7	34.1 ± 13.0	34.4 ± 23.1	23.9 ± 24.8
IR-70	39.8 ± 17.5	37.4 ± 15.1	41.0 ± 21.2	31.3 ± 21.7
IR-60	40.9 ± 16.9	38.2 ± 15.9	47.0 ± 20.9	38.0 ± 18.8
IR-50	41.7 ± 16.8	38.0 ± 15.5	50.0 ± 20.3	45.2 ± 17.9
IR-40	41.7 ± 16.8	36.8 ± 15.0	50.9 ± 19.1	47.3 ± 18.4
IR-30	41.2 ± 15.4	37.4 ± 15.4	51.2 ± 18.5	49.6 ± 17.6
IR-20	39.6 ± 13.6	36.5 ± 14.1	50.7 ± 16.7	50.5 ± 17.3
IR-10	37.3 ± 12.1	36.6 ± 13.5	49.9 ± 15.8	50.5 ± 15.7
IR0	36.6 ± 11.6	36.8 ± 13.6	47.4 ± 16.1	50.2 ± 15.7
IR10	35.6 ± 10.7	36.3 ± 13.0	44.0 ± 15.0	49.1 ± 15.5
IR20	34.7 ± 9.9	35.8 ± 13.2	39.8 ± 14.4	47.1 ± 15.9
IR30	32.9 ± 8.9	34.9 ± 13.2	33.8 ± 14.7	42.7 ± 17.9
IR40	30.7 ± 8.5	34.0 ± 13.3	25.7 ± 14.9	35.7 ± 16.6
IR50	27.1 ± 9.1	32.3 ± 13.2	19.5 ± 11.6	24.9 ± 15.4
ER50	33.9 ± 15.1	32.8 ± 13.0	18.9 ± 14.0	19.0 ± 18.9
ER40	36.9 ± 16.2	35.2 ± 13.9	24.8 ± 17.3	27.6 ± 18.9
ER30	37.5 ± 16.0	35.7 ± 14.0	29.9 ± 17.3	33.7 ± 17.7
ER20	38.0 ± 15.2	35.9 ± 13.7	35.4 ± 15.2	37.8 ± 17.7

Table 2. *Cont.*

Angle (°)	Concentric AST (N.m)		Eccentric AST (N.m)	
	Preferred	**Non-Preferred**	**Preferred**	**Non-Preferred**
ER10	38.0 ± 14.0	36.0 ± 12.6	39.9 ± 14.7	40.6 ± 17.4
ER0	37.9 ± 13.0	35.9 ± 11.5	43.7 ± 14.2	44.6 ± 16.3
ER-10	38.0 ± 12.0	36.2 ± 11.5	46.5 ± 14.1	47.7 ± 16.4
ER-20	37.9 ± 11.1	36.5 ± 11.1	48.1 ± 13.2	50.8 ± 15.6
ER-30	37.8 ± 10.2	36.6 ± 10.5	50.9 ± 13.0	50.8 ± 14.1
ER-40	37.2 ± 9.6	35.6 ± 9.6	49.8 ± 12.9	48.4 ± 13.9
ER-50	35.8 ± 9.0	32.9 ± 8.4	46.4 ± 13.1	43.1 ± 13.2
ER-60	33.9 ± 9.8	29.2 ± 7.1	39.1 ± 14.3	34.4 ± 12.8
ER-70	29.1 ± 8.1	24.1 ± 6.6	29.2 ± 12.0	23.5 ± 12.7
ER-80	23.0 ± 7.9	17.2 ± 9.1	17.9 ± 10.7	14.5 ± 7.8

Concentric side-to-side IR IPT asymmetry was significantly less than AST at −80° ($p = 0.018$), −70° ($p = 0.045$), −50° ($p = 0.029$), −40° ($p = 0.018$), −30° ($p = 0.016$), −20° ($p = 0.027$), 40° ($p = 0.010$) and 50° ($p = 0.001$). Side-to-side ER IPT asymmetry was significantly less than AST at 50° ($p = 0.011$), 40° ($p = 0.013$) and −80° ($p = 0.00017$) (Figure 1). Eccentric side-to-side IR IPT was significantly less than AST at 50° ($p = 0.000024$) 40° ($p = 0.000063$) 30° ($p = 0.00042$), 20° ($p = 0.006$), 0 ($p = 0.037$), −70° ($p = 0.0013$) and −80° ($p = 0.0034$). Side-to-side ER IPT was significantly less than AST at −80° ($p = 0.00042$), −70° ($p = 0.00026$), −60° ($p = 0.0014$), 30° ($p = 0.0076$), 40° ($p = 0.0032$) and 50° ($p = 0.000016$) (Figure 2). Effect sizes are presented for each significant difference (Figures 1 and 2).

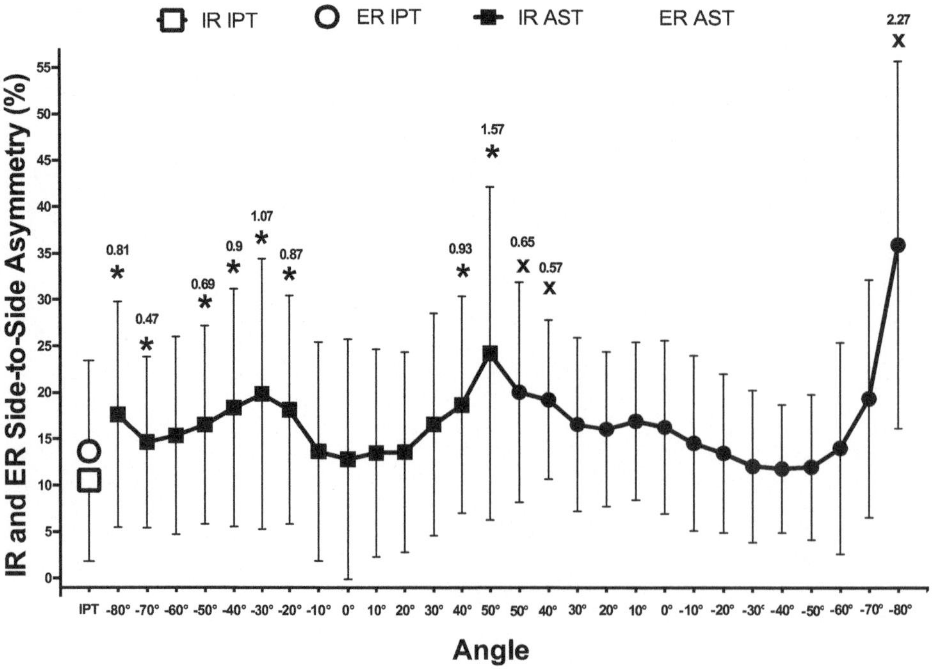

Figure 1. Means ± SD of concentric internal rotators (IR) and external rotators (ER) angle specific torque (AST) and independent peak torque (IPT) side-to-side asymmetry. * Significantly less than IR AST; **x** significantly less than ER AST. Effect sizes are presented for each significant difference.

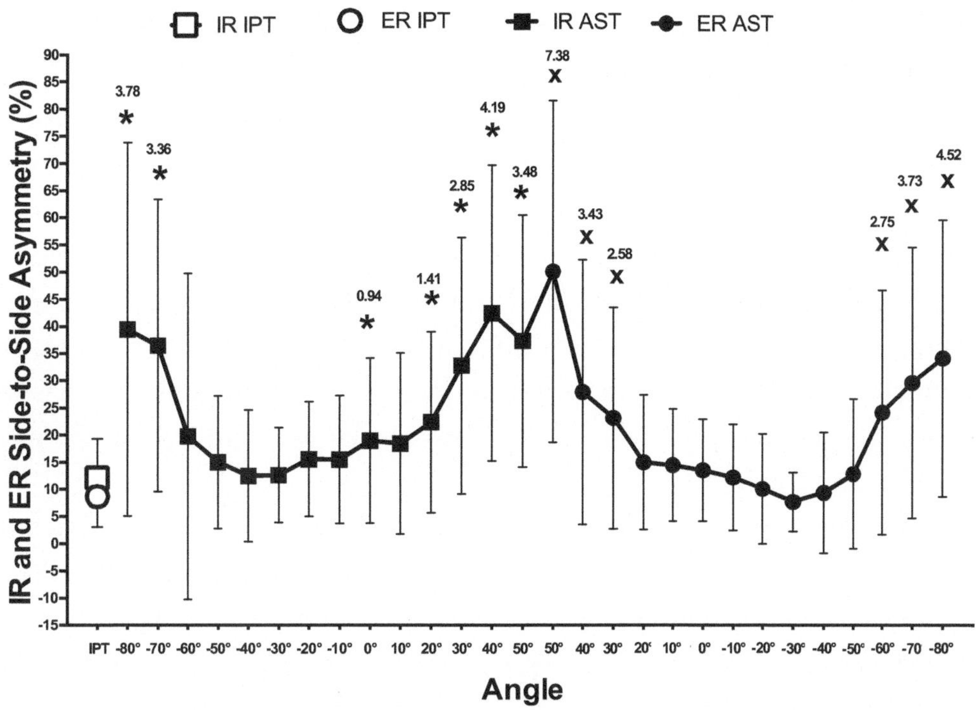

Figure 2. Means ± SD of eccentric internal rotators (IR) and external rotators (ER) angle specific torque (AST) and independent peak torque (IPT) side-to-side asymmetry. * Significantly less than IR AST; **x** significantly less than ER AST. Effect sizes are presented for each significant difference.

5. Discussion

The aim of this study was to compare side-to-side asymmetry of the shoulder rotators between IPT and ten-degree AST methods. Our results revealed that concentric IPT was different than AST at eight angles for IR, and three angles for ER. In addition, eccentric IPT was different than AST at seven angles for IR, and six angles for ER. ER differences were found primarily at the beginning and end points of ROM. This demonstrates that IPT might not be an accurate representation of the entire ROM tested in either testing mode. The AST values allow a more precise estimation of strength asymmetry between shoulder rotator muscles. The use of IPT alone may lead to erroneous interpretations of full ROM side-to-side strength differences.

The reliability of IPT and AST for clinical use has been questioned. Brown *et al.* [13] demonstrated a high test-retest reliability of IPT on the Biodex device over a wide velocity spectrum in the knee flexors and extensors. However, Ayala *et al.* [10] showed that this is not transferred to knee unilateral asymmetry calculations, which presented moderate reliability in strength ratios calculated by IPT, and poor reliability in ratios calculated by AST. This was also confirmed for IPT side-to-side calculations of the shoulder rotators in another recent study [14]. This might be explained by strength imbalance calculations being composed of two measurements, where each can vary in two different directions [14].

The IPT is the highest point of the torque curve across a full ROM [15]. This measurement is widely used to indicate maximum strength levels, as well as the occurrence of possible muscle strength imbalance [1,2,5,15–18]. Previous studies have widely utilized IPT as a measure to calculate side-to-side asymmetry of the shoulder internal and external rotators [2,5,14,19–22]. Ellenbecker and Davies [5] concluded that a 5%–10% IPT difference between arms is normal in recreational level upper-limb sport athletes and non-athletes. Our results are slightly outside this range, as both concentric ER and IR IPT, and eccentric IR IPT demonstrated a 10%–15% difference. This may be due to the specific method we used in our isokinetic testing. We measured participants in a supine position with their arms abducted in the frontal plane. This position was based on Forthomme *et al.* [11], which indicated that it results in greater reliability and reproducibility compared to other testing positions. To our knowledge, this position has not been used to determine side-to-side strength imbalance of the shoulder rotators in a non-athletic population. Therefore, direct comparison of our results to established normative values of previous studies [5] is problematic since shoulder asymmetry is probably position dependent as has been shown in other joints [23,24]. Nevertheless, our eccentric ER IPT results were still within the normal range suggested by Ellenbecker and Davies [5].

Our tested velocity may have also played a role in our results. Even though overhead actions such as throwing can reach speeds up to 7200°/s, especially in sports performance [4], we tested at 60°/s in order to avoid a large load range reduction during isokinetic testing, thereby significantly decreasing the total ROM available for analysis [25–27]. Brown *et al.* [26] have shown that very fast isokinetic velocities significantly affect torque patterns. This may also influence side-to-side asymmetry assessment. Greater repetitive use of the preferred arm in throwing actions in recreational and sporting activities may explain our asymmetry results [2,21]. However, previous studies have used a variety of different speeds in order to provide sport specific information about strength imbalance and injury risk in the shoulder rotators [3,4,9]. The use of a single velocity to describe angle specific strength is a limitation of our study.

The limitation of IPT is that it does not take into account the full ROM [15]. This has also been shown to affect the interpretation of shoulder rotators unilateral strength imbalance [1], and many studies have opted to use an AST approach in order to gain more specific information of joint strength imbalances [1,3,4,6–8]. We have previously demonstrated that shoulder IPT dynamic control ratios are significantly different than AST at several angles when calculated by 10° intervals over a 150° total ROM [1]. Similar to this, our present study also found significant differences between side-to-side asymmetry between concentric and eccentric IPT and AST through many ROM angles, especially for IR. In contrast, ER differences were found primarily at the beginning and end of the ROM.

The beginning shoulder ROM (cocking phase) is critical in overhead activities due to full external rotation, and superior and anterior forces being applied to the shoulder; while the end ROM (deceleration phase) requires the arm to be stopped in a short period of time from high velocities [3,4,9]. These points of the ROM have been suggested as where most imbalances may occur, leading to shoulder muscle and ligament injuries [3,4,9]. Previous reports found there were side-to-side asymmetry differences between these phases in athletes [3,4], and college students [9]. This is in agreement with our results and makes the use of AST especially important. In fact we found that eccentric ER AST at 50°, which represents the last deceleration angle at the end of the ROM, had the greatest difference and magnitude of change across all angles when compared to IPT. While ER strength is important for the preparation and deceleration phases of overhead actions, IR strength is primarily used for the acceleration phase in overhead throwing and racket sports [2,4]. A strength balance of IR and ER between upper limbs across the entire ROM, especially at the beginning and end [3–5,9], may not only help to avoid and rehabilitate injuries, but help determine performance in overhead sports [21]. Although unilateral overhead sports may result in dissimilar side-to-side differences, clinicians have assumed that peak torque value equivalency between shoulders may be used as a target for prevention and rehabilitation of injury in athletes and physically active individuals [5,21]. A strength balance between the upper limbs could be used to precisely identify where primary imbalances are present and prescribe strength exercises to diminish these differences at the affected angles. However, the greatest side-to-side asymmetry differences we found were near the extreme ranges and could be due to muscle sarcomeres being at a disadvantage on the length-tension curve and thereby generating low torques [28].

We also found that although IPT occurred at similar angles for concentric strength, they were at non-corresponding angles for eccentric strength. This could influence decision making of clinicians and physical therapists when interpreting shoulder strength results. Our results demonstrate that AST may provide a more accurate and detailed assessment of side-to-side asymmetry across the full ROM. This information can be used for the prescription of strength training programs based on bilateral equivalency for optimal performance and prevention of injury caused by repetitive sporting activities [20,21].

6. Conclusions

This study demonstrates that IPT is significantly less than AST at several angles when measuring side-to-side asymmetry of the shoulder rotators. IPT represents only one single angle across the entire ROM tested, and may occur at non-corresponding angles for eccentric strength. Therefore, AST is suggested as a new approach, which allows for measurement of the specific angles where strength differences between arms are present. This information could be used to assist in the prescription of strength training programs that focus on the precise angles where asymmetry occurs to enhance performance and reduce risk of shoulder injuries.

Author Contributions

Cassio V. Ruas, Ronei S. Pinto and Lee E. Brown were involved in study design and data interpretation. Cassio V. Ruas and Lee E. Brown were involved in data collection. Cassio V. Ruas, Ronei S. Pinto, Eduardo L. Cadore and Lee E. Brown were involved in manuscript writing and revision.

Conflicts of Interest

The authors declare no conflict of interest.

References

1. Ruas, C.V.; Pinto, R.S.; Hafenstine, R.W.; Pereira, M.C.; Brown, L.E. Specific joint angle assessment of the shoulder rotators. *Isokinet. Exerc. Sci.* **2014**, *22*, 197–204.
2. Gulick, D.T.; Dustman, C.S.; Ossowski, L.L.; Outslay, M.D.; Thomas, C.P.; Trucano, S. Side dominance does not affect dynamic control strength ratios in the shoulder. *Isokinet. Exerc. Sci.* **2001**, *9*, 79–84.
3. Ng, G.Y.; Lam, P.C. A study of antagonist/agonist isokinetic work ratios of shoulder rotators in men who play badminton. *J. Orthop. Sports Phys. Ther.* **2002**, *32*, 399–404.

4. Yildiz, Y.; Aydin, T.; Sekir, U.; Kiralp, M.Z.; Hazneci, B.; Kalyon, T.A. Shoulder terminal range eccentric antagonist/concentric agonist strength ratios in overhead athletes. *Scand. J. Med. Sci. Sports* **2006**, *16*, 174–180.
5. Ellenbecker, T.S.; Davies, G.J. The application of isokinetics in testing and rehabilitation of the shoulder complex. *J. Athl. Train.* **2000**, *35*, 338–350.
6. Kellis, E.; Katis, A. Quantification of functional knee flexor to extensor moment ratio using isokinetics and electromyography. *J. Athl. Train.* **2007**, *42*, 477–485.
7. Dehail, P.; Gagnon, D.; Noreau, L.; Nadeau, S. Assessment of agonist-antagonist shoulder torque ratios in individuals with paraplegia: A new interpretative approach. *Spinal Cord.* **2008**, *46*, 552–558.
8. Evangelidis, P.E.; Pain, M.T.; Folland, J. Angle-specific hamstring-to-quadriceps ratio: A comparison of football players and recreationally active males. *J. Sports Sci.* **2015**, *33*, 309–319.
9. Scoville, C.R.; Arciero, R.A.; Taylor, D.C.; Stoneman, P.D. End range eccentric antagonist/concentric agonist strength ratios: A new perspective in shoulder strength assessment. *J. Orthop. Sports Phys. Ther.* **1997**, *25*, 203–207.
10. Ayala, F.; De Ste Croix, M.; Sainz de Baranda, P.; Santonja, F. Absolute reliability of hamstring to quadriceps strength imbalance ratios calculated using peak torque, joint angle-specific torque and joint rom-specific torque values. *Int. J. Sports Med.* **2012**, *33*, 909–916.
11. Forthomme, B.; Dvir, Z.; Crielaard, J.M.; Croisier, J.L. Isokinetic assessment of the shoulder rotators: A study of optimal test position. *Clin. Physiol. Funct. Imaging* **2011**, *31*, 227–232.
12. Rhea, M.R. Determining the magnitude of treatment effects in strength training research through the use of the effect size. *J. Strength Cond. Res.* **2004**, *18*, 918–920.
13. Brown, L.E.; Whitehurst, M.; Bryant, J.R.; Buchalter, D.N. Reliability of the biodex system 2 isokinetic dynamometer concentric mode. *Isokinet. Exerc. Sci.* **1993**, *3*, 160–163.
14. Edouard, P.; Codine, P.; Samozino, P.; Bernard, P.L.; Herisson, C.; Gremeaux, V. Reliability of shoulder rotators isokinetic strength imbalance measured using the biodex dynamometer. *J. Sci. Med. Sport* **2013**, *16*, 162–165.
15. Brown, L.E.; Weir, J.P. Asep procedures recommendation i: Accurate assessment of muscular strength and power. *J. Exerc. Physiol. Online* **2001**, *4*, 1–21.
16. Ruas, C.V.; Minozzo, F.; Pinto, M.D.; Brown, L.E.; Pinto, R.S. Lower-extremity strength ratios of professional soccer players according to field position. *J. Strength Cond. Res.* **2015**, *29*, 1220–1226.
17. Ruas, C.V.; Pinto, M.D.; Brown, L.; Minozzo, F.; Mil-Homens, P.; Pinto, R.S. The association between conventional and dynamic control knee strength ratios in elite soccer players. *Isokinet. Exerc. Sci.* **2015**, *23*, 1–12.
18. Brown, L.E.; Sjostrom, T.; Comeau, M.J.; Whitehurst, M.; Greenwood, M.; Findley, B.W. Kinematics of biophysically asymmetric limbs within rate of velocity development. *J. Strength Cond. Res.* **2005**, *19*, 298–301.
19. Hurd, W.J.; Kaplan, K.M.; ElAttrache, N.S.; Jobe, F.W.; Morrey, B.F.; Kaufman, K.R. A profile of glenohumeral internal and external rotation motion in the uninjured high school baseball pitcher, part ii: Strength. *J. Athl. Train.* **2011**, *46*, 289–295.

20. Codine, P.; Bernard, P.L.; Pocholle, M.; Benaim, C.; Brun, V. Influence of sports discipline on shoulder rotator cuff balance. *Med. Sci. Sports Exerc.* **1997**, *29*, 1400–1405.
21. Perrin, D.H.; Robertson, R.J.; Ray, R.L. Bilateral lsokinetic peak torque, torque acceleration energy, power, and work relationships in athletes and nonathletes. *J. Orthop. Sports Phys. Ther.* **1987**, *9*, 184–189.
22. Sirota, S.C.; Malanga, G.A.; Eischen, J.J.; Laskowski, E.R. An eccentric- and concentric-strength profile of shoulder external and internal rotator muscles in professional baseball pitchers. *Am. J. Sports Med.* **1997**, *25*, 59–64.
23. Findley, B.W.; Brown, L.E.; Whitehurst, M.; Keating, T.; Murray, D.P.; Gardner, L.M. The influence of body position on load range during isokinetic knee extension/flexion. *J. Sport Sci. Med.* **2006**, *5*, 400–406.
24. Findley, B.W.; Brown, L.E.; Whitehurst, M.; Gilbert, R.; Groo, D.R.; O'neal, J. Sitting *vs.* Standing isokinetic trunk extension and flexion performance differences. *J. Strength Cond Res.* **2000**, *14*, 310–315.
25. Brown, L.E.; Whitehurst, M.; Gilbert, R.; Buchalter, D.N. The effect of velocity and gender on load range during knee extension and flexion exercise on an isokinetic device. *J. Orthop. Sports Phys. Ther.* **1995**, *21*, 107–112.
26. Brown, L.E.; Whitehurst, M.; Findley, B.W.; Gilbert, R.; Buchalter, D.N. Isokinetic load range during shoulder rotation exercise in elite male junior tennis players. *J. Strength Cond. Res.* **1995**, *9*, 160–164.
27. Brown, L.E.; Whitehurst, M.; Findley, B.W.; Gilbert, R.; Groo, D.R.; Jimenez, J.A. Effect of repetitions and gender on acceleration range of motion during knee extension on an isokinetic device. *J. Strength Cond. Res.* **1998**, *12*, 222–225.
28. Huxley, A.F.; Niedergerke, R. Structural changes in muscle during contraction. *Nature* **1954**, *173*, 971–973.

21

The Effect of High Intensity Intermittent Exercise on Power Output for the Upper Body

Leonie Harvey [1,*], Matthew Bousson [1], Chris McLellan [2] and Dale I. Lovell [1]

[1] School of Health and Sport Sciences, Faculty of Science, Health & Education, University of the Sunshine Coast, Sippy Downs, Queensland 4556, Australia;
E-Mails: mattbousson@gmail.com (M.B.); dlovell@usc.edu.au (D.I.L.)

[2] Faculty of Health Sciences and Medicine, Bond University, Robina, Queensland 4226, Australia;
E-Mail: cmclellan@bond.edu.au

* Author to whom correspondence should be addressed; E-Mail: lmh009@student.usc.edu.au;

Academic Editor: Arno Schmidt-Trucksäss

Abstract: The aim of the present study was to examine and measure high intensity, intermittent upper body performance, in addition to identifying areas of the body that affect the variance in total work done during the 5 × 6 s sprint test. Fifteen males completed an upper body 5 × 6 s sprint test on a modified electro-magnetically braked cycle ergometer, which consisted of five maximal effort sprints, each 6 s in duration, separated by 24 s of passive recovery. A fly wheel braking force corresponding to 5% of the participants' body weight was used as the implemented resistance level. Body composition was measured using dual-energy X-ray absorptiometry (DEXA). Percent (%) decrement was calculated as 100 − (Total work/ideal work) × 100. Significant ($P < 0.05$) differences were found between sprints for both absolute and relative (W, W·kg^{-1}, W·kg^{-1} Lean body mass (LBM) and W·kg^{-1} Upper body lean body mass (UBLBM)) peak (PP) and mean (MP) power. The % decrement in total work done over the five sprints was 11.4%. Stepwise multiple linear regression analysis revealed that UBLBM accounts for 87% of the variance in total work done during the upper body 5 × 6 s sprint test. These results provide a descriptive analysis of upper body, high intensity intermittent exercise, demonstrating that PP and MP output decreased significantly during the upper body 5 × 6 s sprint test.

Keywords: upper body; intermittent; high intensity; exercise; 5 × 6 s; sprint, RSA

1. Introduction

There are significant differences in neuromuscular and cardiovascular function between the upper and lower body at rest and during exercise [1,2]. The upper body is reported to have a higher percentage of type II fibers [3] and extract less oxygen during exercise indicating a greater reliance on anaerobic pathways, compared to that of the lower body [2]. Additionally, differences in peak and mean power during the Wingate test have also been reported between the upper and lower body even when normalized for active muscle mass [4]. Taken together these studies would appear to suggest significant differences exist between upper and lower body anaerobic performance. Similarly a recent study also found no correlation between the upper and lower body anaerobic performance in semi-elite rugby league players [5]. These findings are extremely pertinent as a number of sports which are intermittent in nature require intense exercise efforts using predominantly the upper body musculature.

High intensity, intermittent exercise is an important component of many team and individual sports that involve short periods of high intensity exercise followed by periods of rest or recovery [6]. The ability to perform repeated maximal efforts (<10 s) has previously been defined as repeat sprint ability (RSA) [7,8]. RSA has been shown to be an essential determinant in the outcome of match-play, with small decrements in ability resulting in significantly reduced performance [6]. Moreover, it has been suggested that athletes with superior RSA would have an increased likelihood to perform at a higher power output level or speed compared to those athletes who have a reduced ability to perform repeated sprints [6].

While the majority of studies have examined the RSA of the lower body, high intensity, intermittent upper body exercise has also been shown to be an important component of many sports such as rugby league, rock climbing and wrestling [5,9,10]. During both wrestling and rugby league match-play, participants utilise significant upper body musculature to bring their opponent to the ground [11]. Indeed, it has been established that upper body anaerobic power may help to differentiate between successful and less successful wrestlers [12]. However, despite its importance in a number of sports, few studies have examined high intensity intermittent exercise primarily involving the upper body.

Due to a lack of recent studies examining high intensity, intermittent upper body exercise, the purpose of the present study was to measure RSA during the 5 × 6 s sprint test. Additionally, correlations between both active and total muscle mass, and performance measures including peak power (PP) and mean power (MP) were also assessed.

2. Materials and Methods

2.1. Participants

Fifteen males (n = 15, 24 ± 3 years, 83.3 ± 12.1 kg, 174 ± 7 cm) volunteered to participate in the study. Participants were not highly trained in any specific sport but participated in regular physical activity, completing ≤3 activity sessions·wk^{-1}. Regular physical activity included walking, jogging, tennis and recreational sports such as touch football and surfing.

2.2. Study Design

All participants reported to the laboratory on two separate occasions which were separated by a minimum of five days. During the first visit, participants completed a medical history questionnaire and the required pre-screening procedures. They completed pre-screening procedures and medical history questionnaires, indicating that all participants were healthy and free from any cardiovascular or neuromuscular irregularities. Upon the fulfilment of this inclusion criteria, participants were then familiarised with the electro-magnetically braked cycle ergometer and 5 × 6 s sprint test protocol. During the second visit, participants completed an upper body 5 × 6 s sprint test. Prior to participation, the experimental procedures and potential risks were explained to the participants and all provided written informed consent. All relevant research ethic applications have been approved by the University of the Sunshine Coast Ethics Committee application reference number (S/09/233), and performed in accordance with the Declaration of Helsinki.

2.3. The 5 × 6 s Sprint Test Protocol

The upper body 5 × 6 s sprint test was conducted on a modified electro-magnetically braked cycle ergometer (EE) (Excalibur Sport, Lode B.V., Groningen, The Netherlands). The EE was fixed to a table with the table fixed to the ground to prevent any movement of the EE during the 5 × 6 s sprint test, with participants being instructed to keep their feet flat on the ground and remain seated throughout the 5 × 6 s sprint test. The seat height and back rest were adjusted so that with the crank position on the opposite side to the body and the hand grasping the handles, the elbow joint was almost in full extension (165°–175°) and the shoulders in line with the centre of the ergometers shaft. When seated, participants were then restrained at the waist with an adjustable seatbelt in an attempt to minimise any unwanted movement and involvement from the lower body musculature. A fly wheel braking force corresponding to 5% of the participants' body weight was used for the upper body 5 × 6 s sprint test [13].

Prior to the commencement of the 5 × 6 s sprint test, participants completed a 5 min warm-up at 50 W which included three short sprint efforts followed by a 5 min recovery. Following the warm-up participants stretched for approximately 3 min before the commencement of the test. Participants were instructed to arm crank as fast as possible during each sprint performance. The 5 × 6 s consisted of five maximal effort sprints, all of which were set at the above resistance and lasted for 6 s in duration. Between each of the five repeated sprints there was a 24 s passive recovery. Participants were given verbal encouragement to maintain their highest possible cadence throughout each 6 s sprint.

2.4. Performance Measures

Power output was recorded by the Wingate version 1.0.7 software (Lode B.V., Groningen, The Netherlands) during the 5 × 6 s sprint test. The following performance measures were determined for each 6 s sprint: PP was calculated as the highest single point of power output (recorded at 0.2 s intervals). MP was the average power output during the 6 s sprint effort.

2.5. Body Composition

Body composition was assessed using dual-energy X-ray absorptiometry (DEXA (model XR36, Norland, Fort Atkinson, WI, USA). The same licensed and experienced technician operated the DEXA for each participant, which was calibrated before all testing with a multi-step wedge phantom of tissue and bone reference material. The CV was 1.0% at 95% confidence level. Whole body values were presented as total mass (kg) and percent fat of total body mass (%) and lean body mass (LBM) (g). Upper and lower body measurements were determined on the basis of bony landmarks via manual analysis. The total lean mass for the arms and the shoulders and the addition of the muscle groups of the back and chest, was measured and reported as the upper body lean body mass (UBLBM). The UBLBM muscles have been reported as active during upper body arm ergometry [14], and as such are reported and referred to as the ACTIVE muscle mass during the upper body 5 × 6 s sprint test. For the lower body, both legs and gluteal muscle groups were measured and reported as lower body lean body mass (LBLBM) [4].

2.6. Other Calculations

The total work done was calculated as the sum of the work done in each of the 6 s sprints. This was achieved by converting the MP output (W) for each sprint into kilojoules (Kj) using the following formula:

Kj = ((MP output × time)/1000)
Kj = ((watts × 6 s)/1000)
Total Work (Kj) = Sprint 1 (Kj) + Sprint 2 (Kj), Sprint 3 (Kj) + Sprint 4 (Kj) + Sprint 5 (Kj)

After the total work (Kj) done was calculated (see above), the ideal work (Kj) and % decrement was calculated using the formulas below [15,16]:

Ideal work (Kj) = (highest of 6s sprints × 5)
Decrement (%) = (100 − (Total work/ideal work × 100))

2.7. Statistical Analysis

All analyses were performed using the IBM SPSS 19.0 program for Windows (Chicago, IL, USA). Data are reported as means ± standard deviation (SD). The distribution of the data was analyzed by the Shapiro–Wilk test and the results showed a normal Gaussian distribution. A stepwise multiple linear regression analysis was used to establish the most important determinants of peak and mean upper body 5 × 6 s sprint test power. Collinearity diagnostics were used to remove predictor variables with strong relationships. A one-way repeated measures analysis of variance (ANOVA) was performed to determine significance differences between each 6 s sprint of the 5 × 6 s sprint test. A stepwise multiple linear regression analysis was used to establish the most important determinants of total work done measured in kilojoules (Kj) during the upper body 5 × 6 s sprint test. Variables included body mass (BM), total lean body mass (LBM), body fat %, trunk lean body mass (TLBM), arm lean body mass (ARMLBM), upper body lean body mass (UBLBM) which was a total of TLBM and ARMLBM and lower body lean body mass (LBLBM). A level of significance of 5% ($P < 0.05$) was adopted in all analyses.

3. Results

The descriptive and anthropometric characteristics of all participants are displayed in Table 1. Participants were all otherwise healthy, physically active males of a similar age. This selection criteria was enforced to ensure a homogenous participant group and minimize the effect of any potentially confounding variables. Performance data from the upper body 5 × 6 s sprint test are displayed in Table 2. Absolute PP output during sprint 1, 2 and 3 was significantly ($P < 0.05$) higher than the PP measured during sprint 4 and 5 respectively. When expressed in relative terms ($W \cdot kg^{-1}$), PP in sprint 1 and sprint 2 was significantly higher than sprint 4 ($P < 0.05$). When expressed relative to lean body mass (LBM) ($W \cdot kg^{-1}$ LBM) and active muscle mass ($W \cdot kg^{-1}$ UBLBM) sprint 1 PP was significantly higher than sprint 4 ($P < 0.05$) and 5 ($P < 0.05$), while sprint 2 PP was significantly higher than sprint 4. The PP achieved during sprint 3 was significantly higher ($P < 0.05$) than that measured during sprint 5 when expressed relative to UBLBM.

Table 1. The descriptive and anthropometric data of study participants ($n = 15$).

Age (years)	24 ± 3
Height (cm)	174 ± 7
Body mass (kg)	83.3 ± 12.1
Body fat (%)	16 ± 7.9
LBM (g)	6,5305 ± 6905
UBLBM (g)	3,8851 ± 3900
ARMLBM (g)	9120 ± 1428
LBLBM (g)	2,2238 ± 2911

LBM, Lean body mass; UBLBM, Upper body lean body mass; ARMLBM, Arms lean body mass; LBLBM, lower body lean body mass; (cm), centimetres; (kg), kilograms; (%), percent; (g), grams.

Table 2. 5 × 6 s sprint test performance data ($n = 15$).

Performance Measure	Sprint 1	Sprint 2	Sprint 3	Sprint 4	Sprint 5
PP (W)	1098.5 ± 217.0	1074.3 ± 205.9	1061.9 ± 172.7	1027.1±182.3 ^{a,b}	1036.2± 57.5 ^{a,c}
MP (W)	537.2 ± 112.4	516.5 ± 113.7	555.1 ± 135.4	509.6 ± 95.2 ^{a,c}	519.9 ± 87.1
PP ($W \cdot kg^{-1}$)	13.5 ± 2.0	13.2 ± 2.0	13.1 ± 1.4	12.6 ± 1.8 ^{a,b}	12.8 ± 1.5
MP ($W \cdot kg^{-1}$)	6.6 ± 1.1	6.3 ± 1.2	6.8 ± 1.5	6.3 ± 0.9 ^{c}	6.4 ± 1.0
PP ($W \cdot kg^{-1}$ LBM)	16.9 ± 2.1	16.6 ± 2.3	16.4 ± 1.7	15.9 ± 2.1 ^{a,b}	16.0 ± 1.5 ^{a}
MP ($W \cdot kg^{-1}$ LBM)	8.3 ± 1.2	8.0 ± 1.4	8.6 ± 1.5	7.9 ± 1.1 ^{c}	8.1 ± 1.0
PP ($W \cdot kg^{-1}$ UBLBM)	28.5 ± 3.5	27.9 ± 3.9	27.7 ± 3.1	26.8 ± 3.6 ^{a,b}	27.0 ± 2.6 ^{a,c}
MP ($W \cdot kg^{-1}$ UBLBM)	14.0 ± 2.0	13.4 ± 2.3	14.4 ± 2.6	13.3 ± 1.9 ^{c}	13.6 ± 1.7

Active muscle mass for the upper body = UBLBM, upper body lean body mass; LBM, lean body mass; PP, peak power; MP, mean power; (W), watts; ($W \cdot kg^{-1}$), watts per kilogram; Data is displayed as mean ± SD: ^{a} $p < 0.05$ from Sprint 1; ^{b} $p < 0.05$ from Sprint 2; ^{c} $p < 0.05$ from Sprint 3.

In comparison, absolute MP output values were only significantly different between sprint 1 and 4 ($P < 0.05$) and sprint 3 and 4 ($P < 0.05$). The only significant difference in relative ($W \cdot kg^{-1}$) MP values occurred between sprint 3 and 4 ($P < 0.05$). Significant differences in MP where identified when expressed relative to LBM ($W \cdot kg^{-1}$ LBM) and active muscle mass ($W \cdot kg^{-1}$ UBLBM) between sprint 3 and 4 ($P < 0.05$).

Predictors of upper body 5 × 6 s sprint performance are displayed in Table 3. Stepwise multiple linear regression analysis revealed that UBLBM accounts for 87% of the variance in total work done during the upper body 5 × 6 s sprint test. The decrement in total work done over the five sprints was 11.4%.

Table 3. Predictors of upper body 5 × 6 s sprint test performance ($n = 15$).

Variable	Adjusted R^2	F value	Predictors	Standardized β coefficient	P
Total work (Kj)	0.871	$F_{1,20} = 143.1, p < 0.001$	UBLBM	0.937	<0.001

(Kj), kilojoules; UBLBM, Upper body lean body mass.

4. Discussion

To the best of our knowledge, the intermittent high intensity 5 × 6 s sprint test (RSA) for the upper body has not previously been investigated in a group of physically active individuals. Upper body intermittent performance has been shown to be a key requirement for a number of sports [6] and in the workplace [17]. Therefore the aim of this study was to measure RSA of the upper body and to determine key predictors of RSA ability.

The main findings of the present study were that peak power (PP) output decreased significantly during the upper body 5 × 6 s sprint test, with an approximate decrement of 11.4% in total work performed. Furthermore, stepwise multiple linear regression analysis revealed that UBLBM was the best predictor of total work done.

The highest peak power (PP) value occurred during sprint 1 with significantly lower values occurring during sprints 4–5. These significant differences remained even when expressed relative to LBM and active muscle mass (UBLBM). Mean power (MP) values were also found to decrease, however were only significantly different between sprints 1 and 4 and sprints 3 and 4. When LBM and UBLBM were taken into consideration, significant differences emerged for mean power output between sprint 3 and 4. The greater decline in PP compared to MP may be related to the inability of the upper body to replenish phosphocreatine stores which has been show to affect PP during lower body repeat sprints [18]. The ability to maintain MP during the repeat sprints may also be due to a greater reliance on the aerobic pathways which provides less rapid energy for power and has shown to increase from 10% to 40% over five repeat sprints [19].

Our findings that the highest peak power value occurred in sprint one and then significantly decreased thereafter is in contrast with most previous studies which have investigated the 5 × 6 s sprint test for the lower body [20–22] where no significant decreases in PP have been observed. Furthermore, while we found PP output to be significantly lower during sprints 4 and 5 compared to sprint 1, a recent study which implemented a lower body 10 × 6 s sprint protocol reported that PP output was significantly less only after sprints 8, 9 and 10 [20]. These conflicting findings between the upper and lower body may be attributed to a number of factors, including differences in muscle fiber type characteristics [2,3], their respective PCr resynthesis rates [23], and H^+ buffering capabilities of the muscle [24]. This is further supported by findings that arm exercises are more sensitive to performance improvements induced by increased buffering capacity than leg exercises [25].

Taken together, this suggests that the more efficient replenishment of PCr stores and removal of waste products from the leg musculature extends the time taken, or number of efforts required, to produce a significant decrement in power output compared to the upper body musculature. Moreover, the increased day to day reliance on the lower body musculature for ambulation compared to the upper body may induce favourable training adaption's which allow for a reduced decrement in RSA. In support of these findings the present study found the % decrement in total work performed across the five sprints to be approximately 11.4% for the upper body which is in agreement with a recent study conducted using elite cross country skiers [26], however differs compared to previous studies which have reported between approximately 5.4% and 8.5% for the lower body in endurance and team athletes respectively [15]. These findings, in conjunction with reports of a significant correlation between blood buffer capacity and RSA [27] further suggests a reduced buffering capacity of the upper body musculature, which consequently leads to a higher decrement in work performed and thus decreased RSA performance.

The present study also reported that UBLBM was found to be the best predictor of total work performed during the upper body 5 × 6 s sprint test. These findings are in contrast to Weber *et al.*, 2006 [4] who reported that body mass (BM) rather than lean body mass (LBM) or arm lean body mass (ARMLBM), was the best predictor of upper body Wingate power. These differences may be attributed to the start-stop nature of the 5 × 6 s sprint test compared to the continuous effort of the Wingate. As a result the Wingate does not have the opportunity to replenish PCr stores as per the 5 × 6 s sprint test but relies more on the glycolytic and aerobic pathways for energy. Our findings of UBLBM being the best predictor in work performed across the five sprints suggests that peripheral factors, such as localised neuromuscular activation, play an important role in upper body sprint initiation and fatigue. In support of this, it has been reported that when fatigue is substantial, *i.e.*, a decrement in performance of >10%, there is a concomitant decline in mechanical performance and peripheral electromyography (EMG) amplitude [28,29], suggesting an inability to fully activate the targeted musculature. While central fatigue may also play a role in fatigue during intermittent exercise recent evidence suggests that further studies are required to better understand the role of neural drive on the aetiology of fatigue during the 5 × 6 s sprint test [6].

5. Conclusions

In summary, the present study found that PP output significantly decreased during the upper body 5 × 6 s sprint test even after LBM and UBLBM was accounted for. Stepwise multiple linear regression analysis revealed that UBLBM was the best predictor of total work performed, with a decrement of approximately 11.4% in total work done during the upper body 5 × 6 s sprint test. The findings from the present investigation suggest that as a result of the diminished capacity of the upper body to perform short duration, high intensity, intermittent exercise a training approach whereby the desired physiological mechanisms targeted and activated during match play and sports performance may in turn lead to improved upper body performance during such exercise. Furthermore, this study highlights the need to investigate the upper body as an independent region, rather than making comparisons or drawing conclusions from findings obtained during lower body, short duration, high intensity, intermittent exercise.

Author Contributions

Leonie Harvey, Matthew Bousson, Chris McLellan and Dale Lovell were involved in study design, data collection, data interpretation, and manuscript writing.

Conflicts of Interest

The authors declare no conflict of interest.

References

1. Sawka, M.N. Physiology of Upper Body Exercise. *Exerc. Sport Sci. Rev.* **1986**, *14*, 175–212.
2. Calbet, J.A.; Holmberg, H.C.; Rosdahl, H.; van Hall, G.; Jensen-Urstad, M.; Saltin, B. Why do arms extract less oxygen than legs during exercise? *Am. J. Physiol. Regul. Integr. Comp. Physiol.* **2005**, *289*, R1448–R1458.
3. Sanchis-Moysi, J.; Idoate, F.; Olmedillas, H.; Guadalupe-Grau, A.; Alayón, S.; Carreras, A.; Dorado, C.; Calbet, J.A.L. The upper extremity of the professional tennis player: muscle volumes, fiber-type distribution and muscle strength. *Scand. J. Med. Sci. Sports* **2010**, *20*, 524–534.
4. Weber, C.L.; Chia, M.; Inbar, O. Gender differences in anaerobic power of the arms and legs--a scaling issue. *Med. Sci. Sports Exerc.* **2006**, *38*, 129–137.
5. Lovell, D.; Bousson, M.; McLellan, C. Upper and lower body anaerobic performance of semi-elite Rugby League players. *J. Sport Health Sci.* **2013**, *53*, 477–482.
6. Girard, O.; Mendez-Villanueva, A.; Bishop, D. Repeated-Sprint Ability—Part I. *Sports Med.* **2011**, *41*, 673–694.
7. Bishop, D.; Spencer, M.; Duffield, R.; Lawrence, S. The validity of a repeated sprint ability test. *J. Sci. Med. Sport* **2001**, *4*, 19–29.
8. Glaister, M. Multiple sprint work. *Sports Med.* **2005**, *35*, 757–777.
9. García-Pallarés, J.; López-Gullón, J.M.; Muriel, X.; Díaz, A.; Izquierdo, M. Physical fitness factors to predict male Olympic wrestling performance. *Eur. J. Appl. Physiol.* **2011**, *111*, 1747–1758.
10. Koukoubis, T.; Cooper, L.; Glisson, R.; Seaber, A.; Feagin Jr., J. An electromyographic study of arm muscles during climbing. *Knee Surg. Sport Traumatol. Arthrosc.* **1995**, *3*, 121–124.
11. Yoon, J. Physiological profiles of elite senior wrestlers. *Sports Med.* **2002**, *32*, 225–233.
12. Horswill, C.; Miller, J.; Scott, J.; Smith, C.; Welk, G.; Van Handel, P. Anaerobic and aerobic power in arms and legs of elite senior wrestlers. *Int. J. Sports Med.* **1992**, *13*, 558–561.
13. Dotan, R.; Bar-Or, O. Load optimization for the Wingate Anaerobic Test. *Eur. J. Appl. Physiol. Occup. Physiol.* **1983**, *51*, 409–417.
14. Smith, P.M.; Chapman, M.L.; Hazlehurst, K.E.; Goss-Sampson, M.A. The influence of crank configuration on muscle activity and torque production during arm crank ergometry. *J. Electromyogr. Kinesiol.* **2008**, *18*, 598–605.
15. Bishop, D.; Spencer, M. Determinants of repeated-sprint ability in well-trained team-sport athletes and endurance-trained athletes. *J. Sports Med. Phys. Fitness* **2004**, *44*, 1–7.
16. Fitzsimons, M.; Dawson, B.; Ward, D.; Wilkinson, A. Cycling and running tests of repeated sprint ability. *Aust. J. Sci. Med. Sport* **1993**, *25*, 82.

17. Nussbaum, M.A.; Clark, L.L.; Lanza, M.A.; Rice, K.M. Fatigue and endurance limits during intermittent overhead work. *AIHAJ Am. Ind. Hyg. Assoc.* **2001**, *62*, 446–456.
18. Mendez-Villanueva, A.; Edge, J.; Suriano, R.; Hamer, P.; Bishop, D. The recovery of repeated-sprint exercise is associated with PCr resynthesis, while muscle pH and EMG amplitude remain depressed. *PLoS ONE* **2012**, *7*, e51977.
19. McGawley, K.; Bishop, D.J. Oxygen uptake during repeated-sprint exercise. *J. Sci. Med. Sport* **2015**, *18*, 214–218.
20. Billaut, F.; Basset, F.; Giacomoni, M.; Lemaitre, F.; Tricot, V.; Falgairette, G. Effect of high-intensity intermittent cycling sprints on neuromuscular activity. *Int. J. Sports Med.* **2006**, *27*, 25–30.
21. Bishop, D.; Edge, J. Determinants of repeated-sprint ability in females matched for single-sprint performance. *Eur. J. Appl. Physiol.* **2006**, *97*, 373–379.
22. Dawson, B.; Goodman, C.; Lawrence, S.; Preen, D.; Polglaze, T.; Fitzsimons, M.; Fournier, P. Muscle phosphocreatine repletion following single and repeated short sprint efforts. *Scand. J. Med. Sci. Sports* **1997**, *7*, 206–213.
23. Tesch, P.; Thorsson, A.; Fujitsuka, N. Creatine phosphate in fiber types of skeletal muscle before and after exhaustive exercise. *J. Appl. Physiol.* **1989**, *66*, 1756–1759.
24. Holloszy, J.O.; Coyle, E.F. Adaptations of skeletal muscle to endurance exercise and their metabolic consequences. *J. Appl. Physiol. Respir. Environ. Exerc. Physiol.* **1984**, *56*, 831–838.
25. Robertson, R.J.; Falkel, J.E.; Drash, A.L.; Swank, A.M.; Metz, K.F.; Spungen, S.A.; Leboeuf, J.R. Effect of induced alkalosis on physical work capacity during arm and leg exercise. *Ergonomics.* **1987**, *30*, 19–31.
26. Sandbakk, Ø.; Skålvik, T.F.; Spencer, M.; van Beekvelt, M.; Welde, B.; Hegge, A.M.; Gjøvaag, T.; Ettema, G. The physiological responses to repeated upper-body sprint exercise in highly trained athletes. *Eur. J. Appl. Physiol.* **2015**, 1381–1391.
27. Bishop, D.; Lawrence, S.; Spencer, M. Predictors of repeated-sprint ability in elite female hockey players. *J. Sci. Med. Sport* **2003**, *6*, 199–209.
28. Mendez-Villanueva, A.; Hamer, P.; Bishop, D. Fatigue in repeated-sprint exercise is related to muscle power factors and reduced neuromuscular activity. *Eur. J. Appl. Physiol.* **2008**, *103*, 411–419.
29. Racinais, S.; Bishop, D.; Denis, R.; Lattier, G.; Mendez-Villaneuva, A.; Perrey, S. Muscle deoxygenation and neural drive to the muscle during repeated sprint cycling. *Med. Sci. Sport Exer.* **2007**, *39*, 268–274.

22

Kinematics and Kinetics of Youth Baseball Catchers and Pitchers

Gretchen Oliver *, Keith Lohse and Sarah Gascon

School of Kinesiology, Auburn University, 301 Wire Road Auburn, AL 36830, USA;
E-Mails: krl0022@auburn.edu (K.L.); ssg0012@auburn.edu (S.G.)

* Author to whom correspondence should be addressed; E-Mail: goliver@auburn.edu

Academic Editor: Eling de Bruin

Abstract: The purpose of this study was to compare the throwing kinematics and kinetics of youth catchers and pitchers. It was hypothesized that catchers and pitchers would exhibit differences throughout the throwing motion. Descriptive statistics were used to investigate kinematics during the four events of throwing: foot contact (FC), maximum shoulder external rotation (MER), ball release (BR) and maximum shoulder internal rotation (MIR). Additionally, kinetics were investigated within phases of the events: Phase 1 (cocking; FC to MER), Phase 2 (acceleration; MER to BR) and Phase 3 (deceleration; BR to MIR). Results revealed significant difference in torso flexion, lateral flexion, pelvis lateral flexion and segment velocities between the catchers and pitchers. Based on data from the current study, it appears that the youth catchers execute their throw as they have been instructed. It is unclear if the throwing mechanics displayed by these youth are efficient for a catcher, thus further investigation is needed to determine long-term injury susceptibility.

Keywords: baseball; catchers; throwing; upper extremity; youth

---

1. Introduction

Biomechanical analysis of youth throwing continues to evolve and has taken on a new resurgence with the focus on injury prevention. To date, a majority of the available data dedicated to biomechanics of throwing has focused on youth pitchers [1–4]. However, there is another position that requires more throws than the pitcher, the catcher [5]. Additionally, the catcher often has to make all their throws coming up from a squatted position. The catcher not only throws the ball back to the pitcher after every non-hit pitch, but may also throw to any of the three bases as required by a variety of circumstances. Though a majority of the catcher's throws may be submaximal, the throws to hold a runner on base are maximum effort.

The catcher's effectiveness is based on his or her ability to catch the ball, quickly transfer the ball to their throwing hand and throw the ball to another positioned player to make a play. However, when a catcher is attempting to throw out a runner, they may be required to catch, transfer and throw in a rapidly unfolding play; those throws are not as common. Thus, as a catcher more frequently makes that throw to second base to prevent a runner from stealing, it has been speculated that the catcher's throwing mechanics are altered because of the necessity to rush their throw, thus possibly contributing to long-term injury susceptibility [5–7].

2. Context

Recently, due to the increased awareness of injury in youth baseball, the position of catcher has gained interest. In 2011, Fleisig *et al.* published prospective injury data on youth baseball pitchers, and though not statistically significant, those athletes playing dual roles (catcher and pitcher) during the same game were of concern to the authors [2]. Additionally, it was thus recommended that youth who play the position of pitcher not concomitantly play the position of catcher. Thus, with the current recommendations for youth not to play dual positions, in addition to the limited data regarding the catcher's throwing mechanics, it was the purpose of this study to not only examine the mechanics of catchers, but also to compare the throwing kinematics and kinetics of youth catchers and pitchers. It was hypothesized that catchers and pitchers would exhibit differences throughout the throwing motion.

3. Materials and Methods

3.1. Experimental Approach to the Problem

The goal of the experiment was to determine kinematic and kinetic differences in the throwing motion of youth baseball catchers and pitchers. Descriptive statistics were used to investigate kinematics during the four events of throwing: foot contact (FC), maximum shoulder external rotation (MER), ball release (BR) and maximum shoulder internal rotation (MIR). Ball release was estimated as the midpoint between maximum elbow flexion and maximum elbow extension. This estimate was required because we did not have the capability to track the movement of the ball. This method to estimate ball release has been used previously in the throwing literature using electromagnetic tracking, but has yet to be validated [4,5,8]. Additionally, kinetics were investigated within the phases of the events: Phase 1 (cocking; FC to MER), Phase 2 (acceleration; MER to BR) and Phase 3 (deceleration; BR to MIR). Kinetics were averaged within each phase. A mixed-factorial ANOVA was conducted to examine the differences between positions (catcher and pitchers) and throwing events.

3.2. Participants

A total of 50 youth baseball catchers (N = 25; 12.0 ± 2.2 years; 150.3 ± 11.7 cm; 44.9 ± 11.7 kg) and pitchers (N = 25; 11.0 ± 1.3 years; 153.0 ± 8.5 cm; 47.2 ± 8.9 kg) participated. The inclusion criterion was freedom from injury within the past six months; however, none of the participants reported they had ever suffered an injury that prevented them from throwing. Participants were tested during the fall baseball season and had not performed any throwing 24 h prior to arrival into the lab on the day of testing. The Institutional Review Board of the University approved all testing protocols. Prior to data collection, all testing procedures were explained to each participant, as well as to parent(s)/legal guardian(s), and informed consent and participant assent were obtained.

3.3. Procedures

Participants reported to the laboratory on a day that they had abstained from physical activity, as well as any type of throwing. Upon arrival, participants were instructed on the testing protocol. Catchers, dressed in full gear (helmet, chest protector and shin guards), were instructed to catch a pitched ball and throw with maximum effort to a position player on second base at regulation distance (84.85 feet, 25.86 m) as they would if throwing out a runner trying to steal second. The catchers were instructed to catch and throw as quick as possible at maximum effort. Catchers were to throw three maximum effort throws, with the fastest throw being selected for analysis. The pitchers were instructed to throw maximum effort four-seam fastballs, from a regulation mound, for a strike to a catcher regulation distance (46 feet, 14.02 m). The fastest of the three four-seam fastballs for strikes was selected for analysis. The throwing surface was constructed so that the participant's stride would land on top of the 40 cm × 60 cm Bertec force plate (Bertec Corp, Columbus, OH, USA) that was anchored into the floor. Following instruction, participants were given an unlimited time to perform their own specified pre-competition warm-up. Average warm-up time was ten minutes. A JUGS radar gun (OpticsPlanet, Inc., Northbrook, IL, USA) positioned in the direction of the throw determined ball speed.

Kinematic data were collected with The MotionMonitor™ (Innovative Sports Training, Chicago, IL, USA) synched with an electromagnetic tracking system (Flock of Birds Ascension Technologies Inc., Burlington, VT, USA). The Flock of Birds Ascension system has been validated for tracking humeral movements, producing trial-by-trial interclass correlation coefficients for axial humerus rotation in both loaded and non-loaded conditions in excess of 0.96 [9]. The field distortion has been shown to be the cause of error in excess of 5° at a distance of 2 m from an extended range transmitter [10], but increases in instrumental sensitivity have reduced this error to near 10° prior to system calibration and 2° following system calibration [11,12]. Previously-established techniques were used to calibrate the system prior to data collection [10–12]. Following calibration, pilot data collected prior to testing indicated that the magnitude of error in determining the position and orientation of the electromagnetic sensors within the calibrated world axes system was less than 0.01 m and 3°, respectively.

Electromagnetic sensors were affixed to the participant's skin using PowerFlex cohesive tape (Andover Healthcare, Inc., Salisbury, MA, USA) to ensure that the sensors remained secure throughout testing. Sensors were attached to the following locations: (1) the posterior/medial aspect of the torso at C7; (2) posterior/medial aspect of the pelvis at S1; (3–4) bilateral distal/posterior aspect of the upper arm; (5) the flat, broad portion of the acromion of the scapula; (6–7) bilateral distal/posterior aspect of the forearm; (8–9) bilateral distal/posterior aspect of the lower leg; and (10–11) bilateral distal/posterior aspect of the upper leg [4,13–16]. A twelfth sensor was attached to a stylus that was used for digitization of the bony landmarks described by the International Shoulder Group of the International Society of Biomechanics [17]. Two points described the longitudinal axis of the segment, and a third point described the plane. Participants stood in anatomical position during digitization to guarantee accurate bony landmark identification. The digitization of the bony landmarks allowed transformation of the sensor data from the global coordinate system to the anatomically-based local coordinate system (Table 1).

Table1. Description of bony landmarks palpated and digitized.

Bony Landmark	Bony Process Palpated and Digitized
Thorax	
Seventh Cervical Vertebra (C7)	Most dorsal aspect of the spinous process
Eighth Thoracic Vertebra (T8)	Most dorsal aspect of the spinous process
Suprasternal Notch	Most cranial aspect of sternum
Humerus	
Medial Epicondyle	Medial/distal aspect of condyle
Lateral Epicondyle	Lateral/distal aspect of condyle
Glenohumeral Joint Center of Rotation	Rotation method *
Forearm	
Radial Styloid Process	Lateral/distal aspect of radial styloid
Ulnar Styloid Process	Medial/ distal aspect of ulnar styloid

* The center of glenohumeral rotation was not digitized. The rotation method estimated joint center using the least squares algorithm for the point moving the least during a series of short rotational movements.

Data describing the position and orientation of electromagnetic sensors were collected at 100 Hz. Raw data were independently filtered along each global axis using a 4th order Butterworth filter with a cutoff frequency of 13.4 Hz [4,15]. Neutral stance was the Y-axis in the vertical direction; horizontal and to the right of Y was the X-axis; and posterior was the X-axis [16].

Euler angle decompositions were used to determine humeral and scapular orientation with respect to the thorax. Humeral orientation was determined as rotation about the Y-axis of the humerus (plane of elevation), rotation about the Z-axis (elevation) and rotation about the y-axis (axial rotation) (Table 2). Rotations were based on the recommendations of the International Shoulder Group [17]. Elbow and shoulder kinetics were computed using a linked chain "bottom-up" model as previously described [18]. Force and moment data are normalized by dividing joint forces and moments by the participant's body weight (mass * gravity).

Table 2. Angle orientation decomposition sequences.

Segment	Axis of Rotation	Angle
Torso		
Rotation 1	Z	Flexion (−)/Extension (+)
Rotation 2	X′	Left Lateral Tilt (−)/Right Lateral Tilt (+)
Rotation 3	Y″	Right Rotation (+)/Left Rotation (−)
Shoulder		
Rotation 1	Y	Plane of Elevation (0 = Abduction; 90 = Flexion)
Rotation 2	X′	Elevation
Rotation 3	Y″	Internal Rotation (+)/External Rotation (−)
Elbow		
Rotation 1	Z	Flexion (+)/Hyperextension (−)
Rotation 2	X′	Carrying Angle
Rotation 3	Y″	Pronation (+)/Supination (−)

Prime (′) and double prime (″) notations represent previously-rotated axes due to the rotation of the local coordinate system resulting in all axes within that system being rotated. Rotation about the X-axis also results in rotation of both Y- and Z-axes, resulting in a new system of X′, Y′, Z′. Subsequent rotations are then about those axes.

3.4. Statistical Analysis

Statistical analyses were conducted using IBM SPSS Statistics 22. All kinematic variables were analyzed using a mixed-factorial ANOVA that included event (FC, MER, BR, MIR) as a within-subject factor and position (pitcher *versus* catcher) as a between-subject factor. The analysis of velocity included an additional within-subject factor of segment (hip, torso, humerus or forearm), and the analysis of knee flexion included an additional within-subject factor of side (left *versus* right).

The kinetic variables of the Y-axis force and Z-axis moments were analyzed using a mixed-factorial ANOVA that included phase (Phase 1, Phase 2, Phase 3) and joint (shoulder *versus* elbow) as within-subject factors and position (pitcher *versus* catcher) as a between-subject factor.

Mauchly's test of sphericity was conducted prior to all analyses, and a Greenhouse–Geisser correction was imposed when sphericity was violated. Quantile-quantile plots were constructed at each event/phase for each dependent variable to ensure that data at all time-points were approximately normally distributed. As phase × position interactions were largely exploratory, rather than multiple *post hoc* tests, we have presented 95% confidence intervals for each position at each time point in the figures [19].

4. Results

4.1. Analysis of Kinematic Measures

The results for the kinematic variables of catchers and pitchers are supplied in Table 3. Results revealed a significant difference between catchers and pitchers averaging across the different events/phases (as a main effect, ME) for: torso flexion, torso lateral flexion, pelvic lateral flexion and segment velocity (Figures 1–4, respectively). In addition, significant event by position interactions for torso flexion, pelvis lateral flexion and segmental velocity were also revealed. The meaning of the difference between catchers and pitchers changes over time and may only be statistically significant for a subset of the events. For velocity, there was also a significant main effect of segment, $F(1.67,80.32) = 1851.0$, $p < 0.001$, $\varepsilon = 0.56$, and a segment by phase interaction, $F(3.47,166.68) = 385.4$, $p < 0.001$, $\varepsilon = 0.38$, such that the change in velocity over time was dependent on the segment; see Figure 4a,b.

Table 3. Summary of ANOVA results for kinematic variables. ME, main effect.

Variable	ME of Event	ME of Position	Event × Position Interaction
Torso Flexion	$F(1.28, 61.59) = 115.18$, $p < 0.01$, $\varepsilon = 0.43$	$F(1,48) = 19.51$, $p < 0.01$	$F(1.28, 61.59) = 13.08$, $p < 0.01$, $\varepsilon = 0.43$
Torso Lateral Flexion	$F(1.36, 65.16) = 202.06$, $p < 0.01$, $\varepsilon = 0.45$	$F(1,48) = 14.90$, $p < 0.01$	$F(1.36, 65.16) = 0.\ 13$, $p = 0.79$, $\varepsilon = 0.45$
Torso Rotation	$F(1.99, 95.56) = 1081$, $p < 0.01$, $\varepsilon = 0.66$	$F(1,48) = 0.38$, $p = 0.54$	$F(1.99, 95.56) = 2.55$, $p = 0.08$, $\varepsilon = 0.66$
Pelvic Lateral Flexion	$F(1.33, 63.76) = 14.03$, $p < 0.01$, $\varepsilon = 0.44$	$F(1,48) = 6.61$, $p = 0.01$	$F(1.33, 63.76) = 3.86$, $p = 0.04$, $\varepsilon = 0.44$
Pelvic Rotation	$F(1.65, 78.87) = 1060.08$, $p < 0.01$, $\varepsilon = 0.55$	$F(1,48) = 0.97$, $p = 0.33$	$F(1.65, 78.87) = 2.86$, $p = 0.07$, $\varepsilon = 0.55$
Elbow Flexion	$F(1.38, 66.19) = 20.\ 83$, $p < 0.01$, $\varepsilon = 0.46$	$F(1,48) = 1.84$, $p = 0.18$	$F(1.38, 66.19) = 1.88$, $p = 0.17$, $\varepsilon = 0.46$
Plane of Elevation	$F(2.01, 96.35) = 153.38$, $p < 0.01$, $\varepsilon = 0.67$	$F(1,48) = 0.77$, $p = 0.38$	$F(2.01, 96.35) = 0.02$, $p = 0.97$, $\varepsilon = 0.67$
Humeral Elevation	$F(2.13, 102.08) = 13.83$, $p < 0.01$, $\varepsilon = 0.71$	$F(1,48) = 0.56$, $p = 0.46$	$F(2.13, 102.08) = 1.59$, $p = 0.97$, $\varepsilon = 0.71$
Humeral External Rotation	$F(2.43, 116.64) = 476.33$, $p < 0.01$, $\varepsilon = 0.81$	$F(1,48) = 0.23$, $p = 0.63$	$F(2.43, 116.64) = 1.29$, $p = 0.28$, $\varepsilon = 0.81$
Velocity *	$F(2.57, 123.43) = 273.04$, $p < 0.01$, $\varepsilon = 0.86$	$F(1,48) = 8.37$, $p < 0.01$	$F(2.57, 123.43) = 5.88$, $p < 0.01$, $\varepsilon = 0.81$

* Velocity included an additional factor of segment (hip, torso, humerus, forearm). See the main text for the main effects and interactions of these factors.

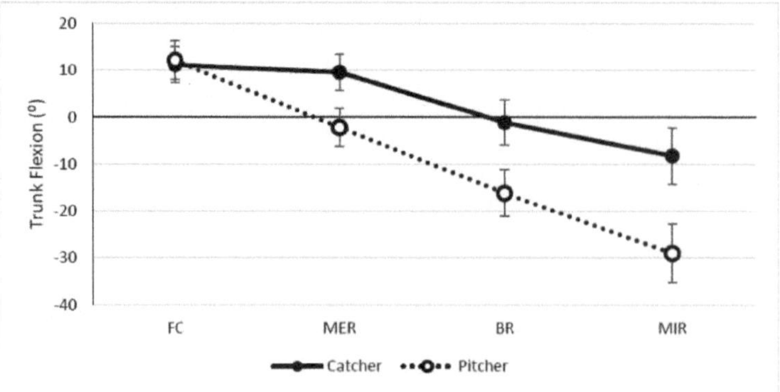

Figure 1. Torso flexion. (+) = extension; (−) = flexion. Flexion expressed as torso relative to the world axis. FC, foot contact; MER, maximum shoulder external rotation; BR, ball release; MIR, maximum shoulder internal rotation.

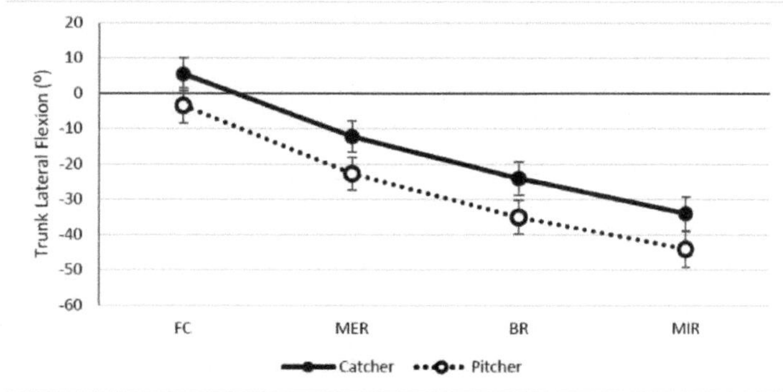

Figure 2. Torso lateral flexion. (+) = toward throwing arm side; (−) = toward glove side. Lateral flexion expressed as torso relative to the world axis.

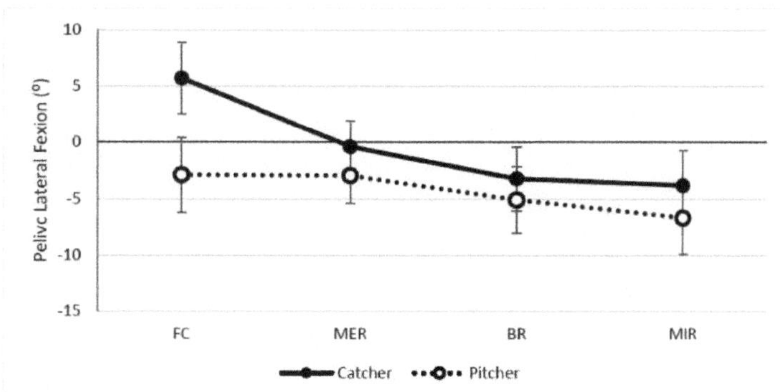

Figure 3. Pelvis lateral flexion. (+) = toward throwing arm side; (−) = toward glove side. Lateral flexion expressed as torso relative to the world axis.

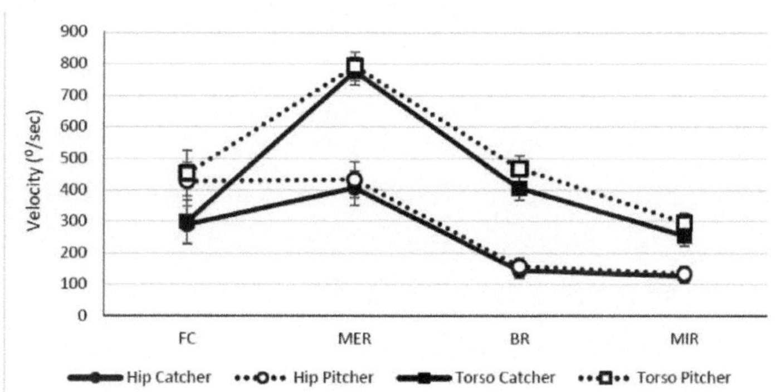

(a)

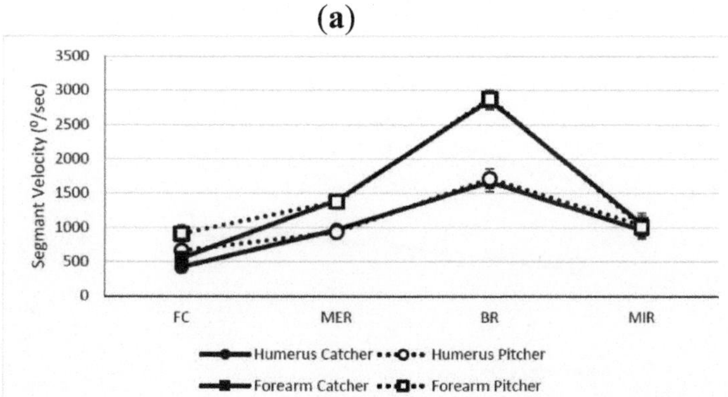

(b)

Figure 4. (**a**) Velocity of hip and torso; (**b**) velocity of humerus and forearm.

4.2. Analysis of Kinetic Measures

For Y-axis force (distraction force), there were significant main effects of phase and position (Table 4). Although the main effect of joint was not significant, there was a significant joint by phase interaction, $F(1.70,81.52) = 63.76$, $p < 0.001$, $\varepsilon = 0.85$, such that shoulder forces decreased more from the arm cocking though arm deceleration phase than did elbow forces (Figure 5).

Table 4. Summary of ANOVA results for kinetic variables.

Variable	ME of Phase	ME of Position	Phase × Position Interaction
Y Force *	$F(2, 96) = 61.34$, $p < 0.01$	$F(1,48) = 6.76$, $p = 0.01$	$F(2, 96) = 1.29$, $p = 0.30$
Z Moment *	$F(1.60, 75.26) = 31.27$, $p < 0.01$, $\varepsilon = 0.80$	$F(1,47) = 0.45$, $p < 0.51$	$F(1.60, 75.26) = 0.37$, $p = 0.64$, $\varepsilon = 0.80$

* Y force and Z moment analyses also included an additional factor of joint (shoulder *versus* elbow). See the main text for the main effects and interactions of these factors.

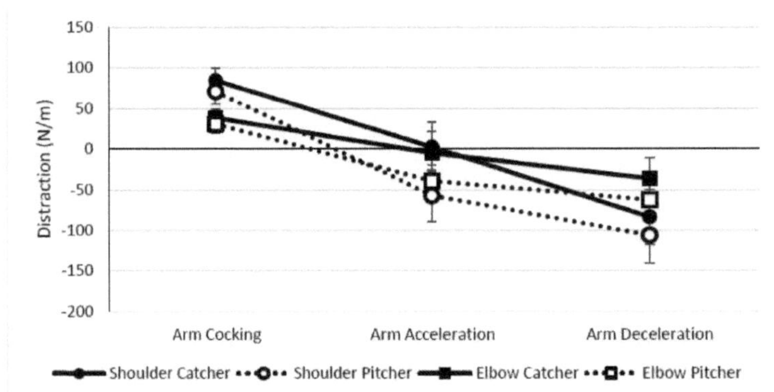

Figure 5. Shoulder and elbow distraction force. (+) = compressive force; (−) = distraction force.

For Z-axis moments (adduction moment at the shoulder and varus moment (resists valgus opening) at elbow), there was a significant main effect of phase (Table 4) and joint. These main effects were complicated by a significant joint by phase interaction, $F(1.39, 65.58) = 3.78$, $p = 0.04$, $\varepsilon = 0.70$. As shown in Figure 6, this interaction reflects the fact that elbow moments tended to change more over time than did shoulder moments.

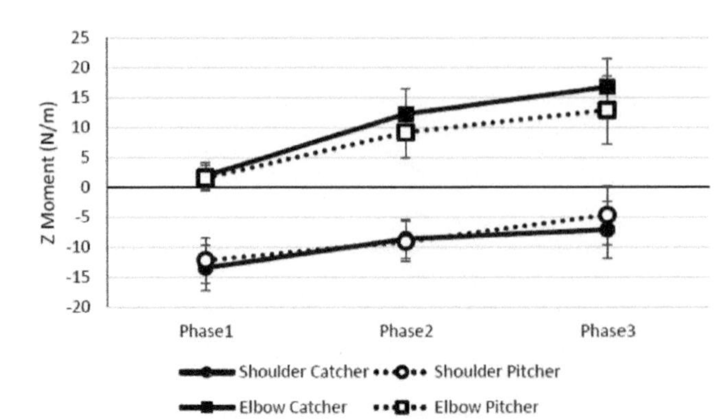

Figure 6. Z axis moments. (+) = varus moment; (−) = valgus moment.

5. Discussion

As many youth are involved in baseball, the need for understanding the throwing motion is important. The literature has documented the mechanics of youth pitchers [1–4,8,20,21]; however, data regarding the mechanics of catchers is only beginning to become available [5]. With both the catcher and pitcher performing multiple throws throughout the course of a game, it is important to understand not only the mechanics of the throw, but also to determine if differences exist. It was hypothesized that catchers having to make a longer throw as quickly as possible would exhibit mechanical differences from those of the pitchers.

Based on the results of the current study, the catchers displayed significant difference in their mechanics, particularly at the pelvis and torso, throughout the throwing motion. This finding of both pelvis and torso differences reiterates the effect of how the body moves as a series of interdependent links working proximal to distal for ball propulsion [22]. As the pelvis laterally flexes, so does the torso in a sequential fashion. Thus, the results of pelvis and torso differences are not surprising; however, if only torso or only pelvic differences were exhibited, then it would be a more alarming find. However, as the body works as a linked system and the pelvis and torso are working in the same plane of movement, differences exhibited at both segments are expected. The youth catchers in the current study exhibited greater pelvis and torso lateral flexion than the pitchers. The greatest difference in pelvis lateral flexion occurred at FC, and then the motion progressed to MER, BR and MIR; their torso flexion continued to increase. These results are in opposition to what has previously been published; however, those data were of collegiate catchers and pitchers [7]. In the previously-published proceeding of catchers and pitchers, it was the pitchers who displayed the greater pelvis and torso lateral flexion. Conversely, the forward flexion of the catchers in the current study was in agreement with the previously-mentioned study [7]. It should be mentioned that other than the experience level of the participants in the current and previously-mentioned study, the catchers in the Fortenbaugh [7] study were not in their catching gear while throwing [7]. The protective gear of a catcher is a part of their position; thus for the current study, we feel that youth wearing gear that could possibly not fit as well as desired could definitely factor into the throwing mechanics.

The decreased torso flexion displayed in the current study could possibly be indicative of the catcher trying to rush their throwing release and keeping their torso more upright toward the target *versus* continuing forward in their throw; however, further investigation is needed to make this assumption. The current study did note that as the catcher's progressed through the throwing motion, they were able to rotate about their hip forward and over their stride leg for completion of the throw. This technique is often see in long toss [7] and is considered correct.

When examining the segmental velocities of the catchers and pitchers, the main difference occurred at the event of FC for the hip and torso, as well as humerus and forearm. This finding was not unexpected, as it has previously been reported with collegiate-level catchers and pitchers [7] with the exception that our youth had a greater difference in velocities of the pitchers at FC. This could be a result of the catcher's technique of ball transfer up from their squat to the position for FC *versus* already being more vertical as pitchers position into FC with pitching off the mound. Once a catcher receives the pitch, they quickly strive to get the ball out of their glove and into throwing position for the best opportunity for a quick and efficient throw; while a pitcher typically begins in his or her optimal throwing position.

Thus, the discrepancies in segmental velocity could be attributed to the catcher having to come up out of a squat to initiate the throw.

Though not statistically significant, the authors thought it was important to discuss elbow flexion (Figure 7). The catchers in the current study displayed extreme ranges of elbow flexion. It should be noted that exaggerated elbow flexion coincides with how catchers are typically taught to transfer the ball from the glove to a throwing position of MER [6]. Ideally, a catcher wants to have the ball out of their glove and approaching MER when they make FC. As in the current study, it was the position of MER where the youth catchers displayed maximum elbow flexion, similar to what has been reported in collegiate catchers [7].

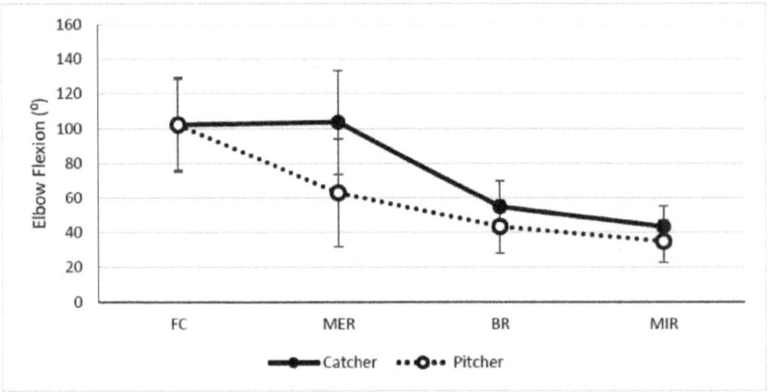

Figure 7. Elbow flexion.

Examining the kinetic data, the stresses about the shoulder and elbow in the current study were similar in magnitude, as well as comparable to those previously reported [7]. Additionally, it has been reported that elbow varus moments are lower when the elbow is more flexed [20,23]. As displayed in the current data, our findings also reiterate lower varus moments when the elbow is more flexed, and then, as the motion progresses through the phases, the moment increases. These findings of equivalent magnitudes are not surprising as there was no significant difference in the ball velocity between the catchers and pitchers (45.3 ± 8.2 mph and 48.4 ± 5.9 mph, respectively). However, it should be noted that ball velocity is not the only variable affecting upper extremity kinetics.

6. Conclusions

Based on data from the current study, it appears that the youth catchers execute their throw as they have been instructed [6]. It is unclear if the throwing mechanics displayed by these youth are efficient for a catcher or if catchers should try to throw with mechanics similar to pitching or long tossing. However, the implementation of long toss throwing mechanics is not known, since those mechanics are similar to pitching, sacrificing the quick ball release that a catcher is trying to employ. Additionally, further research should examine if the altered mechanics that catchers are utilizing predispose them to injury after prolonged throwing.

Author Contributions

G.O. conceived of and designed the experiments. G.O and S.G. performed the experiments. G.O. analyzed the data. G.O and K.L. contributed reagents/materials/analysis tools. G.O. and S.G. wrote the paper.

Conflicts of Interest

The authors declare no conflict of interest.

References

1. Dun, S.; Loftice, J.; Fleisig, G.; Kingsley, D.; Andrews, J. A biomechanical comparison of youth baseball pitches is the curveball potentially harmful? *Am. J. Sports Med.* **2008**, *36*, 686–692.
2. Fleisig, G.S.; Andrews, J.R.; Cutter, G.R.; Weber, A.; Loftice, J.; McMichael, C.; Hassell, N.; Lyman, S. Risk of serious injury for young baseball pitchers: A 10-year prospective study. *Am. J. Sports Med.* **2011**, *39*, 253–257.
3. Dun, S.; Fleisig, G.S.; Loftice, J.; Kingsley, D.; Andrews, J.R. The relationship between age and baseball pitching kinematics in professional baseball pitchers. *J. Biomech.* **2007**, *40*, 265–270.
4. Oliver, G.D.; Keeley, D.W. Pelvis and torso kinematics and their relationship to shoulder kinematics in high-school baseball pitchers. *J. Strength Cond. Res.* **2010**, *24*, 3241–3246.
5. Plummer, H.; Oliver, G.D. Quantitative analysis of kinematics and kinetics of catchers throwing to second base. *J. Sports Sci.* **2013**, *31*, 1108–1116.
6. Stallings, J. Chapter 16: Stopping opponents with solid defense. In *The baseball coaching bible*; Kindall, J., Winkin, J., Eds.; Human Kinetics: Champaign, IL, USA, 2000.
7. Fortenbaugh, D.; Fleisig, G.; Bolt, B. Coming down: Throwing mechanics of baseball catchers. In Conference Proceedings of the International Society of Biomechaincs in Sports, Volume 28. Marquette, WI, USA, 19–23 July, 2010.
8. Oliver, G.D.; Keeley, D.W. Gluteal muscle group activation and its relationship with pelvis and torso kinematics in high-school baseball pitchers. *J. Strength Cond. Res.* **2010**, *24*, 3015–3022.
9. Ludewig, P.M.; Cook, T.M. Alterations in shoulder kinematics and associated muscle activity in people with symptoms of shoulder impingement. *Phys. Ther.* **2000**, *80*, 276–291.
10. Day, J.; Murdoch, D.; Dumas, G. Calibration of position and angular data from a magnetic tracking device. *J. Biomech.* **2000**, *33*, 1039–1045.
11. Meskers, C.; Fraterman, H.; Helm, F.; Vermeulen, H. Calibration of the flock of birds electromagnetic tracking device and its application in shoulder motion studies. *J. Biomech.* **1999**, *32*, 629–633.
12. Perie, D.; Tate, A.J.; Cheng, P.L.; Dumas, G.A. Evaluation and calibration of an electromagnetic tracking device for biomechanical analysis of lifting task. *J. Biomech.* **2002**, *35*, 293–297.
13. Myers, J.B. Scapular position and orientation in throwing athletes. *Am. J. Sports Med.* **2005**, *33*, 263–271.
14. Myers, J.B.; Oyama, S.; Hibberd, E.E. Scapular dysfunction in high school baseball players sustaining throwing-related upper extremity injury: A prospective study. *J. Shoulder Elb. Surg.* **2013**, *22*, 1154–1159.

15. Oliver, G.D. Relationship between gluteal muscle activation and upper extremity kinematics and kinetics in softball position players. *Med. Biol. Eng. Comput.* **2013**, doi:10.1007/s11517-013-1056-3.
16. Oliver, G.D.; Plummer, H. Ground reaction forces, kinematics, and muscle activations during the windmill softball pitch. *J. Sports Sci.* **2011**, *29*, 1071–1077.
17. Wu, G.; van der Helm, F.C.T.; Veeger, H.E.J.; Makhsous, M.; Van Roy, P.; Anglin, C.; Nagels, J.; Karduna, A.R.; McQuade, K.; Wang, X.; *et al.* Isb recommendation on definitions of joint coordinate systems of various joints for the reporting of human joint motion—Part II: Shoulder, elbow, wrist and hand. *J. Biomech.* **2005**, *38*, 981–992.
18. Gagnon, D.; Gagnon, M. The influence of dynamic factors on tri-axial net muscular moments at the l5/s1 joint during asymmetrical lifting and lowering. *J. Biomech.* **1992**, *25*, 891–901.
19. Cummings, G. *Understand the New Statistics: Effect Sizes, Confidence Intervals and Meta-Analysis*; Routledge Taylor and Francis Group: New York, NY, USA, 2013.
20. Sabick, M.B.; Kim, Y.K.; Torry, M.R.; Keirns, M.A.; Hawkins, R.J. Biomechanics of the shoulder in youth baseball pitchers: Implications for the development of proximal humeral epiphysiolysis and humeral retrotorsion. *Am. J. Sports Med.* **2005**, *33*, 1716–1722.
21. Fleisig, G.S.; Barrentine, S.W.; Zheng, N.; Escamilla, R.F.; Andrews, J.R. Kinematic and kinetic comparison of baseball pitching among various levels of development. *J. Biomech.* **1999**, *32*, 1371–1375.
22. Kibler, W.B.; Wilkes, T.; Sciascia, A. Mechanics and pathomechanics in the overhead athlete. *Clin. Sports Med.* **2013**, *32*, 637–651.
23. Werner, S.L.; Murray, T.A.; Hawkins, R.J.; Gill, T.J. Relationship between throwing mechanics and elbow valgus in professional baseball pitchers. *J. Shoulder Elb. Surg.* **2002**, *11*, 151–155.

Permissions

All chapters in this book were first published in Sports, by MDPI; hereby published with permission under the Creative Commons Attribution License or equivalent. Every chapter published in this book has been scrutinized by our experts. Their significance has been extensively debated. The topics covered herein carry significant findings which will fuel the growth of the discipline. They may even be implemented as practical applications or may be referred to as a beginning point for another development.

The contributors of this book come from diverse backgrounds, making this book a truly international effort. This book will bring forth new frontiers with its revolutionizing research information and detailed analysis of the nascent developments around the world.

We would like to thank all the contributing authors for lending their expertise to make the book truly unique. They have played a crucial role in the development of this book. Without their invaluable contributions this book wouldn't have been possible. They have made vital efforts to compile up to date information on the varied aspects of this subject to make this book a valuable addition to the collection of many professionals and students.

This book was conceptualized with the vision of imparting up-to-date information and advanced data in this field. To ensure the same, a matchless editorial board was set up. Every individual on the board went through rigorous rounds of assessment to prove their worth. After which they invested a large part of their time researching and compiling the most relevant data for our readers.

The editorial board has been involved in producing this book since its inception. They have spent rigorous hours researching and exploring the diverse topics which have resulted in the successful publishing of this book. They have passed on their knowledge of decades through this book. To expedite this challenging task, the publisher supported the team at every step. A small team of assistant editors was also appointed to further simplify the editing procedure and attain best results for the readers.

Apart from the editorial board, the designing team has also invested a significant amount of their time in understanding the subject and creating the most relevant covers. They scrutinized every image to scout for the most suitable representation of the subject and create an appropriate cover for the book.

The publishing team has been an ardent support to the editorial, designing and production team. Their endless efforts to recruit the best for this project, has resulted in the accomplishment of this book. They are a veteran in the field of academics and their pool of knowledge is as vast as their experience in printing. Their expertise and guidance has proved useful at every step. Their uncompromising quality standards have made this book an exceptional effort. Their encouragement from time to time has been an inspiration for everyone.

The publisher and the editorial board hope that this book will prove to be a valuable piece of knowledge for researchers, students, practitioners and scholars across the globe.

List of Contributors

Daisy Bond, Laura Goodson, Samuel W. Oxford and Michael J. Duncan
Centre for Applied Biological and Exercise Sciences, Coventry University, Coventry CV1 5HB, UK

Alan M. Nevill
Faculty of Education, Health and Well-Being, University of Wolverhampton, Walsall WS1 3BD, UK

Kristen C. Cochrane, Terry J. Housh, Ethan C. Hill, Cory M. Smith, Nathaniel D.M. Jenkins, Joel T. Cramer, Glen O. Johnson and Richard J. Schmidt
Department of Nutrition and Health Sciences, 211 Ruth Leverton Hall, University of Nebraska-Lincoln, Lincoln, NE 68583, USA

Nicole C. Dabbs
Biomechanics and Sport Performance Laboratory, Department of Kinesiology, California State University, San Bernardino, 5500 University Parkway, San Bernardino, CA 92407, USA

Jon A. Lundahl and John C. Garner
Applied Biomechanics Laboratory, Health, Exercise Science, and Recreation Management Department; The University of Mississippi, P.O. Box 1848, Oxford, MS 38677, USA

Bryce Dyer
Faculty of Science & Technology, Bournemouth University, Fern Barrow, Poole BH12 5BB, UK

Adebisi Bisi-Balogun and Firdevs Torlak
Clinical Exercise Science, Faculty of Health Science, University of Potsdam Out-Patient Clinic, Potsdam 14469, Brandenburg, Germany

Nathaniel D. M. Jenkins, Terry J. Housh, Kristen C. Cochrane, Cory M. Smith, Ethan C. Hill, Richard J. Schmidt and Joel T. Cramer
Department of Nutrition and Health Sciences, 211 Ruth Leverton Hall, University of Nebraska-Lincoln, Lincoln, NE 68583, USA
Samuel L. Buckner
Department of Health, Exercise Science, and Recreation Management, University of Mississippi, Oxford, MS 38677, USA

Haley C. Bergstrom
Department of Kinesiology and Health Promotion, University of Kentucky, Lexington, KY 40506-0219, USA

Dean Culpepper
Department of Health and Physical Education, Eastern New Mexico University, Portales, NM 88130, USA
Department of Health and Kinesiology, Texas A and M University-Kingsville, Kingsville, TX 78363, USA

Gretchen D. Oliver
School of Kinesiology, Auburn University, Auburn, AL 36849, USA

Audrey J. Stone
Heart and Vascular Institute Penn State College of Medicine, Hershey, PA 17033, USA

Wendi H. Weimar and Jessica K. Washington
School of Kinesiology, Auburn University, Auburn, AL 36849, USA

Lawrence Lemak
Lemak Sports Medicine and Orthopedics, Birmingham, AL 35213, USA

Christopher P. Dougherty
Agility Center, Orthopedics, Bentonville, AR 72712, USA

Matthew D. Cook, Stephen D. Myers, John S. M. Kelly and Mark E. T. Willems
Department of Sport & Exercise Sciences, University of Chichester, West Sussex PO19 6PE, UK

Aneliya V. Manolova, Samuel Crequy, Philippe Lestriez, Pierre Debraux and William M. Bertucci
Groupe de Recherche En Sciences Pour l'Ingénieur (GRESPI, EA4694), Université de Reims-Champagne-Ardenne (URCA), Moulin de la Housse 51687 Reims cedex 2, France

Rachel Massie, Brett Smith and Keith Tolfrey
School of Sport, Exercise and Health Sciences, Loughborough University, Loughborough, Leicestershire LE11 3TU, UK

Frank R. Noyes and Sue D. Barber-Westin
Cincinnati Sportsmedicine and Orthopaedic Center and the Noyes Knee Institute, 10663 Montgomery Road, Cincinnati, OH 45242, USA

Frank R. Noyes and Sue D. Barber-Westin
Cincinnati Sportsmedicine and Orthopaedic Center and the Noyes Knee Institute, 10663 Montgomery Road, Cincinnati, OH 45242, USA

Taylor S. Thurston, Jared W. Coburn, Lee E. Brown, Albert Bartolini, Tori L. Beaudette, Patrick Karg, Kathryn A. McLeland, Jose A. Arevalo, Daniel A. Judelson and Andrew J. Galpin
Center for Sport Performance, Department of Kinesiology, California State University, Fullerton, CA 92834, USA

Hayley C. Russell
Department of Kinesiology, The Pennsylvania State University, Altoona Campus, Altoona, PA 16601, USA

Diane M. Wiese-Bjornstal
School of Kinesiology, University of Minnesota, Twin Cities, Minneapolis, MN 55455, USA

Hossein Hassani
The Statistical Research Centre, Business School, Bournemouth University,
Bournemouth BH8 8EB, UK
Institute for International Energy Studies (IIES), 65 Sayeh St., Vali-e-Asr Ave., Tehran 1967743 711, Iran

Mansi Ghodsi and Mehran Shadi
The Statistical Research Centre, Business School, Bournemouth University,
Bournemouth BH8 8EB, UK

Siamak Noroozi and Bryce Dyer
School of Design, Engineering and Computing, Bournemouth University, Poole House P124, Talbot Campus, Fern Barrow, Poole, Bournemouth BH12 5BB, UK

Andrea Braakhuis and Tea Williams
Discipline of Nutrition/Dietetics, Faculty of Medical and Health Sciences,
The University of Auckland, Private Bag 92019, Auckland, 1142, New Zealand

Elizabeth Fusco and Shawn Hueglin
United States Olympic Committee, 2800 Olympic Parkway, Chula Vista, CA 91915, USA

Alex Popple
High Performance Sport New Zealand, Avantidrome, Hanlin Road, Cambridge 3283, New Zealand

Alfred Nimmerichter and Mathias Steindl
Faculty of Sport and Exercise Sciences, University of Applied Sciences Wiener Neustadt, Johannes Gutenberg Str. 3, Wiener Neustadt A-2700, Austria

Craig Anthony Williams
Children's Health and Exercise Research Centre, Sport and Health Sciences, University of Exeter, St Luke's Campus, Heavitree Road, Exeter EX1 2LU, Devon, UK

Cassio V. Ruas, Ronei S. Pinto and Eduardo L. Cadore
Physical Education School, Federal University of Rio Grande do Sul, Brazil, Felizardo Street, 750—Jardim Botânico, Porto Alegre/RS 90690-200, Brazil

Lee E. Brown
Department of Kinesiology, KHS 233 800 N. State College Blvd., California State University, Fullerton 92831, CA, USA

Leonie Harvey, Matthew Bousson and Dale I. Lovell
School of Health and Sport Sciences, Faculty of Science, Health & Education, University of the Sunshine Coast, Sippy Downs, Queensland 4556, Australia

Chris McLellan
Faculty of Health Sciences and Medicine, Bond University, Robina, Queensland 4226, Australia

Gretchen Oliver, Keith Lohse and Sarah Gascon
School of Kinesiology, Auburn University, 301 Wire Road Auburn, AL 36830, USA